COMPANION BIRD MEDICINE

COMPANION BIRD MEDICINE

EDITED BY **Elisha W. Burr**

IOWA STATE UNIVERSITY PRESS ● AMES, IOWA U.S.A.

DEDICATED TO
LOUISE

who enabled this book to
progress by maintaining my
communication as my job
took me to all corners
of the world

Elisha W. Burr, D.V.M., B.V.Sc. (Hons.),
M.R.C.V.S., grew up on a wild animal farm in
Bethlehem, Connecticut. He has studied and
worked in many countries as an exotic-animal
practitioner and avian consultant for international companies. He is currently working as an
exotic-animal-medicine consultant for a Scan-
dinavian firm and an avian specialist in New
Zealand.

© 1987 Iowa State University Press,
Ames, Iowa 50010
Chapters 5, 26 © 1987 Christine Davis
All rights reserved

Composed by Iowa State University Press
Printed in the United States of America

First edition, 1987

Library of Congress Cataloging-in-Publication Data

Companion bird medicine.

    Includes index.

    1. Cage-birds—Diseases.   I. Burr, Elisha W.
SF994.2.A1C66   1987   636.6′86   86–27606
ISBN 0–8138–0362–4

CONTENTS

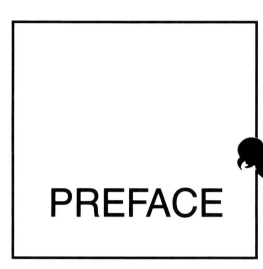

PREFACE

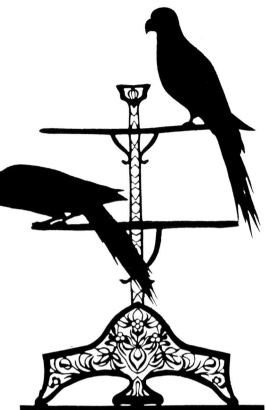

SEVERAL YEARS AGO the idea of doing a multiauthor text, *Companion Bird Medicine,* was prompted by the lack of concise information on the subject. In coordinating and editing such a book I was guided by veterinarians on specific points, in an endeavor to increase the value of the text and keep it up-to-date.

A book such as this owes much to those who offer the benefit of their experience to enhance the knowledge of avian medicine. The field has grown by leaps and bounds over the last decade. Journals now devote whole sections to avian medicine, and research programs have developed rapidly. Suddenly a vast amount of information has become available on the subject in journals, magazines, books, and research publications. This book brings together this widely dispersed material into a text for the practicing veterinarian and student.

Because of the financial value of psittacine birds, much of the research and literature available chiefly concerns this order. This book has attempted to fill the information gap about other orders. Each subject area covered in the book reflects the individual author's specialty or area of interest. The individual chapters have been edited, as space does not allow in-depth discussions of disease conditions and treatment. This book is intended to be a comprehensive reference that gives the practitioner valuable information on disease diagnosis, treatment, and preventive medicine.

This book has several chapters on subjects not usually covered in avian medicine publications: Caging and Environment, Captive Breeding, Avian Behavior, Mutations and Hereditary Disorders, Avian Sex Identification Techniques, and Quarantine and Isolation. These areas are included because of their importance to the veterinarian in treating patients.

The problems encountered in coordinating a book of this magnitude, diversity, and number of international authors are immense. Most practitioners have a limited amount of time to write, and my travels about the world caused numerous communication delays. After four years and several updates of the manuscript, the book is complete. I can only express my thanks to all the authors who contributed to this text, which should be exceedingly valuable to those requiring a comprehensive reference in the field of companion bird medicine. Any information or comments that will benefit future editions are welcomed by the editor.

Without the help of several people this text would have never come to completion. Acknowledgments go to Pat M. Baker, Killarney Heights, Australia, who interpreted my handwriting and transformed my codes into a typewritten page. Many kind thanks to Dr. Ross Perry, Forestville, Australia, for being a critic to the text. Appreciation also goes to Lester Natt, South Plympton, Australia, for help in organizing the original draft. I am grateful to David Alderton, Brighton, England, for providing the research materials used in several sections. The final acknowledgment goes to all the others who helped make this work possible; they are not forgotten—my warm thanks to them.

CONTRIBUTORS

David Alderton, M.A.
158 Balfour Road
Brighton, East Sussex BN1 6NE
England

Gordon F. Bennett, Ph.D.
Professor and Head
International Reference Centre for Avian Haematozoa
Memorial University of Newfoundland
St. John's, Newfoundland
Canada

Arden Bryan Bercovitz, Ph.D.
Avian Reproductive Physiologist
Research Department
Zoological Society of San Diego
P.O. Box 551
San Diego, California 92112-0551

Charles E. Blass, D.V.M.
Department of Clinical Sciences
College of Veterinary Medicine
Louisiana State University
Baton Rouge, Louisiana 70803

Henri Brugère, Dr.V.
Professor
Agrégé de Physiologie et Thérapeutique
L'Ecole Nationale Vétérinaire d'Alfort
94704 Maisons-Alfort
France

Jeanne Brugère-Picoux, Dr.V.
Professor
Agrégée de Pathologie Médicale du Bétail et des Animaux
    de Basse-cour
L'Ecole Nationale Vétérinaire de Lyon
B.P. 31-69752 Charbonnières
France

**Elisha W. Burr, D.V.M., B.V.Sc. (Hons.),
    M.R.C.V.S.**
5 Larkey Road
Oxford, Connecticut 06483

Raymond Butler, B.V.Sc., M.A.C.V.Sc.
Veterinary Consultant
Exotic and Wild Animal Specialist
P.O. Box 54
Applecross, Western Australia 6153
Australia

**Cherukuri Choudary, M.Sc., Ph.D.,
    F.R.C.V.S.**
Pathologist
B-56, F-2 P.S. Nagar Vijayanagar Colony
Hyderabad, Andhra Pradesh
India

Garry M. J. Cross, M.V.Sc., Ph.D.
Special Veterinary Officer, Poultry Health
Department of Agriculture, New South Wales
Central Veterinary Laboratory
Roy Watts Road
Glenfield, New South Wales 2167
Australia

Christine Davis
P.O. Box 816
Westminster, California 92684

Robert E. Dolphin, D.V.M.
Alaska Bird and Cat Clinic
3605 Arctic Boulevard, number 348
Anchorage, Alaska 99503

Graeme J. Eamens, B.V.Sc. (Hons.)
Veterinary Research Officer
Department of Agriculture, New South Wales
Central Veterinary Laboratory
Roy Watts Road
Glenfield, New South Wales 2167
Australia

Murray E. Fowler, D.V.M.
Professor
School of Veterinary Medicine
Department of Medicine
University of California
Davis, California 95616

Jack M. Gaskin, D.V.M., Ph.D.
Associate Professor
Department of Preventive Medicine
College of Veterinary Medicine
J. Hillis Miller Health Center
Box J-138, University of Florida
Gainesville, Florida 32610

Robert F. Giddings, D.V.M.
Cheshire Veterinary Hospital
1572 South Main Street
Cheshire, Connecticut 06410

Paul T. Gilchrist, B.V.Sc., F.A.C.V.Sc.
Chief, Division of Animal Production
Department of Agriculture, New South Wales
P.O. Box K220
Haymarket, New South Wales 2001
Australia

E. Gwyn Harry, M.Sc., B.Pharm., Ph.D.
60 Hartford Road
Huntingdon, Cambridgeshire PE18 6RP
England

Patrick N. Humphreys, M.Sc., M.R.C.V.S.
Department of Zoology
University College
P.O. Box 78
Cardiff CF1 1XL
Wales

Lester Mandelker, D.V.M.
Community Veterinary Hospital
1631 West Bay Drive
Largo, Florida 33540

Scott E. McDonald, D.V.M.
Midwest Bird and Exotic Animal Hospital
Westchester, Illinois 60153

Marilyn Monahan-Brennan
Animal Health Technician
Animal Medical Centre of Lawndale
4473 West Rosecrans Avenue
Hawthorne, California 90250

Anthony B. Olszewski, B.A.
Avante-Garde Aviculture
P.O. Box 3362
Jersey City, New Jersey 07303

Guru P. Patgiri, Ph.D.
Associate Professor, Department of Microbiology
College of Veterinary Science
Khanapara, Gauhati, Assam 781 022
India

Ross A. Perry, B.Sc. (Vet.) (Hons.), B.V.Sc. (Hons.), M.A.C.V.Sc.
Forestville Veterinary Hospital
635 Warringah Road
Forestville, New South Wales 2087
Australia

Rodney L. Reece, B.V.Sc., M.Sc., M.A.C.V.Sc.
Veterinary Pathologist, Avian Diseases
Department of Agriculture and Rural Affairs
Veterinary Research Institute
Park Drive
Parkville, Victoria 3052
Australia

Brian G. Rich
Manager, Veterinary Clinic
30 Belair Road
Hawthorn, South Australia 5062
Australia

Walter J. Rosskopf, Jr., D.V.M.
Animal Medical Centre of Lawndale
4473 West Rosecrans Avenue
Hawthorne, California 90250

William D. Russell, B.V.Sc., M.R.C.V.S.
Veterinary Surgeon
Bryanston Veterinary Clinic
99 Grosvenor Road
P.O. Box 67853, Bryanston 2021
Republic of South Africa

David J. Schultz, B.V.Sc.
Veterinary Surgeon
30 Belair Road
Hawthorn, South Australia 5062
Australia

S. Reuben Shanthikumar, B.V.Sc., D.T.V.M.
S number 2 Orchard Park
Davis, California 95616

Milan Stehlík, M.V.Dr.
Zoo Veterinarian, East Bohemian Zoo Garden
Dvůr Králové n.L.
P.O. Box 38
Nymburk, Czechoslovakia

G. Vincent Turner, B.V.Sc., D.V.P.H., M.Med.Vet., Ph.D., M.R.C.V.S., Dipl. A.C.V.P.M.
Senior Lecturer, Department of Veterinary Public Health
Faculty of Veterinary Science
University of Pretoria
Onderstepoort 0110
Republic of South Africa

Anne S. Williams, D.V.M.
San Anselmo Veterinary Clinic
780 Sir Francis Drake Boulevard
San Anselmo, California 94960

Genevieve M. Wilson, M.A.
Medical Illustrator
P.O. Box 1616
Ross, California 94957

Raymond D. Wise, D.V.M., Dipl. A.B.V.P.
Scottsdale Animal Clinic
7953 South Cicero Avenue
Chicago, Illinois 60652

Richard W. Woerpel, D.V.M.
Animal Medical Centre of Lawndale
4473 West Rosecrans Avenue
Hawthorne, California 90250

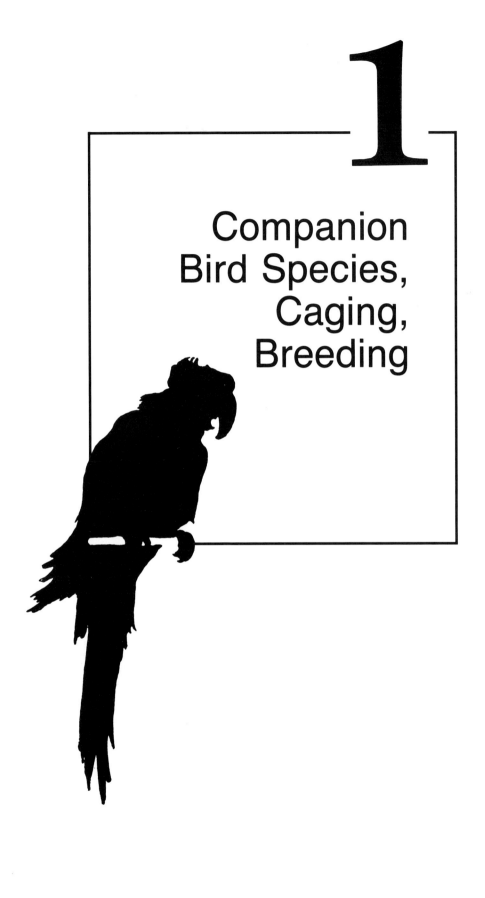

1

Companion
Bird Species,
Caging,
Breeding

1

Common Cage and Aviary Birds

WILLIAM D. RUSSELL

AVICULTURE has made rapid and momentous advances during the past decade with more aviculturists becoming involved with the preservation and propagation of the various species of birds distributed throughout the world. With the advance of civilization, the habitat of many bird species has been and is being destroyed and many species are facing extinction. This fact has raised the value of birds. Some aviculturists have specialized in certain species with the aim of building up aviary-bred strains and increasing the genetic pool in order to prevent the extinction of many of the rarer species.

Avian medicine has been the last link in the chain to develop, but during the past few years it has made some marked advances in order to keep up with avicultural progress. Pressure has been brought to bear on veterinarians by aviculturists in particular and by pet bird owners to upgrade the standard of veterinary services available to bring them in line with those offered to other species. Many veterinarians are themselves capable aviculturists and thus have contributed greatly to knowledge in avian medicine.

Avian medicine is a relatively new science and therefore more research still is necessary to enhance the knowledge that is already available. The variety of species, ranging from the minute hummingbird to the large hornbill and ostrich, means vastly different anatomies, digestive systems, and methods of reproduction. Bird species, which are dwellers of dense forests, open savannahs, semideserts, and arctic and antarctic regions, require diverse methods of husbandry, making the role of the aviculturist even more difficult. One can imagine the different ailments and diseases encountered in the various species. Bird anatomy depends on whether flight is relied on for feeding and/or escaping predators and enemies, and it varies with the type of food eaten (e.g., strong hooked beaks for cracking nuts, sharp strong beaks for tearing meat, strong small beaks for eating seeds, varying types of beaks for eating insects or fruit).

All veterinarians who wish to practice avian medicine should learn about the various common species encountered in practice. A brief study of areas of occurrence, habitats, feeding habits, and breeding can assist considerably in understanding how to treat and care for any species. Species in the following orders might be encountered in practice: Passeriformes, Piciformes, Columbiformes, Psittaciformes, Galliformes, Gruiformes, Anseriformes, Ciconiiformes, Strigiformes, Falconiformes, Struthioniformes, Rheiformes, Casuariiformes, and Sphenisciformes.

Order Passeriformes. This group is by far the largest, most complex, and most highly developed order of birds. This order numbers approximately 5100 species, all land birds. They vary in size from small finches to the large ravens. Perching feet is their outstanding characteristic. Four unwebbed toes join at the same level, three pointing forward and one backward; the hind toe is usually the strongest and best developed. Many are singing birds. The young are usually naked when hatched and are always reared in the nest. They occur throughout the world on all continents except Antarctica.

Seedeaters. These have short, stout, conical seedeating bills. The exposed portion of the upper bill is relatively long. They are small to medium-sized and are usually extremely colorful. The more common New World species (family Fringillidae) include buntings and cardinals. Among the more common Old World species (family Ploceidae) are Australian and African finches, European and Asian goldfinches, bullfinches, Asian mannikins, weavers, whydahs, and canaries.

Tanagers (Family Thraupidae). This family comprises 222 species confined mostly to tropical and subtropical regions. They are common from Mexico through South America, and 1 species, the Scarlet Tanager, occurs in North America. They are small to medium in length. Their diet consists mainly of fruit, nectar, and insects.

Thrushes (Family Turdidae). This family contains some of the most highly regarded songbirds. They are typically plump birds, and their diet consists mainly of fruit and insects. They occur throughout the world.

Leafbirds (Family Irenidae). There are 14 species in this family, all forest dwellers. The males are always colorful, in contrast to the dull-colored females. They occur in Asia and the Philippine Islands.

Starlings (Family Sturnidae). These jaunty, active medium-sized birds with straight or slightly down-curved bills occur worldwide. They have strong, stout legs and feet and walk cockily with a waddling gait. The tail is square and short in most species, but pointed and long in a few. They are generally dark-colored with a metallic sheen, although a few are brightly colored. Many are crested, and a few have prominent wattles on their cheeks or bare patches of skin on their heads. Their basic diet is insects and fruit, although those in suburban areas have a varied diet. The Hill Mynah is the most popular species kept in captivity.

Bulbuls (Family Pycnonotidae). The birds in this family are better known for their song. They range from Africa through Asia. Of moderate size and plainly garbed, they are gregarious, inquisitive, and fairly bold and noisy. The family comprises 119 species. Their necks and wings are short, their tails medium to long. Their bills are slender and slightly down-curved. Most are clad in brown, gray, black, or dull green, with patches of yellow, red, or white about the head and undertail coverts. Their basic diet is insects, fruit, and soft seeds.

Other Families. Other groups in this order include antbirds, babblers, birds of paradise, bowerbirds, broadbills, cotingas, crows, jays, flycatchers, larks, mannikins, orioles, troupials, pittas, shrikes, sunbirds, honeycreepers, swallows, martins, and wrens.

Order Piciformes. This group of birds occurs mainly in the tropical regions of the world, with the exception of the woodpeckers, which are widely distributed in temperate and tropical regions. The barbets have large heads, thick conical beaks, stocky bodies, and short broad tails. The wings are short and rounded and the flight is weak. The toucans, toucanets, and acaris are arboreal birds with fast flight despite short, rounded wings. The tails are usually long and wedge-shaped (except the genus *Ramphastas*). The body plumage and beak are usually brightly colored. The beak is enormous and appears clumsy, but in fact is made out of

spongy, bony fibers and is extremely light. Woodpeckers occur throughout the world but are not widely kept aviary birds.

Barbets (Family Capitonidae). This family consists of 76 species. They are small to medium-sized. They occur in America, Africa, and Asia and are most abundant in tropical and semitropical Africa. Their diet includes insects and small animals and plant material, including fruit and berries.

Toucans, Toucanets, and Acaris (Family Ramphastidae). This family comprises 41 species, confined to the tropical regions of America. They are medium to long birds. Their diet consists mainly of fruits and palms, ficus, and other plants.

Order Columbiformes

Pigeons and Doves (Family Columbidae). Pigeons and doves are stout-bodied with short necks and small heads. They have short, slender, rounded bills, thickened toward the tip and thinner in the middle. They have a fleshy cere at the base, through which the nostrils emerge. Most are sleek and fast-flying with strong-shafted feathers. Their voices are a soft, plaintive cooing or booming, usually repetitive. They occur throughout the world. Their greatest development is in the Orient and Australia.

Sandgrouse (Family Pteroclididae). Sandgrouse vaguely resemble squat, short-legged grouse but have pigeonlike heads and necks. Their short, pointed bills lack the pigeon cere, however. Their wings and tails are long and pointed, and their short legs are feathered down to the toes. They are medium-sized, 9–16 in. (23–41 cm) long. They are protectively colored in brown and gray, dappled with orange, black, white, and chestnut, which camouflages them in their semidesert surroundings. They occur in Africa, southern Europe, and central and southern Asia.

Order Psittaciformes. This order, which consists of approximately 353 species, are the best-known group found in aviculture and as pets in homes. Australia, New Guinea, and the Philippine Islands have 109 species, Africa and India 34 species, South America 192 species, and North America and Mexico 18 species. Psittacines occur throughout the world, mainly in the southern hemisphere, and are most prevalent in tropical regions. Strong hooked bills are characteristic of this order. They have a down-curved upper maxilla that is flexible on the skull and fits neatly over a broad, up-curved lower mandible. Parrots have a strong, thick, fleshy tongue. In the Loriidae, the tongue is tipped with brushlike papillae used for gathering pollen. They have strong feet, with two toes pointing forward and two backward to grasp while perching.

Lories and Lorikeets (Family Loriidae). This family comprises 55 species of brightly colored, extremely active birds. They are primarily nectar feeders, hence the brushlike tongue used to harvest pollen. They occur mainly in Australia and the surrounding Indonesian islands. Lories usually have short, square tails and are large-bodied, while the lorikeets have long, pointed tails and are smaller with slender bodies. The largest of this family is approximately 13 in. (33 cm), the smallest 6 in. (15 cm).

Cockatoos (Family Cacatuidae). There are 18 species in this family. Most are white but some are pink or black. The erectile crest is their most obvious feature. They have extremely strong, heavy bills. The largest is the Black Palm Cockatoo of 28 in. (71 cm); the commonly known Cockatiel is the smallest at 13 in. (33 cm). Sexual dimorphism is present in some species. Males have black eyes and females brown ocher eyes. Cockatoos predominate in Australia and the surrounding Indonesian islands.

Parrots (Family Psittacidae)

Amazons (*Amazona* spp.). There are 27 species of amazon parrots. They vary in color, with green predominating. The Blue-fronted and Double-yellow-headed amazons are the most common species found in aviculture and as pets. They vary in size from 12 in. (30.5 cm) to 20 in. (51 cm). Amazons are stocky birds with heavy bills and short, rounded tails. They have a naked cere. This group occurs mainly in South America, the West Indian islands, Central America, and Mexico.

Pionus Parrots (*Pionus* spp.). This genus of parrots is very similar to the amazons. They are medium-sized with short, square tails. There are 8 species in this group. They are fairly colorful, with a variety of colors on their heads, and have a complete orbital ring. They occur mainly in South America, but 1 species, the White-capped Parrot (*P. senilis*), occurs in Panama and southeast Mexico.

Macaws (*Ara, Cyanopsitta,* and *Anodorhynchus* spp.). This group comprises 18 species. They have large, heavy, strong bills to crush hard nuts.

Their most conspicuous feature is a bare facial area. They have long, graduated tails. They vary in size and color; the largest, the Hyacinth Macaw, is 40 in. (102 cm) long and cobalt blue, while the smallest, the Red-shouldered Macaw, is only 12 in. (30.5 cm) long and basically green with red on the point of the shoulder. They all occur in South America.

Conures (*Aratinga, Cyanoliseus,* and *Pyrrhura* spp.). There are 45 species in these genera. They are small to medium-sized parrots with graduated tails and proportionately broad, heavy bills. They have a prominent naked or partly feathered periophthalmic rings, but the lores and upper cheeks are fully feathered. The species have a large variety of colors, especially the smaller varieties. The basic color is green, with an assortment of different-colored heads or necks. In the smaller species the head, neck, throat, and even the body may show barring of varied colors. Conures occur almost entirely in South America.

Rosellas (*Platycercus* spp.). This parakeet genus has 8 species, which vary in color—crimson red, yellow, green, yellow and red, blue and yellow, and red and green. They are approximately 15 in. (38 cm) long, some slightly larger and others slightly smaller. They are swift fliers. They occur in Australia and have recently been introduced into New Zealand.

Budgerigars (*Melopsittacus* sp.). The Budgerigar is by far the best-known of the parrot family. This small parakeet has been bred from the original light green color to the wide range of colors found in aviculture today. The wild Budgerigar occurs in Australia.

Grass Parakeets (*Neophema* spp.). This genus comprises 7 species of brightly colored parakeets, approximately 8 in. (20 cm) long. The common Bourke Parakeet is basically blue and pink, while the other species have green on the back and neck and vary in color on the abdomen and chest. They are found only in Australia.

African Gray Parrots (*Psittacus* spp.). These are well-known parrots and are commonly kept as pets. The nominate race and two subspecies occur. The nominate (Ghana) race, which is mainly dark gray with a bright scarlet tail, occurs in Ghana, Uganda, Kenya, the Congo, and Angola. The Timneh race (*P. e. timneh*), which is powdery gray with a dark red tail, occurs from Guinea to Sierra Leone and Liberia. The Princeps race (*P. e. princeps*), which is dark gray overall with purple-tipped underparts, is confined to the islands of Principe and Fernando Po in the Gulf of Guinea.

Cape, Jardine's, Rüppell's, Meyer's et al. Parrots (*Poicephalus* spp.). This genus comprises 9 species. The largest are the Cape and Jardine's parrots, 14 in. (35.5 cm) long, and the Rüppell's and Meyer's parrots, 10 in. (25.5 cm) long. Their colors are usually somber brown and green interspersed with yellow, blue, and orange. They are found only in Africa.

Lovebirds (*Agapornis* spp.). The genus comprises 9 species and are common pet birds. The naked periophthalmic ring is present in 4 of the species, while the remaining 5 species have feathers around the eye. They all vary in color; their basic color is green, with a variety of gray, black, and orange heads and black cheeks. They occur throughout Africa.

Hanging Parrots (*Loriculus* spp.). There are 10 species of these beautiful little parrots, which measure approximately 5 in. (13 cm) long. Their basic color is green, with variations on the head, throat, rump, and back. Their tails are short and square. They occur throughout southern Asia.

Ring-necked Parakeets (*Psittacula* spp.). These large, mainly Asiatic parakeets comprise 15 species. The Alexandrine Parakeet is the largest at 24 in. (61 cm) and the Blossom-headed Parakeet is the smallest at 12 in. (30.5 cm). They have either a colorful ring around their necks or different-colored heads. They have long, elongated tails. Most species occur on the Indian subcontinent.

Fig Parrots (*Opopsitta* and *Psittaculirostris* spp.). These genera comprise 5 species of highly colorful parrots that occur in Australia, Indonesia, and other Southeast Asian islands. They vary in size from 4 to 8 in. (10–20 cm) and have short, square tails.

Order Galliformes

Curassows and Guans (Family Cracidae). This
species has long, slightly hooked bills and four long slender toes with well-developed hooked claws and a hind toe longer than the others. To amplify the voice, they possess an extended trachea, usually looped with the curve sometimes reaching the abdomen before it enters the thorax. Large birds with short wings and long tails, they spend much of their time in trees. There are 7 species of curassows and 11 species of guans. They occur in South America.

Quails, Partridges, Pheasants, Peafowl, Guinea Fowl, and Turkeys (Family Phasianidae). This family, which comprises 178 species, contains many of the most beautifully colored birds in the world. The males are usually adorned with brightly colored feathers of varying lengths, which give them their striking appearance. The quail and partridge are small to medium-sized rotund birds with short tails. They have three long forward toes, with one hind toe. Their usual somber color enables them to hide in the undergrowth to avoid predators. The pheasants are the brightly colored cousins. Most have long tails with fourteen feathers, and some have extremely long tails, twice the length of their bodies. Some pheasants have a few feathers for a crest, while others have a number of feathers curving upward from the ear coverts to above the head that gives them the appearance of long ears. These species occur worldwide.

Order Gruiformes

Cranes (Family Gruidae). The 14 species of
cranes occur in North America, Africa, and Australia, with the most number of species in Europe and Asia. They are large, long-necked, long-legged waders with toes connected at the base by a membrane. Their bills are straight and long, although the length can vary with the species. The lower mandibles are grooved, with the nostrils placed halfway down the upper mandible. The general coloring is gray or white with black primaries. Some have ornamented plumes on the head, and the secondary feathers are greatly elongated.

Order Anseriformes

Ducks, Geese, and Swans (Family Anatidae)

Ducks (*Anas, Aythya, Tadorna, Aix* et al. spp.). There are 72 species of ducks, which occur throughout the world. They all have webbed feet but vary in color and patterns. The Mandarin and Carolina ducks are the most colorful of those occurring in captivity and the most commonly kept.

Geese (*Anser, Branta* et al.). There are 27 species of geese, which occur in Europe, Africa, Asia, Hawaii, and along the arctic coasts. Geese are medium-sized waterfowl with fairly long erect necks and webbed toes. Their color variation depends on the species. Most are brown, gray, black, and white, with different patterns. The Red-breasted Goose is one of the most beautiful.

Pygmy Geese (*Nettapus* spp.). There are 3 species of pygmy geese, which occur in Africa, Australia, and Asia. They are small birds, approximately 14–16 in. (36–41 cm) long. They have variations of chestnut brown, gray, black, white, and green in various patterns.

Whistling Ducks or Tree Ducks (*Dendrocygna* spp.). There are 8 species of whistling or tree ducks. They occur in South America, southern North America, the West Indies, Asia, and Africa. They are small-sized to medium ducks, approximately 16–20 in. (41–51 cm) long. They have short tails and long necks and legs. Their name comes from their shrill, whistling cry.

Swans (*Cygnus* and *Coscoroba* spp.). There are 8 species of swans, which occur worldwide – the Black Swan in Australia, the Black-necked and Coscoroba swans in South America, the Trumpeter and Whistling swans in North America, and the Mute, Whooper, and Bewick's swans in Europe and Asia. Swans are large birds with long erect necks. Like other waterfowl, they have webbed toes for swimming. They are mainly white, with the exception of the Black and Black-necked swans.

Order Ciconiiformes

Flamingos (Family Phoenicopteridae). There are 4 species of Flamingo. They occur in South America, southern Europe, Asia, and Africa. These are large birds, with long, elongated necks and long legs. Their plumage is pink and red. The bill is larger than the head, sharply decurved at the center. The lower mandible is larger than the upper and deeply channeled, the upper mandible fitting into it like a lid; both bills are lined with fine, hairlike lamellae, except for the Greater Flamingo (*P. ruber*), which has localized lamellae along the mandibles.

Order Strigiformes. Owls have a worldwide distribution. This order contains 143 species of nocturnal birds of prey, ranging from the Pygmy Owls of 5½ in. (14 cm) long to the Eagle Owls 30 in. (76 cm) long. Their eyes are directed forward, and their angle of vision would be restricted were it not for the ability to turn their heads almost 180° in either direction, making it possible to see in all directions without moving their bodies.

Barn Owls (Family Tytonidae). This group has heart-shaped facial disks and long, slender legs only lightly covered with minute feathers.

Typical Owls (Family Strigidae). This family includes the Tawny Owls, Eagle Owls, Snow Owls, and Eared Owls. They have circular facial disks and short, stout legs thickly feathered in nearly all species.

Order Falconiformes. This order comprises the largest number of birds of prey in the world. The eagles, hawks, and falcons have powerful, hooked bills and toes and short, sharp claws (talons) for grasping prey. Their wings are powerful, and they are able to reach tremendous speed in flight.

New World Vultures and Condors (Family Cathartidae). There are 6 species worldwide.

Old World Vultures, Hawks, and Falcons (Family Accipitridae). There are more than 40 species.

Secretary Bird (Family Sagittariidae). There is only 1 species (*Sagittarius serpentarius*).

SUPERORDER RATITAE

These orders comprise the largest living birds. They are primitive, flightless, and without any keel to the sternum. They have small wings, no stiff contour feathers or oil feathers, and powerful legs with which they defend themselves.

Order Struthioniformes

Ostrich (Family Struthionidae). This is the largest living bird, reaching over 8 ft (244 cm) and weighing over 300 lb (137 kilos). The hens are slightly smaller than the males. The ostrich has two toes, one smaller than the other. The egg is the largest produced by birds but is one of the smallest in relation to the size of the bird. Ostriches occur throughout Africa.

Order Rheiformes

Rheas (family Rheidae). Rheas are similar to ostriches but are smaller, standing 4–5 ft. (122–152 cm). Their thighs, head, and neck are feathered, unlike the ostrich. Their wings are longer than those of the ostrich. Rheas only occur in South America.

Order Casuariiformes

Cassowaries (Family Casuariidae). They are heavy-bodied birds with short, stout legs. They have no tail feathers. They have rudimentary wings hidden beneath their plumage and a large, bony helmet on the forehead. The skin of their featherless heads and necks combines vivid reds, blues, purples, and yellows. Decorative wattles hang from the throats of 2 species. Cassowaries occur in Australia, New Guinea, and adjacent islands.

Emus (Family Dromaiidae). Emus are 5–6 ft (152–183 cm) tall and weigh approximately 120 lb (55 kilos). Their heads and necks are feathered, except for two bare spots on either side. They have a broad back and coarse, drooping, heavy plumage. Emus occur only in Australia.

Order Sphenisciformes

Penguins (Family Spheniscidae). There are 14 species of penguins. They occur only in the southern hemisphere, especially on the African, South American, and Australian continents. Penguins are an ancient, primitive group, highly specialized for a marine existence. They are distinctive in their coloring and have flipperlike wings that are useless for flying but make them extremely strong swimmers. These flippers are stiff and lack a flexible "elbow." On land penguins are handicapped by the position of their short legs, which are set far back on their bodies.

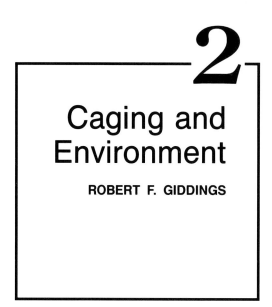

2

Caging and Environment

ROBERT F. GIDDINGS

WHEN WE KEEP birds caged in our homes we drastically alter their entire lives. What were creatures with unlimited freedom to come and go whenever and wherever they pleased are now closely confined, in the constant presence of the humans they once knew as "danger," under the complete control of well-intentioned but often unthinking and poorly informed owners. Captivity offers safety from most predators, from hunger, and from the elements. We place our caged birds in places of prominence in our homes, treat their parasites and diseases, and offer them many toys and amusements to occupy their time and minds. We also house them in cages that are poorly designed and too small, offer them limited and nutritionally incomplete diets, expect that our presence is an adequate substitute for the fellowship of their own kind that we deprive them of, and provide them with no means of escape from the attentions we lavish on them. If we insist on keeping birds caged, we must see that their physical and psychological needs are met as fully as possible. Even species such as the Budgerigar and canary, which have been raised in captivity for generations and are accustomed to the restrictions imposed on them, do better when properly caged. The fact that so many birds apparently do well in our care is not necessarily an indication that our husbandry practices are optimal but rather reveals the resilience, strength, and adaptability of birds.

Cages. People own birds for many reasons, not the least of which is their beauty. It is only natural, therefore, that we should try to house them in such a way as to display that beauty to the greatest extent possible. Unfortunately most commercially available cages, while they look attractive, display birds fully, and complement the decor of our homes, are seldom ideally suited to their occupants' well-being. In general, the more ornate the cage the poorer it probably is for the bird it houses. Tall narrow cylindrical cages and irregularly shaped model bamboo "houses" are two examples of decorative cages that should be particularly avoided.

The most important factor to be considered in providing adequate housing for a bird is the provision of sufficient useful space. Ideally, a cage should provide a bird with enough space for exercise, a "security" area where it can hide from commotion and prying eyes, feeding and bathing areas located so as not to be contaminated by droppings from perches situated above, and space for toys and other amusements.

It is impossible to provide too much space for a captive bird, whether the smallest finch or the largest macaw. The opposite situation usually exists, and we offer far too little room for a comfortable, healthy existence. The reasons for this are basically lack of space in homes and the fact that large cages are very expensive. The important considerations therefore are the minimal amount of space needed by each bird and the arrangement of that space so as to be as useful as possible to the bird occupying it. There should be ample room for a bird to turn completely around in the cage or to extend and flap its wings without touching the top or sides. Table 2.1 lists some suggested minimal cage dimensions and volumes; space in excess of these values is recommended.

Another very important consideration, al-

Table 2.1. Recommended minimum cage sizes

Approximate Bird Size	Minimum Cage Size	Dimensions
Finch, canary, Budgerigar	2 ft³ (.19 m³)	1 ft × 1 ft × 2 ft (30 cm × 30 cm × 60 cm)
Cockatiel, lovebird	12 ft³ (1.11 m³)	2 ft × 2 ft × 3 ft (60 cm × 60 cm × 90 cm)
Small parrot	18 ft³ (1.67 m³)	2 ft × 3 ft × 3 ft (60 cm × 90 cm × 90 cm)
Larger parrot	24 ft³ (2.23 m³)	2 ft × 3 ft × 4 ft (60 cm × 90 cm × 120 cm)
Macaw	32 ft³ (2.97 m³)	2 ft × 4 ft × 4 ft (60 cm × 120 cm × 120 cm)

Source: R. Dean Axelson, *Caring for Your Pet Bird,* Canaviax Publications Ltd., Willowdale, Ontario, Canada, 1979.

ready mentioned, is the shape of the cage. A rectangle with the longest dimension horizontal (Fig. 2.1) provides much more usable space than does a rectangular or cylindrical cage oriented vertically (Fig. 2.2). A vertical cage is basically wasted space because it allows the bird no movement except climbing; flight is either impossible or very awkward and limited in scope. This type of cage also makes proper placement of food and water very difficult. A horizontal rectangular cage, on the other hand, allows food containers to be easily placed in such a way that contamination by droppings from above is minimized. It also allows maximum space for flight or at least jumping from perch to perch.

The expression "to live in a goldfish bowl" has come to signify life in the public eye, with no time or place for privacy. Commercial bird cages allow their occupants no privacy either; they are fully open on all sides and usually the top as well. The bird can see all that goes on around it at all times and can be seen at all times. For a creature that is partly reclusive by nature and that is equipped both physically and psychologically to fly away and hide when danger approaches, this is doubly upsetting. The bird can neither hide nor flee, and a variety of disorders can result, such as stereotyped movements and feather chewing. The goldfish is usually provided some plants and rocks in its aquarium, which serve as decoration but also function as a barrier behind which the fish can hide. We should do more for our caged birds and provide each cage with some specific area where the bird can be visually shielded from its surroundings. This can be accomplished in several ways. The cage can be located in the corner of a room or behind a large piece of furniture that shields it from the rest of the room. The cage can be left partly covered at all times. If the cover method is used there should be a perch in the covered area so the birds can make use of it. A third method of providing a privacy area is the placement of a box or barrier inside the cage so the bird can get in it or behind it. A nesting box can serve this function, or a metal or wooden box can be built. It should be large enough so the bird fits comfortably inside, and it should either have a perch placed inside or have a bottom; it is unnecessary to have both. If the box has a perch but no bottom, cleaning it becomes a much easier job. Note that when this method of providing privacy is used, space is taken from the interior of the cage. Therefore it should be used only if the cage is already larger than the minimum suggested size.

Placement of the box within the cage should be tailored to the bird for which it is designed. Parrots and finches usually prefer it

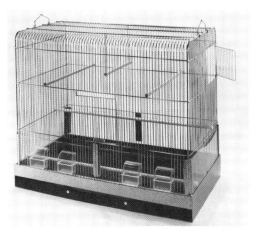

Fig. 2.1. Cage for finches, parakeets, canaries, with dimensions of 24 in. (61 cm) × 20¼ in. (51.5 cm). Its horizontal orientation makes it a good choice. (*Courtesy of Prevue Metal Products, Chicago, Ill.*)

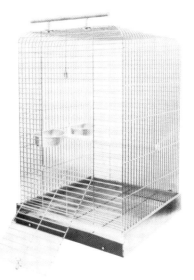

Fig. 2.2. This cage is advertised as a macaw/cockatoo cage. Its dimensions are 26 in. (66 cm) × 26 in. (66 cm) × 39 in. (99 cm), making it more suitable for a Cockatiel (*Nymphicus hollandicus*). (*Courtesy of Prevue Metal Products, Chicago, Ill.*)

high in the cage, while mynah birds accept it more readily on the cage floor. For mynahs and finches a paper bag or cardboard box may suffice, since they will not chew and destroy it as would a psittacine. These paper items should be discarded and replaced when they become soiled.

The problems of cage shape, cage size, and security areas can all be solved by the use of a box or semibox cage rather than the common wire cage. Box cages are much less readily available, but when the welfare of the bird is the prime concern it is well worth the time and effort to search for one or to make one. When making a box cage several points should be kept in mind. Materials must be nontoxic and not susceptible to damage by the bird (which can be a major challenge with a large parrot). They should be easy to clean and disinfect. No sharp edges or points on which a frightened bird could injure itself should protrude into the cage. Provision must be made for easy access to food and water containers and to the cage bottom so daily cleaning and changing of papers does not become such a chore that it is neglected. If wire is used for the front of the cage, the mesh or openings between the bars should be small enough that the occupant cannot get its head through. Latches should be strong and placed so a bird cannot reach them and open them or catch a toe in them. The exterior of the cage can be finished or decorated so that it becomes a tasteful addition to the room in which it is placed, as well as being a safe and comfortable home for its inhabitant.

Perches. Except for the times when a bird is flying or incubating, its weight is entirely supported by its feet and legs. For captive birds this means that the feet are weight bearing almost constantly, yet the perches they are forced to stand on are rarely of a type that is good for them. Usually they are either a wooden dowel or rigid ribbed plastic, both of which are hard, unyielding, of uniform diameter, round, and smooth. Sometimes they are covered with sandpaper, which helps soften them a little and which improves the bird's ability to grip them securely. But the problems caused by sandpaper far outweigh the benefits; not only does it fail to keep the nails worn down as it is supposed to do, but it is impossible to disinfect, it provides ideal cover for parasites such as *Cnemidocoptes* mites, and the grit it contains is very irritating to the plantar surfaces of the feet. The perches mentioned cause other foot problems as well. Because they are of uniform diameter the feet are always held in the same semiclenched position, get almost no exercise, and always have pressure applied to the plantar surfaces in the same location. Birds often sit on the edges of their food containers or on a mineral block or hang on the bars of the cage as a way of getting some relief from the discomfort.

There are several ways of solving the poor perch situation. Covering existing perches with pieces of heavy cloth or rubber tubing will help, or tubing or rope can be used alone. Cloth covers have some of the same drawbacks as sandpaper, since cloth can shelter parasites and must be removed frequently for cleaning and disinfection. If rope is used, especially in a parrot cage, the bird must be watched to make sure it does not eat it, since a crop impacted with ingested fibers could result. Different sizes and shapes of perches can be put in the cage. Oval, flat, and rectangular shapes can be used. By supplying perches of differing shapes and diameters the bird can exercise its feet and legs more and can change the distribution of weight on its feet. An even better solution to the problem is to provide freshly cut living branches as perches. Fruit trees are excellent, as are most deciduous trees such as oak, ash, maple, willow, and poplar. Toxic plants such as rhododendron and yew must be avoided. Coniferous trees such as pine, spruce, and hemlock are nontoxic but tend to ooze pitch when cut and are therefore less desirable. The bark should be left on to provide improved footing. Many birds will chew and shred the bark, and this should not be discouraged because it provides exercise and some emotional outlet for the bird and also helps keep the beak properly worn. Branches of varying diameters should be used. One disadvantage to the use of natural perches is that they cannot be cleaned and disinfected well, so they have to be discarded and replaced frequently. This is a minor inconvenience compared with all the benefits the bird derives from this type of perch.

The number of perches and their placement in the cage are important. At least two should be provided; more can be added if there is sufficient room in the cage. If only two are used, they should be placed approximately parallel to each other, as far apart as possible, and at similar heights to allow the bird maximal exercise as it moves from perch to perch. They should not be so near the ends of the cage that the bird's tail rubs when it turns around. Care should also be taken that they are not placed above food and water containers, to avoid the problem of contamination. In a large cage with multiple occupants the perches must be placed so that birds sitting on a low perch do not have droppings land on them.

Many birds enjoy a moving perch such as a swing. This type of perch gives slightly when the bird lands on it and thus cushions the landing somewhat, approximating the soft landing experienced in landing on the small outer branches of a tree. Commonly available swing perches are made of a dowel suspended from the top of the cage by a U-shaped rod. The dowel can be replaced with a piece of branch or other material. Alternatively, a moving perch can be constructed by stringing rope or rubber tubing across the cage.

Food and Water Containers. Containers for food and water are available in a variety of shapes, sizes, and materials and are satisfactory in most cases. Birds readily accept either open dishes or hopper-type feeders. The size of the feeder should be appropriate to the bird using it, with 1 oz (30 g) adequate for birds up to the size of a Budgerigar, 2–4 oz (60–120 g) for smaller parrots, 4–6 oz (120–180 g) for larger parrots, and 12–18 oz (360–540 g) for the large macaws. Similar size ranges can be used for soft-bills. Containers should be of nontoxic, nonporous material such as plastic, glass, ceramic, or metal. There should be no sharp edges or protruding points. Perches to be used during feeding should be placed close enough to the feeder so the bird can comfortably reach the food or water but not so close that a leg or head can get caught between the perch and the feeder. If metal is used it must not have any soldered joints, since lead poisoning can result either from leaching of lead into the food or water or from the bird's chewing at the solder and eating it. Feeders may be placed either high or low in the cage for psittacines and finches and should be placed on or near the cage bottom for ground-feeding birds such as doves. In general the higher the feeder is placed in the cage the less contamination there will be from droppings but the more mess there will be around the cage from scattered seeds and hulls.

Several different food containers should be present in the cage to allow a variety of foods to be offered. While it is not harmful to place moist, highly perishable foods such as fruits in the same container with less perishable items such as seeds, it is wasteful, since many seeds will be wetted and have to be discarded. There is no best number of food containers, but separate dishes for seed, grit, and perishables should be present. More can be added if desired. Some owners prefer not to mix seeds and offer each seed variety in a separate container.

Sanitation. Cleanliness is extremely important for the continued health and well-being of caged birds. Since the space they occupy is so confined, contaminants build up rapidly; unless cages are cleaned frequently, the birds are constantly exposed to excessive numbers of pathogens, resulting in chronic illness and stress. These pathogens are principally the bacteria and fungi that can grow in and on food or accumulated droppings. Even dried droppings are unsafe to leave in the cage, since pathogen-containing dust can form, leading to the possibility of respiratory disease. Some of the ways to help prevent this problem have already been mentioned but are worth repeating: frequent washing or changing of perches; proper placement of perches and food containers to minimize contamination by droppings; and the use of nonporous, easily cleaned materials for cages and dishes. Cage design features such as bottom trays removable for cleaning also help. In addition, food and water containers should be thoroughly cleaned daily, the cage paper should be changed daily or even more frequently for birds with soft watery droppings (lorikeets, mynahs), and any grids on the cage bottom should be scrubbed daily. The entire cage and all its contents should be cleaned at least weekly with hot soapy water and a mild disinfectant such as hypochlorite, Lysol, or a quaternary ammonium product.

The most practical material to keep on the cage bottom is an inexpensive, readily replaced paper such as newspaper. By cutting several pieces to fit the cage bottom and stacking them there, changing the cage paper becomes no greater chore than removing the top piece of paper. This simplicity helps ensure that it will in fact be done daily. Gravel paper offers no advantage over newspaper other than appearance, and it has the disadvantage of expense. Other materials sometimes used as cage floor coverings that are easy to remove and clean (e.g., plastic) are therefore acceptable. Sand, gravel, or wood shavings are generally used only in aviaries. They are impossible to disinfect properly and must be removed and replaced periodically; this must be done less frequently in an aviary since the droppings there are "diluted" by the larger area of the enclosure, thus lessening exposure to contamination. Even in an aviary, though, certain areas such as those around feeders and under favorite roosts should be cleaned daily.

Toys. Toys are often placed in cages to amuse and distract the birds. Whether they in fact do this, or whether they are no more than convenient objects on which to vent aggression or frustration, will not be argued here. (Is the Budgerigar that constantly courts its reflection in a mirror better or less well off than it would be without the illusion of a mate?) Providing either amusement or an outlet for frustration can be psychologically beneficial, though, so toys and other distractions may be provided without undue worry as to why they are used by the bird.

The main factors to consider when providing toys should be safety, appropriateness, and numbers. Many cages are so cluttered with toys that there is no room left for free movement by the bird. This situation can be avoided if restraint and common sense are used. Beads on a wire or a small plastic bird may be fine for a Budgerigar or Cockatiel but entirely unsuitable for a larger parrot that could destroy or ingest the toy. Balls, bells, ladders, mirrors, keys, and chains are all objects that are readily available and acceptable to use with smaller birds such as Budgerigars, Cockatiels, and canaries. However, it should always be kept in mind that toes may get caught or the toy may be chipped and become dangerously sharpened, or the bird may ingest small pieces of it. These dangers are even more pronounced when dealing with the larger parrots and macaws with their very powerful beaks and their propensity to chew. More appropriate toys for these birds are fresh twigs and branches, bones, rawhide dog chewies, and metal spoons or bells. In any case, amusements should be left in the cage only if the bird actually uses them. If a toy does not appeal to a particular bird it is better to remove it and either replace it with a different object or do without it, thus removing unnecessary cage clutter.

Environmental Factors. Birds cannot remain healthy in even the largest, best-maintained cage if the environment the cage is placed in is not properly controlled and healthful. Such factors as photoperiod (the number of hours that a bird is exposed to light in a 24-hour period) and wavelength of light provided are important, as are temperature, humidity, and general air quality.

In the wild, birds are very strongly influenced by changes in the hours of light and dark per day. As hours of daylight gradually increase or decrease birds may be prompted to molt, migrate, sing, and begin courtship and mating. In both birds and mammals photoperiod affects body temperature, eosinophil count, adrenal gland function, blood sugar levels, and central nervous system activity, among other things. Changes in photoperiod are smallest near the equator and largest at the poles, but over many thousands of years, birds living at a particular latitude have adapted to the changes that take place there. Such regularity of change does not occur in our homes with their artificial lights and television sets. Therefore a bird's biological clock, or circadian rhythm, is constantly disrupted, with resulting stress, abnormal molts and egg laying, and poor health. Rather than try to mimic nature's changes, it is better to give a bird a regular 10–12 hours of uninterrupted darkness and quiet per day by covering the cage with a dark cloth or by darkening the entire bird room by drawing curtains and closing doors. The bird will soon adapt to the regular routine and should be less stressed and healthier. Developing some sort of pattern also makes it possible to alter that pattern in certain ways in an attempt to stimulate or stop egg laying or molting.

Sunlight provides the entire spectrum of light wavelengths, from short (ultraviolet) to long (infrared). This broad-spectrum light provides many health benefits, especially ultraviolet stimulation of the skin to produce vitamin D. Birds that are maintained indoors are deprived of most of the benefits of sunlight, since window glass filters out the ultraviolet portion of the light spectrum. Incandescent and ordinary fluorescent lights do not adequately replace the missing wavelengths. It is therefore a good idea to expose the bird at least periodically to broader-spectrum lights (e.g., Gro-Lux or Vita-Lite), which are available at department stores, garden and nursery supply houses, and some pet stores. Suggested exposure is 8–10 hours per week.

Birds can tolerate a wide range of temperatures if they are healthy and not stressed by other factors such as poor diet, insufficient rest, and disease. Simply because a bird is present in the home is no reason to keep the temperature elevated. In general, if humans are comfortable in a house, a bird will be also, once it is acclimatized. A hardy soul who keeps the thermostat at 60°F (16°C) and purchases a bird that has been maintained at 75°F (24°C) should keep the bird at the higher temperature until it has adjusted to the move and only then begin to decrease the cage temperature gradually to that of the rest of the house. If chilled, a bird will sit with its feathers fluffed out; this is a sign that immediate steps should be taken to warm it up. A quartz heater is excellent for this purpose, since it is safer than a heating pad, does not give off any fumes or combustion products as kerosene heaters can, and does not alter photoperiod as drastically as heat lamps do. Moving the bird to a small room provided with an electric heater is also satisfactory. But it cannot be emphasized too strongly that no matter what heating device is used, an accurate thermometer should be placed in or near the cage to monitor the temperature so as not to overheat the bird. A sick bird should be maintained at 85°–90°F (29°–32°C).

It is also important to control humidity. Birds will fare better if the humidity is over 40%, and it is better to err by keeping the humidity too high rather than too low. Since many parrots kept as pets originate in tropical or subtropical regions with high humidity and frequent rainfall, maintaining high humidity and giving frequent baths can be very beneficial to their general well-being and especially to their plumage.

Birds are much more sensitive to fumes and other air pollutants than are humans, and care must always be taken to minimize or prevent such exposure. Cigarette smoke is harmful to all lungs, and birds should not be exposed to it if possible. Kerosene space heaters have become very popular because of their efficiency, but their safety is being increasingly questioned since they are not vented to the outside of the house. Until that matter is settled it is best not to use them near birds. Gas ranges are generally safe, but a faulty pilot light or some other leak could be dangerous. The fumes of scorched or overheated nonstick cookware are rapidly fatal to birds, while practically unnoticed by humans. And birds should be protected from the fumes of paint, lacquer, solvent, shellac, and aerosol cans, since what is mildly irritating to humans could be serious or even fatal to them. (See the discussion of toxic conditions in Chapter 32.)

Drafts seem to be the greatest fear of many bird owners, a fear that is often shared by pet shop owners and veterinarians. Yet wild birds, birds maintained in outdoor aviaries, and even escaped cage birds remain healthy when subjected to wind. If the bird is not overly stressed by other factors such as inadequate diet, insufficient space, lack of rest, or temperature fluctuations, drafts should be of no concern; any draft that is not bothersome to the humans in the house should have no ill effects on the birds kept there, either.

Freedom from the Cage. Many people allow their birds the freedom to leave their cage at will or remove them from the cage for certain periods of the day, and this practice can be safe and worthwhile. It allows the bird much more exercise and the opportunity for exploration and psychological fulfillment. But it can also result in escape, injury, or death if strict precautions are not observed. Only well-tamed birds should be allowed to fly free outside their cages, as they are less likely to become frightened and crash into furniture or walls and injure themselves. They will also be far easier to capture when it is time to return them to their cages. If birds cannot fly well (e.g., after their wings have been clipped), they need not be so tame, since they cannot move fast enough to injure themselves severely. Before any bird is freed from its cage, the room or rooms in which it will be free should be carefully inspected for hazards; fans should be turned off, and there should not be any hot surfaces that the bird could land on (cookstoves, wood or coal stoves, kerosene or electric heaters). No valuable or poisonous plants should be present. Doors should be closed and windows shielded with shades or curtains for at least the first few times the bird is freed, until it gets accustomed to the confines of its new, larger "cage." Aquariums and other bird cages should be covered. No other pets, including other birds, should be present, and the owner should be there to supervise, especially at first. Obviously as the bird becomes more accustomed to freedom from the cage these restrictions can be relaxed somewhat, but they should never be disregarded altogether or disaster may result.

Keeping a bird outside the cage but chained to a perch is worse than keeping it restricted to a small cage, since movement is still strictly limited and it can be badly injured by the chain. Therefore this practice should never be followed. It is far better to set up two or more perches separated from each other by a few feet so the bird can fly between them. Most larger parrots are fairly sedentary anyway, and if the perches are comfortable and if food and water are supplied on them, the birds may restrict themselves to the perches voluntarily. (See the discussion of perch training in Chapter 5.)

Aviaries. Many people dream of keeping their birds in an aviary rather than in cages, and there is much to be said for the advantages afforded birds that are housed in a large space. Flight becomes possible, as does a more natural environment complete with live plants, areas for seclusion, and enough space so that some of the larger birds such as macaws may reproduce. Different varieties of birds can be kept, including the galliforms. The advantages of captivity are also present, including protection from predators and drastic weather changes and a constantly available food supply.

Aviaries have their disadvantages as well. They are really nothing more than very large cages, and all the caveats concerning sanitation, fresh food and water, uncluttered flight space, proper perches, and so on must be observed. This is especially true with respect to sanitation, since the dirt or gravel floors often used in outdoor aviaries are virtually impossible to disinfect. Concrete would be better, but it is more expensive and less "natural" and therefore less esthetically pleasing. The temptation to house too many birds in an aviary must also be avoided at all costs. Overcrowding compounds sanitation problems and leads to additional stresses as territories are constantly infringed on by other birds. Of course many psittacines cannot be housed together in the first place because of fighting.

Outdoor aviaries have some other disadvantages, including the potential for invasion by vermin such as rats and mice and the diseases and parasites carried by wild birds that sometimes enter the aviary by squeezing through the wires or simply contaminate it with their droppings from above. The most obvious reason for concern for birds housed in outdoor aviaries is their exposure to cold and inclement weather. Therefore some provision for shelter and heat should always be made. The sheltered area must be set up like a small aviary in its own right, since in many areas of the world birds must be housed inside for long periods of time during the winter months.

Indoor aviaries offer another method of successfully housing birds and combine all the best features of cages and outdoor aviaries. They are large, easy to keep clean, protected from invasion by wild birds or other pests, and a constant protection from bad weather. They need not be expensive to construct. Nonpoisonous potted plants can be used to enhance their appearance and can be of great benefit to the birds, as well. On the other hand, indoor aviaries do take up a great amount of space. But for the serious aviculturist, or even a pet owner who wishes to house birds in a manner that puts the birds' welfare first and foremost, an indoor aviary is an excellent choice.

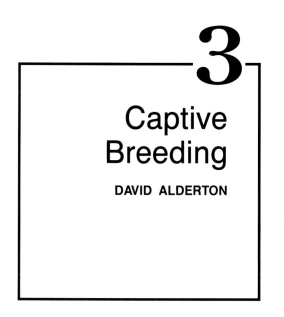

3

Captive Breeding

DAVID ALDERTON

IT IS IMPORTANT for the veterinarian to know about breeding behavior of major captive species to advise clients of normal and abnormal conditions. This chapter provides some of the basic information a veterinarian should have on the subject.

During recent years, many species have reproduced successfully under controlled conditions, and hopes of maintaining viable breeding populations of exotic local species and endangered species are being realized. The incubation period for some of the common avian species is listed in Table 3.1.

Reintroduction of avian species using captive-bred stock has proved successful in certain instances. One of the most successful schemes involved the Red-fronted Parakeet (*Cyanoramphus novaezelandiae*) coordinated by the New Zealand government. This species had been pushed to the edge of extinction as a result of persecution by farmers. Permission was granted for this species to be kept by aviculturists; from an initial population of 103 individuals in 1958, their numbers had increased to 2500 by 1964, indicating the fecundity of this species when kept under controlled conditions. Release schemes in selected areas have since followed, with the government paying aviculturists for their birds.

An increase in captive bird numbers is only possible with a large number of aviculturists having breeding success and holding stock. With many governments encouraging breeding and release schemes, the veterinarian's role in captive breeding programs has greatly increased.

Under a semi-intensive system of management with some species, the first clutch of eggs can be removed for artificial incubation, causing the birds to lay again. This technique, called "double clutching," provides a simple means of increasing the number of potential chicks that can be produced by a pair during the breeding season. An approximation of the reproductive performance of a flock is shown in Table 3.2.

Breeding Stimuli. Various diverse factors act as breeding stimuli. Budgerigars and other Australian parakeets breed naturally at the onset of rainy periods, which stimulate the growth of the grasses on which they feed. Many species are nomadic, moving in search of food and disappearing from areas for long periods of time until local conditions are more favorable.

Photoperiodism is of minor significance to birds coming from tropical areas, where little variation in day length occurs. The availability of food is a more significant factor; however, artificial modification of day length can lead to increased reproductive activity. Various species

Table 3.1. The incubation period for some common avian species

Common Name	Scientific Name	Incubation Period
Domestic Chicken	*Gallus domesticus*	21 days
Turkey	*Meleagris gallopavo*	28 days
Pheasant	*Phasianus colchicus*	23–28 days
Japanese Quail	*Corturnix corturnix japonica*	17 days
Bob-white Quail	*Colinus virginianus*	24 days
Domestic Duck	*Anser platyrhynchos*	28 days
Domestic Goose	*Anser anser*	28–34 days
Muscovy	*Cairina moschata*	35 days
Domestic Pigeon	*Columba livia*	17 days
Canary	*Serinus canaria*	13–14 days
Zebra Finch	*Taeniopygia castanotis*	12 days
Budgerigar	*Melopsittacus undulatus*	18 days
Sulphur-crested Cockatoo	*Cacatua galerita*	30 days
Ostrich	*Struthio camelus*	35–43 days

Source: Dr. R. L. Reece, Parkville, Victoria, Australia.

Table 3.2. An approximation of the reproductive performance of a flock of fifty pairs of breeding canaries (*Serinus canarius*)

Hatchlings Produced per Pair	Number of Pairs Laying Eggs								Total Pairs	Total Hatchlings Produced
	0 egg	1 egg	2 eggs	3 eggs	4 eggs	5 eggs	6 eggs	>6 eggs		
0	2	2	1	1	2	1	0	1	10	0
1	0	2	1	1	1	0	0	0	5	5
2	0	0	4	2	2	1	0	0	9	18
3	0	0	0	7	1	1	0	0	9	27
4	0	0	0	0	9	2	1	0	12	48
5	0	0	0	0	0	4	0	0	4	20
6	0	0	0	0	0	0	1	0	1	6
Total pairs	2	4	6	11	15	9	2	1	50	...
Hatchlings Produced	0	2	9	26	44	33	10	0	...	134

Source: Dr. R. L. Reece, Parkville, Victoria, Australia.

of conures, which prove only single clutched if kept outside in Britain throughout the year, will start laying in January if housed indoors in unheated surroundings on an unchanged diet (the only difference being the increased photoperiod generated by artificial light). Best breeding success can be expected by a progressive increase in the photoperiod, using weekly increments.

In an outside aviary with nestboxes available, the more prolific species of psittacines, notably the Budgerigar (*Melopsittacus undulatus*), Cockatiel (*Nymphicus hollandicus*), and Peach-faced Lovebird (*Agapornis roseicollis*), will attempt to nest throughout the year. Imported birds generally adapt to breed in the warmer months of the year in temperate climates, but some retain a preference for nesting during the autumn and winter. The Madagascar Lovebird (*Agapornis cana*) and *Poicephalus* parrots are often included in this category. The risk of failure and associated problems such as egg binding, are significantly increased if birds are allowed to breed outdoors during cold periods.

Diet modifications (e.g., raising the protein level) help to condition birds for breeding and ensure increased egg hatchability. A seed diet is deficient in essential amino acids and vitamins; pelleted diets and feed supplements offer a more balanced alternative.

Pairing. Pair bonding is important for breeding success in many species. Even the prolific Budgerigar often shows a distinct preference for a certain mate, although mating with other individuals in a colony may occur. Gregarious flock birds may not breed, or fertility may be reduced, if a single pair are kept on their own, out of sight and sound of other Budgerigars. With other species, such as the *Brotogeris*

parakeets, the best results have been obtained by housing pairs individually, in adjoining flights, with double wiring used to prevent fighting. Knowledge of the species is essential to achieve the highest results.

Birds should be placed together well in advance of the anticipated breeding season when possible. Cock birds tend to come into breeding condition slightly earlier than hens and can harass new mates severely if they fail to respond in the appropriate manner or are not compatible partners. Clipping the flight feathers of one wing of a cock should help the hen lead a less traumatic existence until after the breeding season, when they molt. It is not unknown for cock birds to kill intended mates. Molting usually leads to a cessation of reproductive activity, but in a few species, such as eclectus parrots, breeding may continue with the feathers being shed in the nest itself.

Some larger psittacines, such as Little Corella (*Cacatua sanguinea*), become aggressive toward humans at this stage, especially if hand reared.

Failure to Lay. The age of sexual maturity is variable, and while Budgerigars may lay as early as 5 months old, the large macaws may not start laying until their fourth year. Provision of inadequate breeding facilities can be an important factor in cases of reproductive failure.

The provision of adequate wood for chewing purposes is an important stimulant for certain species, particularly the larger psittacines such as cockatoos. The preparation of the nesting site can take a month or longer. Chunks of soft wood placed in the nestbox meet the birds' urge to gnaw and enable them to produce their own nest litter.

Actual nesting material is not used by the

majority of psittacines, with exceptions of hanging parrots (*Loriculus* spp.) and certain lovebirds (*Agapornis* spp.). The majority of passerines require suitable fibers to construct a nest. The construction of a nest is not indicative of immediate breeding behavior. Weaver birds, for example, often build elaborate nests that are never occupied. Pigeons and doves build loose, sloppy nests as a rule and therefore a suitable platform is recommended. Certain species will not lay if their nestboxes are placed in an exposed position. *Poicephalus* parrots generally favor nestboxes placed in dark, secluded surroundings. The cock bird can also play an important role in stimulating the female to produce eggs. With eclectus parrots, separation of a pair followed by reintroduction often stimulates the hen to lay within 3 weeks.

Broken Eggs. Broken eggs can result from disturbances (e.g., rough inspection of the nestbox) and from rodents. Long or misshapen claws can puncture the eggshell. If minor shell punctures are patched with nail varnish, in some instances the egg will hatch.

In certain species, some individuals are obviously egg eaters; sequential clutches are destroyed, the eggshell has a chewed appearance, and the bird may show traces of yolk around its beak. Pheasant breeders often keep infertile eggs from one season to the next, and substitute them under a hen known to be an egg eater. The foul taste of the addled egg discourages further egg eating. Alternatively, and more hygienically, "pot" eggs made of plastic or clay are used to break this abnormal behavior. Otherwise, eggs are saved by modifying the nestbox, providing a concave area raised off the floor, with a hole in the center. When the hen lays, the egg rolls down the concave area and falls through the hole to a soft bed of sawdust beneath, where it is out of reach. Egg breaking usually occurs in the early stages of incubation. Occasionally, if the incubation period is past and the eggs have failed to hatch, the hen will break the eggs.

Failure to Hatch. Incubation often does not begin in earnest until two or more eggs have been laid. Most pairs normally carry out this task without problem, although some individuals may prove nervous and ready to leave the nest if disturbed. Only birds such as quail, some pigeons, and doves are likely to neglect eggs after laying. Although pigeons and doves can be hatched artificially, foster parents are preferable to ensure that the resulting offspring receive the protein-rich "crop milk" secreted by members of this order for their chicks.

It is possible to detect the presence of an embryo in the egg by "candling" (viewing the egg with a light behind it). An egg that has not been fertilized appears translucent (sometimes described as "clear"). Egg examination can yield reliable results from about 8 days after the egg was laid, although in some species, such as the Slender-billed Conure (*Enicognathus leptorhynchus*), the developing embryos may not be visible until the 2-week stage.

In prolific species, infertility commonly results from the hen spending too much time in the nestbox immediately prior to laying, so that mating does not take place. This is likely to occur when eggs are laid before the first round of chicks have left the nestbox. In such a case, the nestbox should be closed for a length of time when the birds are first introduced.

In species in which the female is dominant, such as the Ring-necked Parakeet (*Psittacula krameri*), the male sometimes does not possess sufficient courage to achieve mating. If this is suspected, a change of partners is necessary. Some species, notably cockatoos, mate through the year but do not actually nest. The mating ritual seems merely intended to reinforce the pair bond.

Failure of fertile eggs to hatch is increased during periods of cold and wet weather because both the growth of the embryo and the rate of evaporation via the egg's pores are reduced. Studies suggest that, on average, most eggs lose about 15% of their initial weight during the incubation period, although this figure may be increased in eggs of species naturally occurring at high altitudes. By means of artificial incubation, losses of this nature can be kept to a minimum.

Disease and reproductive problems causing failure of eggs to hatch are discussed in Chapter 15.

Failure to Rear. In the first day or so of life, the chick is largely dependent on its yolk sac reserves. In some cases (notably cockatoos, which usually produce two chicks in a clutch), it is not unusual for one chick, usually the youngest, to be neglected by its parents. This chick will almost certainly die unless removed for hand rearing.

Early losses of chicks can result from infectious causes. In the case of Cockatiels, *Candida* can often be implicated in these deaths. A heavy parasitic burden is also likely to be significant, with red mite (*Dermanyssus gallinae*) causing anemia, weakness, and ultimate death of the chicks. Other infections, such as air-sac mite (*Sternostoma tracheacolum*) in Gouldian Finches (*Chloebia gouldiae*), may be acquired by nestlings from their parents.

Particular pairs may be poor parents and

simply allow their chicks to die. African Gray Parrots (*Psittacus erithacus*) are often neglectful if they are persistently disturbed. In temperate climates, birds that nest early in the year may cease to brood their chicks at night and losses from cold can be anticipated. Plumhead Parakeets (*Psittacula cyanocephala*) often lose their chicks for this reason and are rarely double-brooded, unlike related species such as the Alexandrine (*Psittacula eupatria*). A well-insulated nestbox positioned in a sheltered environment is necessary for such birds. Some breeders use low-wattage heating pads in the bottom of the nest to reduce chick losses.

The diet of many species is modified during the breeding season, and failure to meet the demands of the parent birds for additional protein is likely to lead to a low chick-survival rate. Many seedeating finches (e.g., waxbills) become highly insectivorous when rearing chicks. Pack-eted rearing foods for use with various species are available commercially.

Parental Aggression. The main period for danger from parental aggression is immediately prior to and after fledging. While chicks can be left safely with their parents in some instances, it is often safer to remove them once they are feeding independently.

Chicks may be killed while still in the nest; the nape of the neck is the common site of assault. Vicious behavior of this nature is most prevalent in rosellas (*Platycercus* spp.), Red-rumped Parakeets (*Psephotus haematonotus*), *Forpus* parrotlets, and lovebirds (*Agapornis* spp.). A cock known to be aggressive should be removed from the nest at least 1 week before the expected fledging time, or alternatively, the chicks taken away for hand rearing.

2

Cage Bird
Management

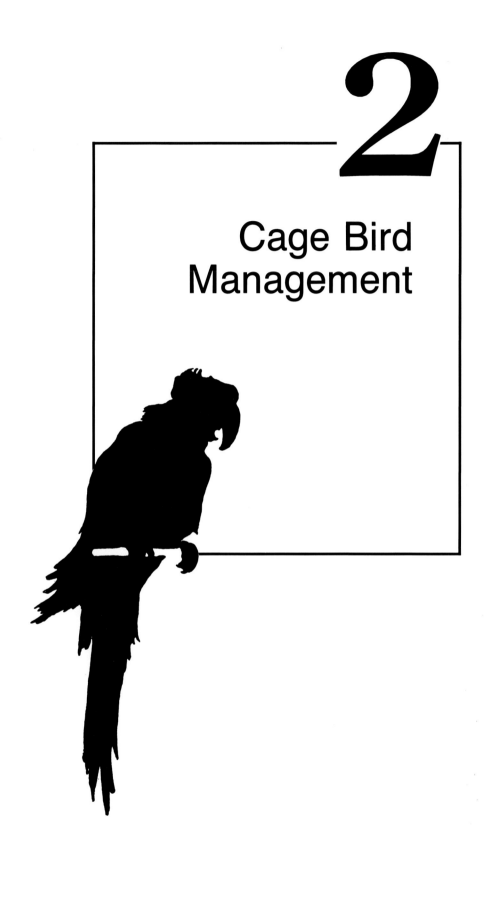

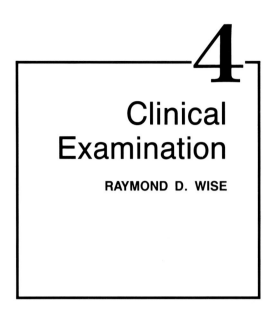

4

Clinical Examination

RAYMOND D. WISE

WHEN AN AVIAN PATIENT is scheduled for an appointment, to expedite the clinical evaluation the following instructions should be given to the owner. The bird is likely to be more at ease in its regular cage, so unless it is very awkward to do so it should be used. The cage should not be cleaned nor should anything be removed from it except the water, because direct observation of the bird's usual environment can be very helpful in diagnosing problems. Samples of all feedstuffs should be brought along because the diet can indicate possible origins of clinical problems. Food samples should include seed mixtures, grit, oyster shell, mineral blocks, cuttlebones, and vitamin and other supplements. Any current or previous medications (or a list) should be included.

History. When the client presents the avian patient for evaluation, taking the history is essential. This should include the species, color, age, and sex, if known. Using the name of the patient generally places the owner more at ease, and occasionally using the name can calm the bird during the examination. If the bird is not in its regular cage, a description of the cage and its components should be requested. The history should also indicate the original source of the bird, the length of ownership, whether the bird is the only one owned by the client, and where and how any other birds are caged in relation to the patient. Other birds on the premises should be characterized by species, source, and duration of ownership. Recent deaths or sicknesses of pet birds at or near the client's address should be recorded. Questions pertaining to the presenting complaint are then asked. (What signs of illness are currently present? How long

have these signs been noted? Were any other signs present earlier? Does the bird have a history of other illnesses?) All signs should be characterized as to frequency of occurrence, duration of occurrence, and time of day noted. Environmental changes may cause feather-picking disorders and can also be important in physical or metabolic problems. These changes may include cage movement, smoke, and the use of any aerosol sprays, fumigation, paint, or chemicals.

Information concerning other pets in the household may reveal trauma to the bird. Free-flighted birds also have more opportunities for trauma and poisoning. Because of better physical stamina, free-flying birds may not appear ill when confined to a cage. Masked respiratory problems can mislead the examiner, but evidence of disease may occur when the bird is stressed with either capture or flight. Confined birds usually have less-massive pectorals and can be expected to have greater feather damage. Confined birds can also be expected to show more foot pathology, as the variability of perches is likely to be small. Pet birds develop a relationship with their owners, and therefore behavioral alterations are more readily noticed. An observant owner can make decisions about the bird's health based on its vocalizations, food consumption, activity, and interaction, as well as physical appearance.

Capture and Restraint. Seldom is one faced with examining a well-trained and calm bird. It is necessary, therefore, to take certain precautions for the safety of the examiner as well as the patient. Frightened, sick birds are frequently stressed to the point where any additional stress could prove fatal. It is of benefit to cover a cage so that the bird can adjust to the sound of the examiner's voice before examination. One should slowly approach the cage talking in low, modulated tones. Observations of the bird's carriage, stance, and balance should be noted. The attitude of the bird (flighty, lethargic) as well as its respiratory characteristics (open or closed mouth, tail bobbing, labored or quiet breathing) should be noted before any handling. The condition of the droppings in the cage should be noted (see the section later in the chapter on collecting droppings).

The owner of the bird should always be informed of the stress involved in a physical exam. It is necessary to have the examination room "bird proof." Doors, windows, and exhaust fans must be closed or adequately covered to prevent escape or injury. It is preferable to darken the room before introducing a hand into the cage, box, or sack containing the bird. If the bird is very elusive, flashing a small penlight into the conveyance will help enable capture. It is sometimes helpful to have a low-wattage red light bulb to provide background lighting in a darkened room.

Often it is a good idea to protect the grasping hand when entering a bird's domain. Small and medium-sized psittacines are readily captured with the use of a small cloth, and medium-sized or large psittacines are better captured with a towel or protective gloves (Fig. 4.1). Small passerines, such as finches and canaries, are best captured with the bare hand, while a small towel is usually required to capture large passerines. Following capture it is best to transfer the bird to bare-handed or simple cloth restraint since gloves will not allow perception of the amount of pressure used for restraint. Most waterbirds can be carried by the wings (Fig. 4.2). Taping beaks closed can be a useful procedure (Fig. 4.3).

Restraining most other bird species centers on grasping the head with simultaneous containment of the body. Small and most medium-sized birds can be restrained adequately in an average person's hand (Fig. 4.4). Some medium-sized and large birds require continued use of a cloth for restraint. A small hand towel is wrapped

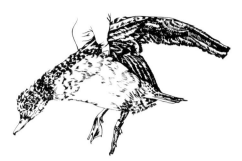

Fig. 4.2. Carrying a waterbird by the wings, holding the humeri near their attachment to the body. (*Drawing by Genevieve M. Wilson*)

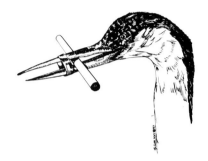

Fig. 4.3. Taping the beak over a dowel during an examination to prevent biting while permitting breathing. (*Drawing by Genevieve M. Wilson*)

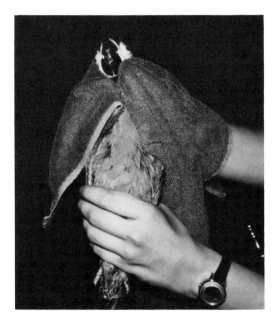

Fig. 4.1. Proper method of restraining a medium-sized to large psittacine, using a towel, with the hand covering the body. (*Courtesy of Steven Wehrmann, Bayshore Veterinary Hospital, Bayshore, Fla.*)

around the bird, with the thumb and forefinger again grasping the head in the vicinity of the bird's ears. The towel contains the wings and gives the feet something to grasp. The bird can then be held to the body of the examiner and the various parts of the bird uncovered and examined as desired. The towel should be loose enough to allow uncompromised respiration and should be unwrapped as much as possible to prevent overheating. It takes two hands to restrain large birds, one for the head and one for the body; therefore it is frequently necessary to have an assistant. It is usually better accepted by the owner if the veterinarian captures the bird and then either transfers the patient to the assistant or has the assistant grasp the necessary portion to free the veterinarian so that the examination can proceed. When transferring a bird to another person for restraint, always pass the head first. Once the head is controlled by the assistant, the examiner may retain the body or have a second assistant take it instead of passing the entire bird.

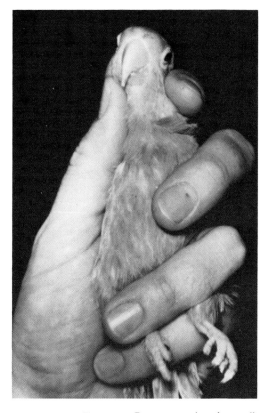

Fig. 4.4. Proper restraint of a small to medium-sized bird. The head is grasped between the forefinger and thumb with the rest of the fingers wrapped lightly around the body. A small bird's feet can also be placed between the fourth and fifth fingers of the restraining hand for better immobilization. (*Courtesy of Steven Wehrmann, Bayshore Veterinary Hospital, Bayshore, Fla.*)

Examination. Once adequate restraint has been implemented, the examination can begin. Determining an accurate gram weight is of extreme importance. Fluctuation in the bird's weight between visits or examinations can be an excellent prognostic sign, one that can call for a change in the therapeutic regime. Several types of weight measurement devices are available.

Start the examination with the bird's head. Running one's fingers over the head of the bird can reveal much about the actual structure of the head and the general shape and contour of the feathers. For examination of the mouth, thumb forceps and hemostats can be used in most birds, varying the size of the instrument to

fit the bird. Metal paper clips of varying sizes can also be used in small species (Fig. 4.5). For safety, in larger species it is best to use a speculum made specifically for the purpose (Fig. 4.6); they are without sharp edges and do not easily collapse.

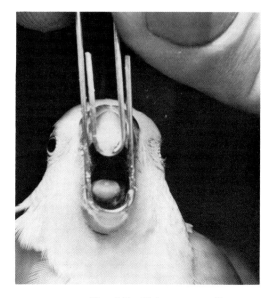

Fig. 4.5. Using a paper clip as an oral speculum. (*Courtesy of Steven Wehrmann, Bayshore Veterinary Hospital, Bayshore, Fla.*)

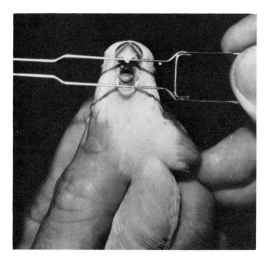

Fig. 4.6. An especially crafted oral speculum for examination of the oral cavity, graduated for use in small to large birds. (*Courtesy of Steven Wehrmann, Bayshore Veterinary Hospital, Bayshore, Fla.*)

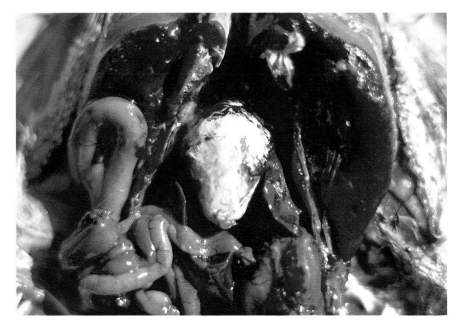

Plate 1. Visceral urate deposition in a pigeon. (*Courtesy of Elisha W. Burr*)

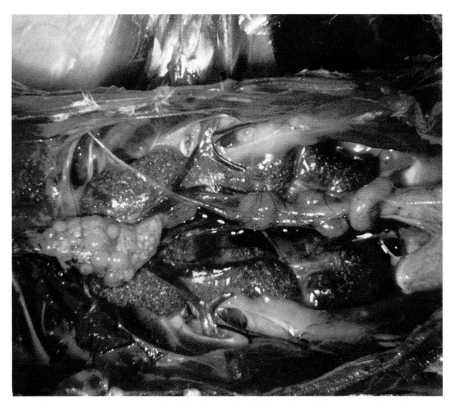

Plate 2. Nephrotoxic visceral urate deposition throughout the kidneys and abdominal viscera.

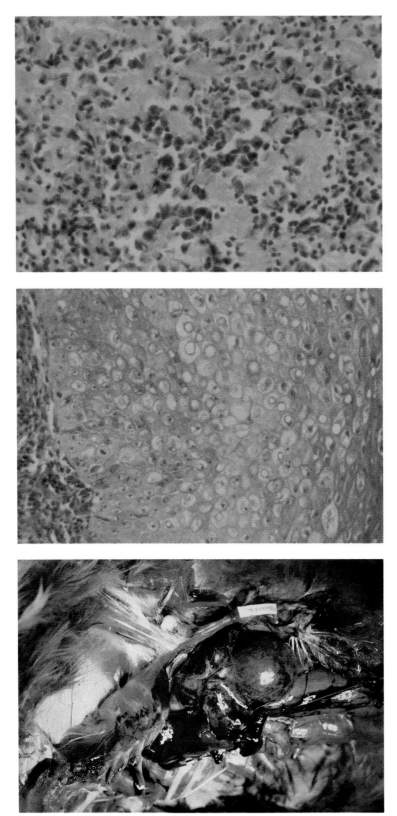

Plate 3. Amyloidosis in the spleen of a Java sparrow (*Padda oryzivora*). (H & E) (*Courtesy of K. E. Harrigan, University of Melbourne Veterinary School, Melbourne, Aust.*)

Plate 4. Poxvirus lesions in a canary (*Serinus canarius*). (H & E) (*Courtesy of K. E. Harrigan, University of Melbourne Veterinary School, Melbourne, Aust.*)

Plate 5. Swollen, inflamed gizzard in a peahen (*Pavo cristatus*). The gizzard wall had been penetrated by a small stick. Antemorten radiography suggested gizzard impaction.

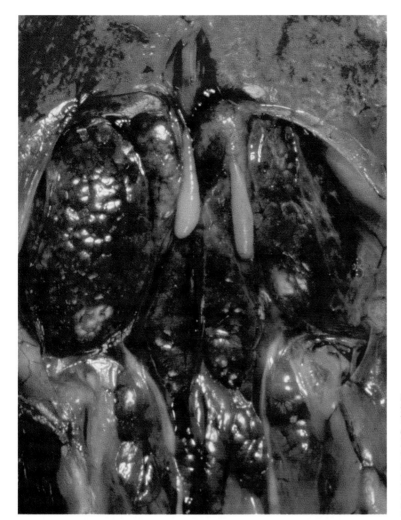

Plate 6. Testes from an immature male. In this bird they are cream-colored and cylindrical. Note their location atop the larger (yellowish) adrenal glands. The reddish-brown kidneys are located laterally, and the pink tissue cranially is the lung.

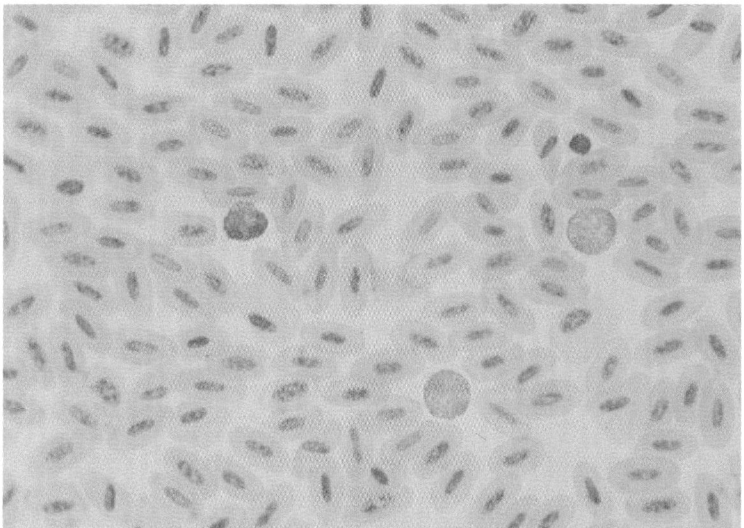

Plate 7. Heterophils, basophils, and thrombocytes from a psittacine blood film.

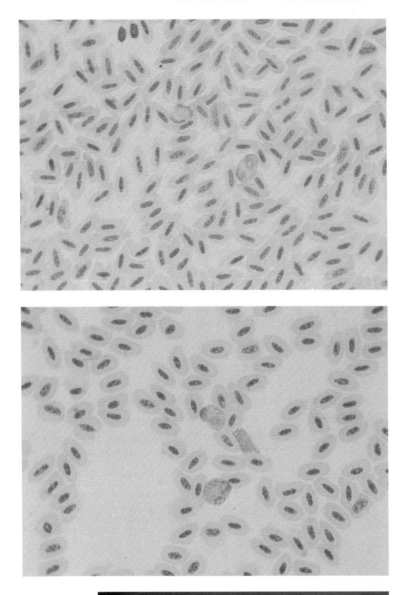

Plate 8. Eosinophils and lymphocytes from a psittacine blood film.

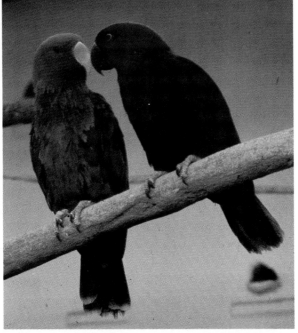

Plate 9. Monocytes and heterophils from a psittacine blood film.

Plate 10. Grand Eclectus Parrots (*Eclectus ornatus*), which exhibit one of the most striking examples of sexual dimorphism in birds. The male is bright green, the female a brilliant red and blue.

Lesions in the mouth may be plaquelike, raised, caseous, or exudative. Occasionally foreign bodies are found (seed hulls, plant awns, small inedible objects).

A decrease in the number of papillae on the surface of the palate, coupled with an atrophied appearance, can indicate a disease state. The tongue varies in shape and function among the numerous avian species. Psittacines (seed-eaters) have a short, round, blunt, and firm tongue, which they use effectively in hulling seeds. Passerines have a narrow, triangular tongue with a flat, malleable surface that rolls slightly. Tongue ulcerations and cuts can be found in the passerines, but they are rare compared to those in the psittacines, who use their tongues to explore objects. Pox lesions, which may be raised, crusty, and inflamed, may be found anywhere in the mouth.

Most birds have colored beaks, which can range from a very light yellow to almost black, with a gradual shade change from the area of growth to the tip of the beak. Although there are exceptions, such as the toucan species, this serves as a rule. In the healthy bird the beak is glossy and smooth; some ridges can be encountered as a result of normal activity but are rare. Alterations of beak structure due to disease and genetics are seldom correctable and may require lifelong intervention to promote proper function. Some birds develop abnormal beaks after reaching maturity, suggesting that environmental factors may be involved. Hemorrhagic, chipped, crumbly, discolored, rippled, splintered, grooved, blunted, and overgrown beaks are all signs of either current or past episodes of disease. Disease states of the beak can include partial or complete sloughing, especially with deep-seated mycotic or bacterial infections. The commissures of the beaks are commonly found to have growths (papules or warts) or cnemidocoptic mange in small psittacines. The cere should be checked for small growths, closure, serous-type discharge, mange (common in Budgerigars), abscessation, and other significant pathology.

An eye check should show the pupil responding to light, as in other species. Lens pathology (cataracts, corneal ulcers) should be looked for. Examination with an ophthalmoscope is possible only in the larger species. Staining and other diagnostics are similar to mammalian techniques. The eye globe should move freely in all directions. Palpation of the closed eye is permittable but should be done gently to avoid corneal denting. The eyes should appear similar in size and shape. Commonly retrobulbar abscesses cause one eye to appear more prominent. Any pronounced ocular discharge is not normal. Clear serous-type discharge is often found when retrobulbar pressure is present but can also indicate corneal trauma or infections.

Budgerigars are prone to cnemidocoptic mange lesions at the lid margins. Canaries are particularly prone to developing feather follicle cysts around the eye, which can result in scarring, abnormal function, and disfiguration. Debris of a white, cheesy nature can occasionally be noted between the third eyelid (nictitating membrane) and the globe, usually indicating a conjunctival infection.

Although seldom encountered, ear pathology can occur and should be looked for. It would require very fine and very pliable fiberoptic equipment to view the tympanic membrane of the bird, so only visual examination of the external ear is carried out.

Following the examination of the head, the structures of the neck are examined. The jugular vein of the right side is easily visualized by parting the feathers along the tracts in the neck. The thin skin of most birds also allows viewing of the esophagus and trachea, which are in close proximity to the right jugular vein. The skin of the lower neck is a frequent victim of feather pickers and must be palpated for cysts and infection in those cases. In the normal bird that has had recent access to food, there should be food visible or palpable in the crop. Especially in young birds, but also in tube-fed birds, crop abscesses can occur and should be looked for. Doughy, hard, or watery texture to the crop can indicate disease. The normal crop of an adult bird on a seed diet should feel pliable, like a small beanbag. Birds on other diets should have an appropriate crop texture. Thickening of the crop can be normal in adult birds rearing young.

Examination of the main body starts with the feathering. Presence of bare skin may indicate an abnormal loss of feathers or emergence of a mass (tumor or cyst). Feather pickers are commonly presented exhibiting large areas of exposed skin. Besides being unsightly, the skin is frequently traumatized and may contain cystic feather follicles and ingrown feathers due to frequent plucking. Chewed feathers are permanently damaged and not able to protect a bird normally because the feather barbules have been altered. Examination should indicate if a skin infection is either a primary or secondary cause of disease. Mite infestations do occur, but usually only in recently acquired birds.

Palpation of the chest gives the clinician an indication of the chronicity and severity of the present illness. The keelbone, which is palpable in most species, should exhibit a prominent muscle mass. Loss of normal muscle mass and the resulting prominence of the keelbone indicates disease. The fatty deposits or growths frequently encountered overlying the keel and clavicle area may require surgical intervention.

Auscultation of the pectoral area with a stethoscope can be useful. Although normal cardiac rates are very high (generally over 300 beats per minute), rhythm and rate are apparent. Respiratory sounds can also be auscultated but are not localized as in mammals. Normal respiratory rate is 85 per minute, but varies widely with stress and species. Alterations in cardiac and respiratory sounds usually take the form of murmurs and chirps, respectively.

Palpation of the abdomen is accomplished with the index fingertip. With the exception of the gizzard, internal structures are not firm. The size of the gizzard varies with the species and is frequently palpable in the caudal abdomen. It should not be mistaken for a growth. In birds with flaccid abdominal musculature the intestines can be palpated by gently rolling the contents between the thumb and index finger. Obese birds or birds with neoplasms are difficult to palpate. If intraabdominal enlargement occurs, the vent may protrude and be subject to trauma. Internal structures may protrude through the vent, especially the reproductive tract of the female bird when egg-bound or diseased. Accumulation of droppings on the feathers around the vent is abnormal and should always be investigated.

Next the back of the bird is examined by rotating the bird slowly in the hand, adjusting the hold accordingly. The majority of problems concerning the back relate to feather loss, either self-inflicted or the result of pulling by a cage mate. Palpation of the back can indicate abnormal growths, infection, or other disease. The tail feathers should be examined for disease and are often found to be damaged. On the dorsum of the tail lies a protruding glandular structure, the uropygial (or preen) gland. This gland may become impacted, infected, or cancerous. Palpation of the normal gland frequently causes secretion of a thick oily material from the orifice, which can be taken to indicate normal function.

When the wing is examined, it should be extended from the body and the feather condition noted. The joints are individually flexed and the integrity of the bones palpated. Feather cysts are frequently present on the wings of young birds (particularly canaries) and occasionally tumors are encountered.

When examining the legs it is easiest to start with the feet. Most caged birds' feet are afflicted with some degree of pathology, particularly those that have been maintained for a long time. Unlike in the wild the caged bird is required to grasp and sit on an extremely limited number of types of perches. Excessive callous formation, overgrown nails, infections, and open sores can be the result.

Caged birds' nails generally receive inadequate wear. This results in overgrowth and trauma, as they can get caught in objects and break easily. Mange mites are very common on the feet of Budgerigars and canaries, causing hyperkeratosis and excessive scale production. Permanent nail damage may be present in longstanding cases.

The joints of the foot are easily viewed and palpated. The blood vessels in the foot are visible and may be engorged when disease is present. Inflammation can be detected by enlargement of the vessels and splotchy, darker foot coloration. The color of the skin over the feet is usually similar to that of the beak. Abscesses can occur in the foot, commonly at the junction of the toes and the tarsal-metatarsal bone, which is the major weight-bearing point in birds. Gout (urate deposits resembling small abscesses) frequently affects the joints of the foot.

After the feet the tibial-tarsal bone, knee joint, and finally the femur and its articulation with the pelvis should be examined. Dark discoloration of the flesh area of the leg may indicate a recent bone fracture.

Collecting Samples

Droppings. As a bird's droppings contain both urine and feces, they must be carefully scrutinized to determine which part may be abnormal. Isolated fresh droppings give the best information. Droppings collected from a nonabsorbable surface (waxed paper, plastic wrap) provide the best sample. Nervous birds often produce poorly formed stools with a larger-than-normal amount of urates (urine). Small psittacines pass a stool characterized as a bull's-eye. These droppings generally are firm with the darker fecal portion appearing on the periphery and the white urate portion located in the center. Color alteration of the urates from the normal white or very pale yellow can be significant. Green, dark yellow, pink, and gray are commonly associated with disease but may also reflect medication or diet. Such a case was encountered by the author when an amazon parrot was presented for passing what appeared to the owner to be blood. It turned out to be food coloring added to a cake the bird had eaten. Liver disorders have been noted to cause discoloration of urates, but this is not a consistent finding.

Several droppings are usually combined for parasitic examination by flotation, with either concentrated sugar or sodium nitrate solution. For culture, sterile swabs should be used to collect fresh droppings from areas that are uncluttered with seed hulls or feathers. These swabs should be directly streaked onto agar plates or placed in sterile broth or media tubes and transported to the lab under refrigeration. Examination of droppings for evidence of psittacosis requires special processing and culture media. Any laboratory providing this service should be consulted in advance concerning sample collection and preparation for culture.

Fecal culture has many benefits for proper selection of antibiotics. Examination of a smear of fresh droppings with a Gram stain as well as a direct unstained smear can be beneficial. The normal gut flora of pet birds has not been adequately characterized, but it is usually considered abnormal for gram-negative rod bacteria to be present in high numbers.

Cloaca. When clean or recent dropping samples cannot be obtained, cloacal samples are taken. Quantity is seldom available, but danger of contamination is minimal if the bird is adequately restrained. To obtain a sample, the feathers must be held away from the orifice and the cloaca everted. Insertion of a standard-sized swab is easily accomplished on medium-sized and large birds; smaller birds such as Budgerigars, canaries, and finches usually require a pared-down swab.

Oral Samples. When taking oral samples a speculum should be inserted to minimize contamination and to facilitate control of the tongue. Pathology is often encountered in the choana, which can be easily swabbed to obtain a sample. To enhance the prospect of a usable sample, a nasal flush can be added to the sampling procedure. A small quantity of sterile saline or other isotonic fluid can be gently directed into one of the nares while the swab is in place in the choana. Cultures can also be made from tracheal swabs or aspirates.

Crop. The contents of the crop can be sampled for examination and culture by passing a sterile feeding tube. Care must be taken to ensure that the tube is in the crop before instilling a small quantity of sterile isotonic fluid. The amount of fluid administered depends on the size of the bird and the amount of air space in the feeding tube. The fluid is then gently aspirated and placed in a sterile container for examination.

Blood. Clipping a toenail short enough to cause a flow of blood has been widely used in small birds (see Table 4.1 for advantages and disadvantages of this method). When trimming the nail, one should make only a moderate cut, taking back the nail to the point that allows ade-

Table 4.1. Advantages and disadvantages of blood collection methods available to the avian clinician

NAIL CLIPPING

Advantages
    Simplest and least stressful to the patient
    Hemostasis quick and simple
    Spares veins for therapy and catheterization
    Enables clinician to properly monitor a case when repeated blood sampling is necessary
    Clinical pathology parameters the same as those obtained by venipuncture

Disadvantages
    Low blood pressure or lack of relaxation on the part of the patient can make blood collection difficult and slow
    Urate residues on the nail may cause blood chemistry artifacts
    Some patients may favor foot from which blood was taken
    Occasionally, nail may begin to bleed after hemostatis achieved

VENIPUNCTURE

Advantages
    Collection of relatively large sample in short period of time
    Technique easy for experienced clinician

Disadvantages
    Very stressful to clinically ill bird
    Veins lost for therapy and catheterization
    Hemostasis time-consuming (stressful) with potential for significant extravasation of blood subcutaneously
        (less a problem with jugular venipuncture)
    Repeat sampling difficult

Source: Drs. R. W. Woerpel and W. J. Rosskopf, Jr., and Tech. M. Monahan-Brennan, Animal Medical Centre of Lawndale, Hawthorne, Calif.

quate flow without "milking" the toe. The foot must be cleansed of any potentially contaminating substances before collection, and a means of stopping the blood flow should be available. Following the blood collection, pressure is applied to the toe by gently squeezing it between the fingers, and chemical or electrical cautery applied to the surface. Chemical cautery is quick but potentially toxic if the chemicals are ingested. Silver nitrate sticks, ferric subsulfate, and styptic pencils are commonly used. Application of pressure or a clotting medium such as cotton to the bleeding area avoids the toxic element but is time-consuming and more likely to result in excessive blood loss. The author prefers ferric subsulfate powder, as it is very quick and convenient and the amount used can be easily varied, thereby minimizing the likelihood of ingestion.

Blood collection from venipuncture is possible in almost all birds (see Table 4.1 for advantages and disadvantages of this method). A syringe with an attached microfine needle like those used by human diabetics is best for blood collection in small avians; being hubless, these needles avoid waste and dilution of the sample. An anticoagulant solution, if desired, can be aspirated and expelled through the syringe before blood collection. The most available vein in small birds is the jugular, located along the right side (Fig. 4.7). During restraint the head is ex-

tended with the index and middle finger of the left hand, while the ring and little finger contain the body. The thumb is used to distend the vein. The feathers are easily separated along their respective tracts to allow visualization of the jugular vein. A cotton-tipped applicator dipped in alcohol can be used to cleanse the venipuncture site. The needle is inserted using standard venipuncture technique and the sample slowly aspirated. When the needle is withdrawn the thumb of the left hand should relax the vein's distension and move up the neck to apply pressure to the venipuncture site. After about 30 seconds there is seldom need for further pressure, but the bird should not be released until the bleeding has stopped. Venipuncture of the jugular in the larger birds requires the use of an assistant for restraint but proceeds in a similar manner.

The brachial vein, located on the ventral aspect of each wing, can be used for blood sampling but is better suited for administration (Fig. 4.8). This type of venipuncture requires an assistant, as the wing must be extended as well as the bird contained. Light pressure in the axillary area will distend the vein, as will tension on the skin in the same area. Gentle cleansing of the area and pressure applied to the puncture site is again recommended. One disadvantage following the use of brachial venipuncture is hematoma formation. Other veins may occasionally

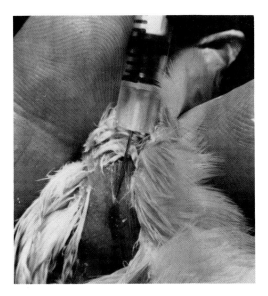

Fig. 4.7. Technique of placing a needle in the jugular vein, located on the right side. (*Courtesy of Steven Wehrmann, Bayshore Veterinary Hospital, Bayshore, Fla.*)

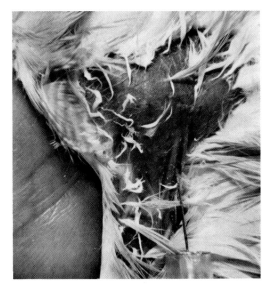

Fig. 4.8. Technique of placing a needle in the brachial vein, located on the ventral aspect of each wing. (*Courtesy of Steven Wehrmann, Bayshore Veterinary Hospital, Bayshore, Fla.*)

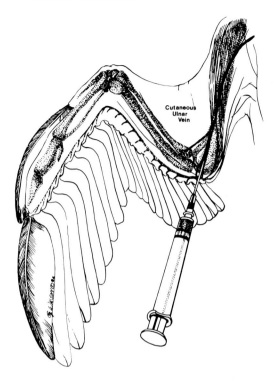

Fig. 4.9. Cutaneous ulnar vein, easily accessible for injection in waterbirds and other species. Injection is made near the point of the elbow on the ventral side of the wing. (*Drawing by Genevieve M. Wilson*)

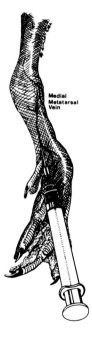

Fig. 4.10. Large, accessible medial metatarsal vein, recommended for blood sampling and injecting medication in waterbirds and some other species, as hematomas are less likely to develop at this site. (*Drawing by Genevieve M. Wilson*)

lend themselves to sampling and should be treated in a similar manner (Figs. 4.9 and 4.10).

Blood is generally collected into heparinized or nonheparinized (depending on the tests to be run) capillary tubes, and should be processed as soon as possible. Smears especially benefit from the use of a fresh sample. Blood collected in unheparinized capillary tubes for serum chemistries should be allowed to clot and then be spun down in a microhematocrit centrifuge. The tube is then broken just above the backed blood cells to obtain the serum for testing. If the sample is to be sent off to a laboratory, both ends of the tube containing the serum should be plugged with clay.

Skin and Feathers. Feathers can be collected for examination and culture. The feather should be firmly grasped and pulled in the direction it grows, employing steady traction until the follicle releases it. Seldom will hemorrhage or tissue tearing occur when a feather is collected in this manner. Feather culture must contain that portion in the follicle (the tip of the quill). Microscopic feather examination can reveal parasitic, nutritional, and environmental problems. Samples are often taken from the beak and feet of birds for parasite, fungus, or bacteria examination. A small flat spatula or similar device should be used to scrape or elevate any scales from the surface. Care must be taken to avoid excessive trauma in collection of samples from these areas, as hemorrhage may be difficult to control.

Other standard tissue sampling techniques can be adapted to avian species as the need arises. Aspirates of body swellings submitted for culture and other analysis can reveal information about disease and prognosis. Samples for histopathology should be handled as are samples from other species but should only be submitted to a laboratory familiar with avian pathology.

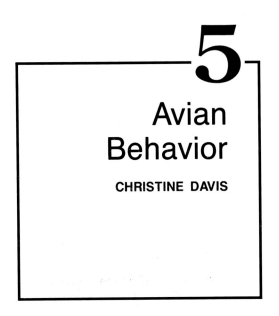

5

Avian Behavior

CHRISTINE DAVIS

BIRDS COMPOSE an extremely unique animal group, and a holistic understanding of their peculiarities should be an integral aspect of ownership. Most clients have to go to their veterinarian for this information, as few are deeply involved in the psychological aspects of avian behavior and its modification. Unfortunately, unless practitioners see many birds on a daily basis, they may not be exposed to the many different aspects of avian behavior and handling. Because psittacines are the most widely kept companion birds and are often handled, much of this section relates to their behavior.

The psittacine patient, in most cases, must be handled with an acute awareness of its unique mental and behavioral makeup. Mishandling of the pet by the owner or the practitioner can lead to permanent negative behavior. Clients unfamiliar with avian behavior will frequently purchase these expensive animals and when they develop problems, turn to the practitioner for assistance. It is necessary to understand these animals not only to treat them in a full capacity medically but also to modify aberrant behavior.

Behavior. It is important to know the basic behavioral idiosyncrasies of various common species of parrots. The younger the pet bird, the tamer and more agreeable it will usually become. An adult must be extremely tame if it is to remain a manageable pet. The bird should show an active interest in the client and display some stability of personality. If the bird is constantly busy—playing, eating, and even bothering the other birds in the cage—it will most likely be an intelligent and active pet but will require more attention than the bird who just sits and does not play. A bird that is too active and aggressive may be too much for the owner to handle. A bird that backs off in caution when talked to or that stays still and listens to the person talking is a good candidate for a steady, reliable pet. A hand-fed pet is preferable to one that is hand-tamed, as the hand-fed bird has usually imprinted on humans and not on other birds. A hand-tamed bird is a previously untamed bird that has been gentled enough to sit on the hand without biting, in contrast to a hand-fed bird, which is one that has been hatched in captivity and left with the mother only for the first 2 or 3 weeks of age (until just before the eyes are open). These fledglings imprint on humans and actually become a little feathered "person." The infant parrot, when hand-fed after its eyes are open, will still be a very good pet but may not be as heavily imprinted on humans.

Basic Behavioral Traits of Various Species

Budgerigars (*Melopsittacus undulatus*). If purchased as very young babies, they can be an absolute joy to own. They can be excellent talkers and entertaining and loving pets.

Cockatiels (*Nymphicus hollandicus*). These are favorite beginners' birds. If purchased as young babies (especially those not exposed to prodding fingers in pet shops), they can make affectionate and gentle pets. Females can be more nervous and nippy, and many do not talk as well as males. The males can speak in muffled tones but not as clearly as larger talking parrots. They are people-oriented, like attention, and make excellent pets.

Gray-cheeked Parakeets (*Brotogeris pyrrhopterus*). These are also good beginners' pets if acquired young. They can be quite noisy, but feisty and cute with lots of personality. They speak in a gravelly voice and are very people oriented.

Lovebirds (*Agapornis* spp.). As a rule, lovebirds have a reputation for not making very good pets. However, if these birds are taken from the nest at 10–12 weeks of age, they become loving and affectionate pets.

Conures. There are many different varieties of conures, and some tame into affectionate and enjoyable pets. They are also feisty birds, and the major drawback to the species, as a whole, is their noisiness, especially Half-Moons (*Aratinga canicularis eburnirostrum*) and Nandays (*Nandayus nenday*). Some never tame into good pets and will remain wild. They can be fair talkers, usually with a gravelly voice. It is best to purchase a very young one.

Miniature Macaws (*Ara* spp.). Most of the miniature macaws have strong, inquisitive personalities. They are bright and animated and have the macaw's typical fair talking ability. These can be truly delightful pets.

African Gray Parrots (*Psittacus erithacus*). These can be a bit hard to handle if purchased mature and wild. Frequently shy and suspicious, these birds are often considered one of the most difficult medium-sized birds to tame. African Grays are usually purchased for their talking ability, yet those that never tame well often do not talk well. They have a tendency to talk only after a year or two of age, which may be due to shyness on the part of untamed birds. African Grays talk for life; they pick up household sounds and whistles, as well as their natural extraordinary range of pops, squeaks, clucks, and chirps. When purchased extremely young or as domestically raised, hand-fed babies, they can be delightful pets, being highly intelligent, inquisitive, and excellent talkers. A dark-eyed bird indicates youth and should be chosen over an older one with golden eyes.

Amazons (*Amazona* spp.). There are many different varieties of amazons, each with highly individual traits. Many can be nippers and tend to get worse with age, but as a group they fit the criteria set by most people for a good pet. The most popular good talkers are the Yellow-naped (*A. ochrocephala auropalliata*), Double-yellow-head (*A. o. oratrix*), Blue-crowned (*A. farinosa guatemalae*), and Blue-fronted (*A. aestiva aestiva*) amazons. These, when purchased young, can be incredibly fun pets with exceptional speaking abilities. Young Yellow-napes tend to talk immediately after weaning if exposed to frequent human speech but have a tendency to slow down in their acquisition of new words and phrases after 2 or 3 years of age. Baby Yellow-napes can get aggressive anywhere from 4 to 9 months of age and must be controlled; otherwise they can turn into absolute tyrants.

The smaller amazons can also be extremely enjoyable pets. Finsch's Amazons (*Amazona finschi*) are great talkers, playful and entertaining, as are Green-cheeked Amazons (also known as Mexican Red-heads) (*Amazona viridigenalis*). They also seem to be the strongest and most disease resistant of the large psittacines, making them the ideal choice for the novice parrot owner.

Cockatoos (*Cacatua* spp.). There are many different varieties of cockatoos, which vary in basic personality traits. Most tame cockatoos desire constant attention from their owners. This trait makes them ideal for the person who wants a pet that can be constantly cuddled and loved but a strain for the busy individual. This incessant need for attention can turn into destructive and noisy behavior if not controlled correctly. The Greater Sulphur-crested (*C. galerita galerita*), Triton (*C. g. triton*), medium (*C. g. eleonora* and *C. g. fitzroyi*), Lesser Sulphur-crested (*C. sulphurea sulphurea*), Citron-crested (*C. s. citrino-cristata*), and Umbrella-crested (*C. alba*) cockatoos are the most animated. They usually enjoy displaying, dancing, and screeching and also are fair talkers but may get noisy if ignored.

The Moluccan Cockatoo (*C. moluccensis*) can be a joy or disappointment, depending on the individual. For those who want a quiet cockatoo, this is the one to have. They are the most docile of the cockatoo family and often do nothing more than sit on their perches, eat, and defecate. In general, cockatoos are better at imitating sounds (e.g., chickens and dogs) than they are at talking. The smaller varieties, such as Red-vented (*C. ducorps*) and Goffin's (*C. sanguinea sanguinea*) cockatoos do not seem to live as long as the others. Cockatoos can also suffer from an endocrine syndrome affecting the feathers that eventually kills them. Cockatoos are demanding, highly intelligent, beautiful, and entertaining pets.

Macaws (*Ara* and *Anodorhynchus* spp.). The Blue-and-gold Macaws (*Ara ararauna*) have a tendency to be playful, raucous, and rowdy. They are intelligent and loyal to their owners. The Green-winged (*Ara chloroptera*), Buffon's (*Ara ambigua*), and majestic Hyacinth macaws (*Anodorhynchus hyacinthius*) are the most congenial species. Young Blue-and-golds and Green-wings occasionally succumb to the macaw wasting syndrome, which makes quarantine station purchase in early life a risk. Little is known about the disease. The very large macaws are like big, gentle Great Danes, and the clownish nature of the Green-wings often makes them personal favorites. Scarlet (*Ara macao*) and Military (*Ara militaris*) macaws can sometimes be nippy and unpredictable and not as much fun to have as pets because of their peevishness. The Red-fronted Macaws (*Ara rubrogenys*) are also nice pets, but not frequently seen. Blue-and-golds, Scarlets, and Green-wings may make good talkers but generally speaking have only limited vocabularies.

Macaws are intelligent, attentive to their owners, and less demanding than cockatoos.

Taming a Bird. There are many ways to tame a bird, and each individual will respond differently to various techniques. The following suggestions can serve as an introduction:

1. The bird's cage should be covered after removing the bird so that its attention is not constantly attracted by the cage.

2. The bird should be worked in short sessions so it does not become angry, frustrated, and tired.

3. The bird will feel fatigued after the first few sessions, so it should be allowed privacy and rest time afterward, as well as a treat (which it may not eat, but the gesture is important).

4. The bird's personal schedule should be considered. It should not be worked when it is tired or sleeping or when it usually eats.

5. A trainer who is tired, in a bad mood, or not feeling well, should not work a bird. A bird can sense when a person is not up to par and will be difficult to work.

6. The handler must always be in complete control. Working birds in a corner, a small room, or a shower stall with solid doors will help to focus their attention on the trainer.

7. One hand can be used to decoy the bird from biting behavior, if necessary.

8. New birds should always be kept separated, not just to quarantine them, but to keep them from imprinting on each other instead of the owner.

Perch and Stick Training. Perch training is a desirable aspect of pet ownership because a bird should be with family members as much as possible. Because of their destructive tendencies, the pet bird's activities must be controlled. As moving a cage to achieve closeness is cumbersome and impractical, the convenience of a perch and subsequent perch training is obvious.

The perch should be high enough to allow the top of the bird's head to reach the center of the owner's chest (see the following section on dominance). It should be 6–9 in. long, with a diameter that fits the bird's feet. The bird is placed on the perch, in a corner where it will not feel threatened and where it can be quickly retrieved. If the bird jumps from the perch, it can be picked up by the fleshy protuberance at the base of the tail and placed gently back (Fig. 5.1). Speed and firmness are extremely important. Too much should not be expected of the bird, and it should not be expected to sit long enough on the perch to become restless.

The next training step is having the bird step from the perch (free-standing, not inside the cage) to a stick and back again. By always offering the perch, the trainer keeps the bird from panicking and it will readily accept gradually lengthening periods of time on the stick. If it leaps from the stick, it can be picked up by the fleshy part of the tail and quickly returned to the stick, and then to the perch again. Birds do not

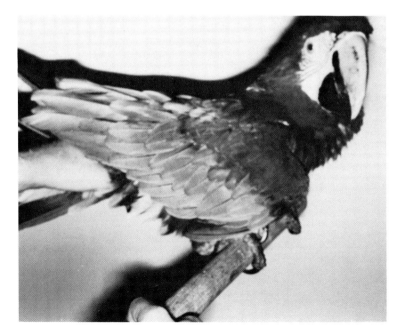

Fig. 5.1. Placing a bird back on the perch by picking it up from the fleshy protuberance at the base of the tail.

like to step down, so it is important to always allow them to step *upward* to the stick or perch. Once a bird accepts the stick readily, arm training can be drilled in the same manner. The handler should wear a tight-fitting, long-sleeved shirt at first, with an elastic bandage under the sleeve if the bird is fractious. Once the arm is accepted the bird can be slowly removed from its area of security in small stages. If a bird leaps or bites the handler, fear of the new environment may be causing the behavior.

Undesirable Behavior

Dominance. This is probably the single most common catalyst for behavioral problems in pet birds. As a wild animal, birds have a natural desire to be a dominant member of a flock. When a bird's head is much higher than mid-chest level, it may become the dominant household member. Conversely, if the top of its head reaches below waist level, it will feel threatened and may become panicky and neurotic in its behavior. Therefore the owner, in order to remain the dominant member of the flock, must remain assertive (but not brutal or "mean") and place perches in the cage no higher than chest level. Signs of a dominance syndrome are many, including chronic skittishness (this may be only fear on the part of the wild bird), a frank inability to be tamed, a tame bird nipping or biting the owner, refusal to be retrieved, blatant or aggressive attack attempts against the owner or other birds, and difficulty in handling.

A bird that refuses to leave the inside of its cage, on the other hand, is not always playing a dominance role. It may actually just be acting out the need for territory of its own. All birds should be allowed a certain amount of personal territory.

Screaming. This is one of the more common complaints as well as one of the most difficult to deal with. Cockatoos, amazons, and macaws can be the worst of the larger parrots, with conures outdoing all of them combined. Most of the complaints with regard to cockatoos come from the fact that they are extremely demanding and make excessive amounts of noise for affection. If they scream at dawn and dusk, they are merely displaying their "pleasure at being parrots," and this often-reinforced behavioral trait of the wild can be difficult to control. Offering food or a new toy a few minutes prior to the time they start yelling helps to control excessive screaming (*never* offer treats after they begin to yell) and sometimes will help to gradually decrease the frequency and intensity. The

alternative is to cover the cage (with a dark cloth) upon the start of screaming and keep it covered until the noisy time has passed. If the owner is away all day and the yelling starts immediately after returning home, the bird can be removed from its cage before the screaming starts.

If these methods do not work, there are always the old standbys of the squirt gun, exile to another room, or avoidance. If the squirt gun is used, care must be taken not to squirt water directly into a bird's eye, ear, or nostril. Exile to another room can be effective, but the bird must be truly isolated. It cannot be allowed to look out of windows, gaze admiringly at itself in mirrors, or be entertained by the sight of other animals or people or by toys, radios, and television.

In summary, any punishment must be quick and consistent. Since early morning and late afternoon screaming is natural and difficult to control, the methods described only work well for the indiscriminate screamers.

Imprinting on One Person. A bird displaying a distinct preference for one person over another within a household is an extremely common occurrence. Aggressive behavior toward lesser-favored members of a household should be curbed, as it can lead to injury to handlers, dominance problems with other birds, and disease problems if something happens to the preferred handler.

Sexual Imprinting. This is a more intense form of fixation, which may also be expressed in large or small birds actually being "in love" with their owners. Sometimes this imprinting manifests itself on an inanimate object, such as a toy, a mirror image, or the perch. The behavior may range from regurgitation to full masturbation by the bird directed to the source of affection.

Sexual frustration in a bird may show itself in aggressive behavior during the breeding season, overzealous preening of a mate or companion bird, or picking its own body bald. Sexual frustration can be treated in some cases by negative reinforcement and also by medical treatment with hormones. No single method is entirely satisfactory.

Feather Picking. Feather picking can be due to infection, boredom, habit, or nutritional deficiency, as well as sexual frustration. Dietary feather pickers often pull the feathers and eat the bloody tips. Diet in these cases must be improved. A mixture of one-half Listerine mouthwash and one-half water sprayed on affected feather areas can sometimes discourage a pet from habitual picking. Toys and entertainment (radio or television) can be provided when the owner is absent if boredom is suspected to be the cause.

Finding a cure for feather picking can be frustrating. Some species (Scarlet Macaws, African Gray Parrots) are more prone to feather picking.

Biting. This can be a difficult behavior to modify unless the root cause is determined. Besides the biting tendencies always found in a wild animal, there are numerous other reasons for birds, especially parrots, to begin or continue biting.

Quick, jerking hand movements can induce a bird to bite. Handlers may be at fault if they offer an arm for the bird to perch on and then, misconstruing the bird's attempt to use its beak for balance, jerk the arm away. An otherwise trusting bird may become distrustful and suspicious and may bite when the arm is presented again.

Some amazon parrots and macaws tend to be nippers by nature, and this behavior is difficult to modify. A bird that is being held and gives the appearance of getting restless (which leads to biting) should be returned to its cage and offered a toy, food, or praise. Such avoidance training does not allow the animal to become aggressive, and the owner can keep control of the situation by watching the bird and giving it a reward before it becomes aggressive.

An owner who has waited too long and sees that the bird is about to lunge at the hand or arm holding it can use the other hand to "decoy" the bird's beak away from its destination. The bird can be touched quickly on its back or tail, or the hand can be presented to its face, moving the fingers to draw away attention until it can be placed on its perch. Sometimes a bird can be discouraged from biting by quickly jolting the arm up and down, giving the bird a slight sense of unbalance to make it forget about biting. A loud verbal reprimand at the same time is also helpful.

In some birds "displaying" behavior is natural but may induce biting (i.e., in amazons, the eyes have pinpoint pupils, the feathers of the tail spread, the neck arches, and the neck feathers stand at attention while the bird becomes quite vocal).

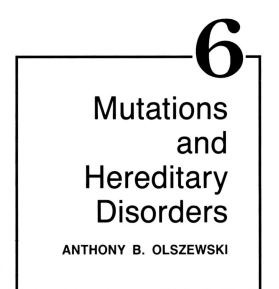

6

Mutations and Hereditary Disorders

ANTHONY B. OLSZEWSKI

AS IN ANY FORM of domestication, mutations in aviculture are of great importance. Even successful initial captive breeding may be as much a matter of selection of a suitable pair as of husbandry. As soon as a first breeding has been accomplished, the aviculturist strives to produce superior or novel strains. "Superior" may mean freer-breeding or steadier strains, or strains resistant to disease or extreme climatic conditions. Novelties are selected most often on the basis of size, feather color, and feather structure.

Mutations are also valuable in the monetary sense. Thus they serve both to create, improve, and vary captive strains and to promote aviculture. The understanding of mutations enables the avian practitioner to separate birds with pathological or metabolic disorders and "artificial" mutations from actual mutations.

Bird breeders must be selective, as in all probability many species will very shortly become extinct as viable wild populations. It is hoped that the normal types of most captive raised birds will not be lost due to unselective breeding.

Hybrids. Hybrids are common in aviculture. Mule breeding, the production of sterile hybrids involving the canary and various finches, is very popular in Europe. The Society Finch is possibly a free-bred blend of several mannikin species. Unfortunately the haphazard production of hybrids has become a liability in aviculture. It took many years for the American stock of lovebirds to become straightened out after various species had been bred together. Often a hybrid is mistaken for a new species or for a mutation. Many "artificial" hybrids and muta-

tions reach the market, which complicates genetic research.

Coloration. The great majority of mutations in aviculture affect plumage color. The appearance of color in the feather is due to two mechanisms, chemical coloration and structural coloration. Biochromes, compounds actually present in the feather, cause chemical coloration. Structural coloration produces an optical illusion by means of anatomical elements in the feather. Orange, red, and yellow are most often caused by carotenoids (lipochromes) deposited in the feather. These compounds are metabolized from plant and animal matter, not synthesized by the bird.

Species that possess carotenoid colors exhibit extreme variation due to changes in the diet. The red of the male Virginia Cardinal (*Richmondena cardinalis*) fades in the northeast United States when fruits, berries, greens, and insects become scarce. The Venezuelan Black-hooded Siskin (*Canduesis cucullatus*) turns yellow if a source of carotenoids is not available.

Yellow ground birds can obtain a sufficient supply of carotenoids from a diet of seed. This is not true for red or orange ground birds, which are frequently supplied with a source of synthetic carotenoids: beta-carotene, apo-carotenol, and canthaxanthin. Canthaxanthin gives the brightest scarlet red, while beta-carotene and apo-carotenol give golden orange shades. Beta-carotene is of limited usefulness, for much is metabolized as vitamin A, which lacks color.

In parrot-type birds the orange, red, and yellow colors are probably not caused by carotenoids. George Smith (1980, 1981) has posited a new class of chemical compounds named "psittacins." In parrot types, color is not clearly a function of the diet.

The black, brown, and gray colors are caused by melanin pigment in the feather. These pigments are synthesized by the bird from amino acids. White is a structural color. All the microstructures of the feather are transparent, including the covering cuticle.

Blue is given by a combination of a transparent cuticle and underlying melanin cells. The transparent cuticle is known in aviculture as white ground. A green effect occurs when yellow carotenoids of psittacins are spread through the cuticle. This is known as yellow ground. If the carotenoids or psittacins of the cuticle are primarily red, a red ground bird results. If no melanins are present, a red or orange hue is observed. Red biochromes do not readily interact with melanin to form structural colors.

Iridescence is given by spectral colors due to light interference. This interference is caused by a twisted and broadened melanin containing barbules or by spherical granules of melanin in close proximity to the cuticle.

Since feather color is governed by only two phenomena, all color mutations may be divided into two classes, mutations of the biochromes or of the microstructures of the feather. The most common mutations are of the chemical colors that affect the melanin granules: inos, cinnamons, fallows, pieds, and yellows.

Sports. Sports are unusual phenotypes of a nongenetic origin. These birds might be afflicted with some sort of metabolic disorder or have suffered a past injury to the skin or growing feather. Splashed or variegated birds are the most common sports. Parrot-type birds sometimes spontaneously develop maroon patches and some Lutino Cockatiels suddenly begin to get a deeper yellow color. Black canaries, sports produced from normal-appearing domestic canary parents, have turned up from time to time.

Lethal Genes. Lethal traits disrupt metabolism of a bird and cause death. Dominant lethals are clearly self-deleting. Recessive and incomplete dominant lethal genes are perpetuated. In cage birds, very few lethal traits have been posited: the crest, hard feather, and dominant white traits in the canary. These traits are all incomplete dominant genes. In one factor, these genes produce an unusual, desirable phenotype in the heterozygous state. In two factors, they cause death in the homozygous configuration.

Frauds. Frauds frequently occur in aviculture. South American Indians have many techniques for treating the growing feathers of parrots to get bizarre and beautiful colors.

The most common fraud is the "Double-yellow-head" Conure. The cheap green conure becomes an expensive peroxide blonde passed off as a juvenile Mexican Double-yellow-head, or Yellow-crowned Amazon (*Amazona ochrocephala*). Dyed finches are often seen in quarantine stations. Similar combinations of dyes and bleaches must always be looked out for by the avian practitioner as a cause of disease (feather abnormalities, skin irritation).

Hereditary Disorders Affecting the Avian Integument

"Feather Duster." This disorder is characterized by continued growth of primary and secondary flight and tail feathers and the various contour feathers. The disease, which affects Budgerigars, results in the bird being unable to

fly (Perry 1984). The feathers often impair the bird's sight and must be regularly trimmed. Affected birds are often unable to make the characteristic sounds of Budgerigars and instead make a barely audible noise. The condition, thought to be due to a recessive genetic fault, was first reported in England in 1966 (Oser et al. 1977). Most birds die at 4–8 months of age in a state of severe muscle wasting caused by a continuous demand on the body for feather growth (Perry 1984). There is no treatment for the disease, and breeding should be discouraged.

Feather Anomalies. Feather anomalies in carrier pigeons may be congenital or hereditary. Some follicles grow normal feathers after the abnormal feathers have been plucked (Hauser 1977). These cases are unlikely to be hereditary.

Micromelic Syndrome. This autosomal, recessive, obligate, lethal mutation in White Peking ducklings (*Anas platyrhynchos*) is described by Kelly and Ash (1976). The disease is characterized by shortening of the upper beak, reduced overall size, shortened limbs, abnormal development of cartilage, reduced bone ash, subcutaneous edema of the neck, absence of preplumulae and prefiloplumulae, a small rachis with a disproportionately small medulla, thickening of the feather sheath, and an increased abundance of pulp cells. Insulin injections given to 5-day embryos produced the same defect.

Feather Cysts. Feather cysts are known as hereditary "lumps" or "hypoteronosis cystica" in genetically predisposed breeds of canaries (Crested, Norwich, and certain other crossbreeds) (Perry 1984). Feather cysts produce a ragged plumage and cause irritation to a bird. Self-mutilation often results, causing hemorrhage, shock, and/or cannibalism. Feather cysts appear to have arisen from artificial selection for feathers with a soft curled or tufted appearance. Feather cysts develop when the young growing feather becomes curled over in its follicle so that the feather sheath fails to erupt. Several such follicles may coalesce and produce a cyst containing abortive feathers, keratin, and a greasy material produced by the subaceous glands of the skin. These cysts rupture, presenting a beige, dry mass with an acrid, fatty smell. The adjacent feathers may become disorganized, giving the bird a bedraggled appearance. The condition worsens at each successive molt. Individual masses can be removed entirely or their contents scraped out, but new cysts tend to develop. The more diffuse type of cyst sometimes responds to treatment with thyroid extract at 1.5 mg/20 g body weight daily, either in liquid or powder mixed with the seed (Perry 1984). This treatment induces a molt and new feather growth. The new plumage is generally paler than normal after such treatment. Affected birds should not be allowed to breed (Arnall and Keymer 1975). Regular manual expression and cleaning usually is adequate to control small cysts. Mosquito forceps are useful for plucking out defective feather shafts. If the cysts are large or numerous, anesthesia is preferred, and all cysts are opened, emptied, and cauterized with strong iodine, phenol, or silver nitrate to destroy the actual feather follicle (Perry 1984). Total surgical excision is also effective but more difficult (Madill 1981). (See Chapter 33 for further information on feather and dermal cysts.)

Overgrown Beaks. Overgrown beaks (upper, lower, or both) can result from hereditary and congenital deformities in a variety of species (Altman 1969). Most documented reports refer to domestic poultry, such as the single, autosomal, recessive, semilethal mutation in White Leghorns called the Donald Duck beak anomaly. The condition is characterized by upturning of the upper beak and buckling of the lower beak, causing an apparent shortening of the lower beak (McGibbon 1973).

References

Altman, R. B. 1969. Conditions involving the integumentary system. In *Diseases of Cage and Aviary Birds,* ed. M. L. Petrak. Philadelphia: Lea and Febiger.

Arnall, L., and I. F. Keymer. 1975. *Bird Diseases.* London: Baillière Tindall.

Harrison, J., and J. Kear. 1962. Some congenital abnormalities in the skulls and beaks of wildfowl. *Vet. Rec.* 74(22):632–33.

Hauser, K. W. 1977. Gefiederanomalien bei tauben. *Prakt. Tierarzt* 58(5):330–31.

Kelly, J. F., and W. J. Ash. 1976. Abnormal feathers of the micromelic syndrome in White Peking Ducks. *J. Hered.* 67(1):63–64.

McGibbon, W. A. 1973. A third Donald Duck beak anomaly in the fowl. *J. Hered.* 64(1):46–47.

Madill, D. N. 1981. Avian surgery. In *Refresher Course for Veterinarians on Aviary and Caged Birds,* pp. 198–218. University of Sydney, Post-Graduate Committee in Veterinary Science, Proceedings no. 55. Sydney, Aust.

Oser, V., G. Routenfeld, and D. Berensvon. 1977. Langfedrigkeit als Anomalie beim Wellensittich [feather dusters]. *Prakt. Tierarzt* 58(6):552.

Perry, R. A. 1984. Unpublished data.

Smith, G. A. 1980. Mutation colours in parrots. *Mag. Parrot Soc.* 14(9):220–22.

_____. 1981. Colour mutations. *Mag. Parrot Soc.* 15(11):307–10.

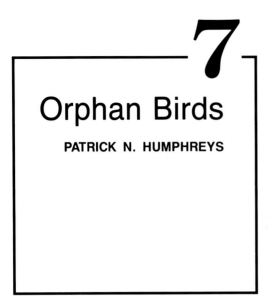

7

Orphan Birds

PATRICK N. HUMPHREYS

THE NEEDS of abandoned young birds brought in from the wild or hatched in incubators can be obtained from studying the nesting behavior, the habitat, and the food of the species in question. Generally speaking, the younger the bird, the more difficult it is to rear (although young passerines old enough to have some feathering and open eyes can be tricky to start with, as they tend to panic when approached and refuse to be fed by hand). If possible, rearing by the young's own parents or foster parents works best; for instance, the male of a pair can often be prevailed on to feed nestlings if the female is lost, although he may lack the brooding instinct and the birds must be kept warm artificially. A female bird with a brood of her own can be induced to foster young of the same or other species, but the introduction must be carried out with extreme care, as near the moment of hatching as possible. Many raptors will rear young of their own or other species when they are placed in their nests (Jones 1981). The period of dependence of young birds is extremely variable, ranging from a few weeks in passerines to many months in birds such as flamingos and some of the large raptors. Some species (e.g., swifts and shearwaters) break the parental tie sharply by the young either leaving the nest when the parents are absent or being abandoned long before fledging (e.g., albatrosses and some other seabirds).

In this chapter, the principal groups of young birds are considered from the point of view of management rather than taxonomic characteristics. Further information on feeding and nutritional disorders and metabolic diseases can be found in Chapters 11 and 12.

Passerines. The passerine group of birds are born in a warm nest, either naked or with a covering of down, with unopened eyes. They must be kept very warm and should first be housed in their own nest or a replica of it, with a thick pad of cotton covering them. If possible, two or more nestlings should be kept together. When the pad is removed the nestlings gape reflexively for food. After feeding, they usually elevate their cloacal regions to the edge of the nest to defecate; the dropping is contained in a thin membrane and should be removed with a teaspoon. Within 2 weeks, most of these chicks can defecate over the edge of the nest. Feeding at first should be frequent; during the daytime as often as every hour, and at night at least every 4 hours. Chicks are fed until they stop gaping. As growth occurs, feeding intervals are lengthened and larger food items given. Young birds are also exposed to the air for longer periods. Chicks grow rapidly and within a few weeks do not require covering except on cold nights; in the daytime they are active, fluttering their wings about the nest. When young birds get to this stage, it is important that the nest be enclosed within a suitable cage so that they cannot fly out and get lost or injure themselves. Once they are independent of the nest, food should be gradually introduced in a feeding dish on the floor of the cage. Live food in the shape of spiders, mealworms, green caterpillars, and aphids should be offered, as young birds have a tendency to peck at moving objects and soon start to feed themselves.

Once young birds begin to eat without aid, they can be introduced to water. A large stone placed in a shallow dish of water gives the birds some security, prevents spillage, and enables them to bathe.

Many young passerines fledge very rapidly and become independent of parental care in a few weeks. Frequently they have to move out of parental territory and disperse while the parents care for a second or even third brood. When only one brood is reared in the wild, however, the young maintain parental contact longer and tend to form itinerant family groups (some tits and tree creepers fall into this category). Orphan birds of these groups, once fledged and feeding, must not be suddenly released into unfamiliar surroundings. They must be allowed to distance themselves by degrees from the rearer.

Most passerines can be reared on foods sold for rearing canaries, usually dried egg–based, with cereal and dried insect added. It is important to add as much live insect food as possible, mealworms being a convenient source. Mealworms fed on cereal containing a high mineral and vitamin content provide the young with a dietary supplement. Hard-boiled egg and/ or scraped raw liver in small quantities can be given if no dried food is available. When the birds grow older, the diet should more closely approximate the adult diet (e.g., more cereal for seed-eating birds).

Raptors. The young of raptors (hawks, owls, vultures) can be reared successfully from the egg. An interesting feature of these birds is that they appear unable to distinguish strange young of their own species introduced into an existing brood of the same age. Some species will also safely adopt the young of other raptorial species, but because of their strong imprinting capacity, this procedure is not recommended.

The first food should consist of chopped neonatal mice, given four or five times a day; as the birds grow, hatchery-waste neonatal chicks and later adult mice and larger pieces of chick can be offered (Bruning et al. 1981). Vitamin and mineral supplements should be added to the diet to prevent deficiencies. Large raptors, such as eagles and vultures, may be fed rabbits or small chickens; pigeons are unsuitable food because of the danger of trichomonas infection (Dornstein et al. 1981). Eventually, young birds must be encouraged to tear up whole carcasses themselves and in due course be released to the wild with food accessible on a post or branch near their home.

No proper nest is made by raptorial birds, and additional heat is only required during the first 10 days or so after hatching; all the young have a profuse coat of down, which is gradually replaced by feathers. Extra drinking water need not be provided. (Care must be taken with birds as they are usually fascinated by water and drowning is common.)

Parrots and Pigeons. Parrots and pigeons initially feed their naked young on a regurgitated crop secretion. It is possible to rear chicks from a tender age by imitating the parents, using a small syringe containing a quantity of milk-based baby food. Young birds should be placed in a small cardboard box and bedded on wood shavings within a cage kept at about 90°F (32°C) for the first 4 or 5 days. To prevent drying and burning of the skin, young birds must be able to move away from the heat source if they wish. The amount of food to give varies with the species. Generally 1 cc will do for a bird of pigeon size, offered every 3 hours during the day. The degree of crop distension indicates the amount of food required. Care should be taken, as overfilling the crop can lead to disease.

Fish-eating Birds. Success in rearing young fish-eating birds is possible if an adequate supply of fish can be obtained. Most species swallow fish whole and may go many hours without food between meals. The very young chicks of gulls and terns need a supply of heat, such as an infrared lamp. On the other hand, keeping arctic and antarctic species cool enough in a temperate climate is the main problem; ice cubes should be placed on the gravel on which they are housed. Whole or sliced fish (preferably whole) should be hand-fed twice daily. Fussy eaters may have to be force-fed until they eat on their own. Most fish contain thiaminase, which destroys vitamin B; therefore it is necessary to feed only certain kinds of fish (trout, eel, minnows) or to add an appropriate amount of thiamin to the food by injecting it into the fish feed (Conway et al. 1977). Another problem encountered is that fish, being oily, easily contaminate the swimming water. Running water or a frequent change of the water is necessary, or the birds will become oiled.

Precocial Birds. Precocial birds are those whose young are hatched covered with down and fully active. The young are not usually fed by the parents (except for the gallinules and grebes). The most convenient heat source for chicks is an infrared lamp (sold for chicken rearing) suspended above a pen. If the young cluster directly under the lamp for warmth, it is hung too high and should be lowered. The ideal is to have the chicks resting separately within the radius of the lamp's rays.

Food and water can be offered in shallow dishes. Water dishes should contain a few stones to prevent immersion. The best bedding is clean sand. Care should be taken not to have too many birds in one pen, as some species are prone to panic and pile up in the corners, with consequent suffocation. Most species start exploratory pecking after the first 24 hours and find by experiment what is palatable. Because most species need a high-protein starter diet and prefer to peck at red, green, and yellow objects, greenfly (shaken off a plant), small earthworms, or mealworms usually start chicks feeding. Commercial chick-crumbs are a suitable basic diet for many species; larger grains and insects can be given as they grow. Young geese of all species need grass early and at 1 week old should be penned in the daytime on short-mown turf (with shelter from sun or rain). Grass should not be cut for them as they manage better when they have to forage for grass shoots themselves. Geese grow rapidly (especially those from extreme latitudes), and once eating grass, they should be taken off chick-crumbs and given an evening meal of crushed whole grain. If goslings are not taken off chick-crumbs, tibial dysplasia may occur because of the excessive rate of body growth compared with mineral absorption.

Quail and Guineafowl. Quail and guineafowl very rapidly become able to fly, and precautions must be taken against losing them due to flight or due to predators such as cats, dogs, and foxes. Half-grown birds, in confined quarters, may turn to pecking each other and even to cannibalism due to boredom and overcrowding. This is difficult to stop once it starts; therefore placement of as few birds in one pen as possible is important, and some occupation, such as picking up scattered grain in earth or sand, should be provided.

Vitamins and Minerals for Young Birds. Young birds are very susceptible to bone deformation when artificially reared, owing to an imbalance of minerals and vitamins in their diets. Conway et al. (1977) refer to insertion of salt and thiamine tablets into fish fed to young puffins and murres. This practice is essential for all species of fish-eating birds. A multiple preparation, such as Vionate (Squibb), is the most useful for routine administration: 25 mg per day for canary-sized birds and up to 250 mg for pigeons. It is safe to give larger doses to young, actively growing chicks in the form of a powder added to the food.

References

Bruning, D., J. Bell, and E. P. Dolensek. 1981. Observations on the breeding of condors at the New York Zoological Park. In *Recent Advances in the Study of Raptor Diseases*, ed. J. E. Cooper and A. G. Greenwood, pp. 49–50. Keighley, Engl.: Chiron.

Conway, W. G., J. Bell, D. Bruning, and E. Dolensek. 1977. Care and breeding of puffins and murres. *Int. Zoo. Yearb.* 17:173–74.

Dornstein, G. M., P. Zwart, J. W. W. Souwman, and J. M. Rens. 1981. Hand-rearing of vultures at the Wassenaar Zoo, The Netherlands. In *Recent Advances in the Study of Raptor Diseases*, ed. J. E. Cooper and A. G. Greenwood, pp. 51–52. Keighley, Engl.: Chiron.

Jones, C. G. 1981. Abnormal and maladaptive behaviour in captive raptors. In *Recent Advances in the Study of Raptor Diseases*, ed. J. E. Cooper and A. G. Greenwood, pp. 52–59. Keighley, Engl.: Chiron.

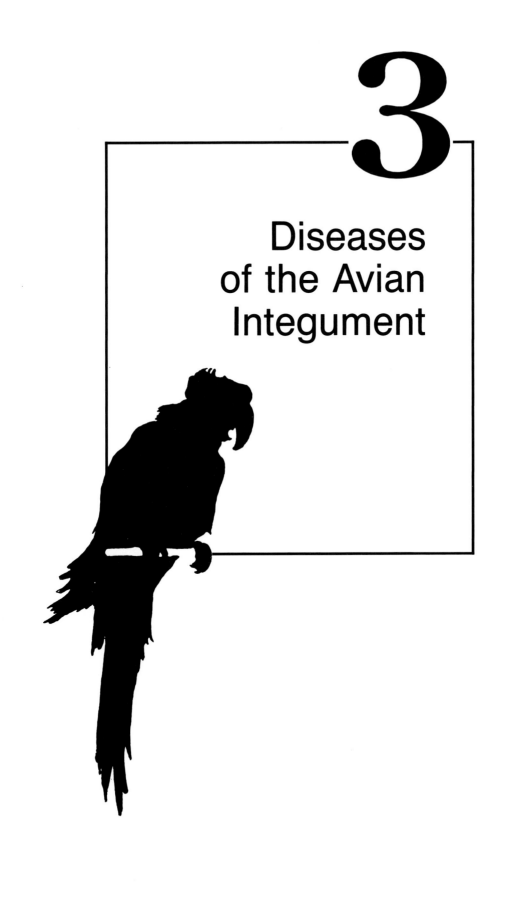

3

Diseases
of the Avian
Integument

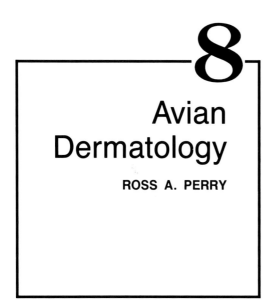

8

Avian Dermatology

ROSS A. PERRY

THE AVIAN INTEGUMENT is a series of highly specialized structures that show extreme variation between species of birds, depending on the interaction of evolutionary processes with the birds' habitat and life-styles. The most important functions of the feathers relate to thermoregulation, a basic requirement for continued life, and to the possibility of flight. Diseases of the avian integument are therefore likely to endanger survival of the individual.

Trauma-associated Disorders of the Avian Integument

Laceration. Serious abrasions and lacerations, with or without mortalities, result when birds run into enclosure fences when panicked by stray animals, especially barking dogs.

Small skin lacerations can be cleaned and treated as open wounds with EDP or antibiotic powders such as Tricin or Terramycin in preference to ointments, which often mat the feathers, decrease insulation, and distress the bird. Healing is very rapid and contraction good. Large lacerations can be debrided and sutured with 4-0 or 5-0 Dexon or similar materials, but even large wounds may heal well without suturing. Avian skin is loose and easily mobilized, and hence quite large defects can be adequately covered.

Scalping. Scalping of female Mallard Ducks in captivity as a result of "gang rape" by

---

For brevity and to avoid repetition, the following topics have been largely omitted from this section: congenital, hereditary, endocrine, parasitic, nutritional, and neoplastic diseases of the avian integument; conditions specific for domestic poultry; iatrogenic, pox-virus-associated, and beak conditions; wing, beak, and claw clipping; and anatomical and physiological features, including molting.

several males is not uncommon. Pinioned birds cannot escape and may suffer from tearing of the skin over the cranium. An extensive injury is difficult to treat, but suturing and application of a gauze netting head cap may assist healing. Commonly it is better to destroy the bird unless of special value because it will be useless for breeding during the remainder of the season. A similar condition is seen in female King Quail in Australia. Excessive grooming and mutilation of the surgical site by the parents of pinioned goslings, ducklings, or cygnets may be minimized by removal of all traces of blood from the wings. See Hymphreys (1978).

Feather Hemorrhage. A blood feather is a newly emerging, immature, actively growing feather. Trauma, either accidental or iatrogenic (as in wing trimming), to the keratin sheath surrounding these blood vessels can produce severe hemorrhage. Hemorrhage inside the follicle often results in death of the feather. The dead feather is retained rather than molted normally and may predispose to feather plucking until it is pulled out. Treatment is best accomplished by grasping the blood feather with pliers or artery forceps and removing it from the follicle in the direction in which it was growing. Firm digital pressure should be maintained on the empty feather follicle until bleeding stops (approximately 3 minutes). Attempts to apply hemostatic compounds to the bleeding end of the blood feather or to clamp it with forceps are likely to prove futile. Owners may be instructed to firmly ligate the proximal end of the broken feather with strong cotton or string, provided the bird is not in shock (Madill 1981). The remaining section will fall off in due course. Stressed and shocked birds should be immediately given appropriate treatment with corticosteroid injections (e.g., 2 mg dexamethasone/ ml Dexadreson, Intervet at 0.15–0.4 ml intramuscularly). In canaries and finches, subcutaneous injections are preferable to intramuscular injections. Fluid therapy (e.g., balanced electrolyte solution and/or 5% dextrose at 1.0– 1.3 ml/100 g body weight, intramuscularly) should also be administered in shock cases (Philip 1981). The bird should be placed in a warm, quiet environment, possibly with added oxygen. Blood can be cleaned from the feathers with hydrogen peroxide.

Breast Blisters. Breast blisters in birds are false bursae; one or more can occur along the sternum, varying in length from 1 to 8 cm. They occur most commonly in male birds of heavy breeds during the growing period. The cause is mechanical, due to pressure on, or injury to, the sternum. Pressure may be caused by the weight of the bird forcing the sternum against wire, slatted floors, or perches. Incising the infected blisters and expressing the contents reduces their size.

Leg Bands. Pressure necrosis of the skin and abrasion from leg bands and leg rings (e.g., chaining cockatoos) is well documented. Once a band or ring becomes immobilized on the leg, a buildup of keratin occurs under the band and this slowly strangulates the circulation to the foot and causes pressure necrosis of the underlying tissues.

Small plastic and metal bands applied to finches, small parakeets, and canaries can be removed easily by either cutting or spreading them apart. Metal leg bands applied to larger birds may require heavy metal shears. General anesthesia facilitates removal of leg bands in birds with swollen feet and in large, fractious birds. The band should be cut away from the numbers and returned to the owner.

Feet. Bumblefoot (pododermatitis) refers to localized and generalized inflammation of the feet. Bumblefoot occurs in species of birds forced to perch or walk on unnatural surfaces (e.g., concrete floors for anseriforms), especially those surfaces heavily contaminated with feces (Butler 1981).

In Budgerigars (*Melopsittacus undulatus*), bumblefoot is a very common cause of bilateral lameness. It develops because of the abrasive action of sandpaper perches or perches that are too smooth or cylindrical (Fig. 8.1). Bumblefoot

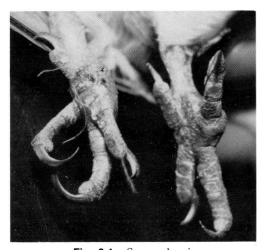

Fig. 8.1. Severe chronic pododermatitis (bumblefoot) in a Budgerigar (*Melopsittacus undulatus*), caused by unsuitable perches, synthetic fibers, and gout.

in Budgerigars may also be predisposed by insufficient vitamin A in the diet (Harrison 1982). In wild pigeons and occasionally in canaries, finches, and other pet birds, tangling of the feet in multifilament synthetics can cause bumblefoot. In raptors, the problem begins as a puncture wound to the foot from the bird's own talons, as a bruise, or as an excoriation from prolonged perching on an unsuitable surface (Arnall and Keymer 1975).

Once a break in the epithelium occurs, *Staphylococcus* spp. or *Streptococcus* spp. invade the foot and result in abscessation. *Escherichia coli, Mycobacterium* spp., and *Candida albicans* have also been encountered (Redig 1981).

Bumblefoot is associated with swelling of the ball or soft pad of the foot, which may not be obvious until the bird is handled. Strangulation and loss of toes is frequently observed.

Prevention and treatment of bumblefoot should include replacement of soiled, abrasive, and/or cylindrical perches with clean, nontoxic tree branches of several diameters. Systemic antibiotics (e.g., chloramphenicol, trimethoprim potentiated sulfas, and tylosin) and topical application of dimethyl sulfoxide (DMSO) or dexamethasone can be used for treatment. Surgical treatment involves curettage or dissecting out of infected caseous material, closing the wound with 5-0 silk, or placing a drain tube to be flushed with antibiotics, allowing the lesion to granulate (Bird 1982).

Talons and Claws. The talons and claws of captive birds are particularly susceptible to traumatic damage and may become secondarily infected with a variety of organisms, including *Staphylococcus aureus, Escherichia coli,* and *Proteus* spp. (Cooper and Lloyd 1974). Regular trimming with a scalpel blade, sharp knife, nail file, or piece of sandpaper will prevent further disease conditions.

Burns. Burns most frequently occur in pet birds when the birds are left unattended with access to chemicals and electrical appliances. Thermal burns require immediate first aid with the application of cold water to affected areas. Severe burn cases can cause extensive tissue necrosis on the feet and lower abdomen (Fig. 8.2). Lotagen or vitamin A/vitamin E creams may be applied every 8 hours. Contamination of affected areas with feces and self-mutilation must be prevented, for example, by bandaging the feet. Antibiotics and intramuscular administration of fluids at 1 ml/100 g body weight may be indicated (Schultz 1981).

Attempts to manage the severely burnt feet of a snowy owl have been described (Gumbs

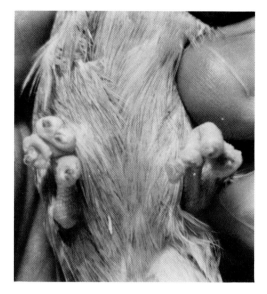

Fig. 8.2. Severely damaged feet with tissue necrosis in a Budgerigar (*Melopsittacus undulatus*) following a mishap with a hot skillet. (*Courtesy of Raymond D. Wise, Scottsdale Animal Clinic, Chicago, Ill.*)

1982). These included the use of a synthetic skin (e.g., Mediski 1, sterile porcine skin) and a silver-based topical antibiotic (silver sulfadiazine). To minimize trauma, feathers along the toes were cut rather than plucked.

Chemical burns should be managed similarly to thermal burns. Acid corrosives must be removed and/or neutralized by washing thoroughly and applying a sodium bicarbonate solution. Dilute white vinegar is useful for neutralizing alkali burns from coal tar products, potash, and most other caustics (Arnall and Keymer 1975). These authors advocate the application of antibiotic cream, preferably containing an antihistamine and/or a corticosteroid to reduce pain and shock, and they state that a humid environment at 70–75°F (21–24°C) is preferable to a higher temperature with low humidity. When toes are lost, the perches should be modified to provide a broad, flat upper surface. Potential sequelae to burns are pneumonia and systemic infections, which may occur a few days after the incident.

Frostbite. Frostbite (distal extremity necrosis) is commonly seen in tropical or subtropical birds (e.g., Whistling Ducks) exposed to inclement weather. A dry gangrene of the exposed terminal phalanges or web develops, and one or more toes may be lost. If possible, these birds should be housed in a frost-proof building at

night in severe weather. Unless extensive tissue damage is done to the affected foot, recovery is usually uncomplicated.

Feather Problems

Self-mutilation of Feathers. This is a common problem in some cage and aviary birds, especially psittacines. Skin irritants and disturbances that may cause self-mutilation and plucking of feathers include boredom, dietary deficiency, psychosis, bacteria, viruses, fungi, parasites, lack of sleep due to household lights being left on, and contact with strangers, dogs, and cats (Peckham 1955; Galvin 1979; Burr 1982). Disturbances, which are regarded as stress factors, most commonly affect newly acquired birds. Stress after capture and initial confinement is experienced by all wild caught birds. Some species calm quickly while others remain nervous in captivity. Excessive feather picking may lead to loss of appetite, resulting in poor plumage and malnutrition.

The etiology of disease may be revealed by a full discussion of the bird's history, environment, and cage size; its social interaction with the family; evidence of displaced behavior or activity; and any change in the life of the bird coinciding with the onset of the feather problem (Galvin 1979; Amand 1982).

Chewing and self-mutilation of feathers must be distinguished from normal grooming and feather sheath removal from growing feathers. Chewed feathers show the ramus of the feather split longitudinally in an irregular, ragged fashion. Mutilated feathers are confined to areas where a bird can chew (flight and contour feathers). Birds with psychologically caused self-mutilation of feathers exhibit the absence of any deformed, discolored, or mutilated feathers on the head and the absence of beak deformity, mites, or lice. Self-mutilation attributed to psychological causes often lacks bilateral symmetry, especially in the early stages (Perry 1981).

When kept together, immature canaries of about 1 month of age sometimes peck one another. Therapy includes separation of offending birds, wound treatment, blood removal, and debeaking (Seneviratna 1969).

Feather plucking of other cage and aviary birds can sometimes be attributed to influences of gonadal hormones (Fig. 8.3), population size and density, genetics, and environmental factors loosely described as "boredom" (Hughes and Duncan 1972; Duncan and Hughes 1973; Hughes 1973).

Excessive biting, preening, or scratching at a particular area warrants investigation and may reveal a tumor, abscess, wound, or hernia.

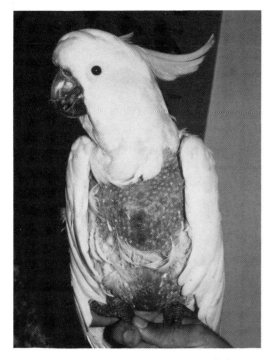

Fig. 8.3. Chronic self-mutilation (feather plucking) in a Sulphur-crested Cockatoo (*Cacatua galerita*) that concurrently exhibits obesity and cutaneous changes due to long-term therapy with medroxyprogesterone acetate. Note that the feathers of the head and neck are normal, as is the beak structure, but the beak has an abnormal glossy sheen due to destruction of powder down feathers.

Gang-gang Syndrome. Gang-gang Cockatoos (*Callocephalon fimbriatum*) are often feather pluckers in captivity when not provided with a constant fresh supply of foliage, such as large *Casuarina* spp. (she-oak) branches laden with nuts, together with fruit and vegetables, as well as the normal seed mixture. Feather picking in unpaired birds during the breeding season or when a mate is taken away or dies are examples of frustration-induced disease. Feather picking (cannibalism type) in canaries can be attributed to overcrowding, unhygienic conditions, and ectoparasitism. Parent birds subjected to such poor management may peck nestlings.

Galah Syndrome. A form of self-mutilation, the Galah syndrome, affects mainly Galahs (*Cacatua roseicapilla*) but also Gang-gangs, corellas (*C. sanguinea, C. tenuirostris*), rosellas (*Platycercus* spp.), and rarely Budgerigars (Schultz 1978).

This condition can affect birds of any age or sex, usually those that are very tame, hand-reared, and kept in a small cage. Birds often start picking when attention paid them is minimal. Flight and tail feathers are first affected, then the contour feathers of the back and breast, producing a fluffy, downy appearance. The feather shafts are often chewed about 3 cm from the skin, leaving a splintered stump, but may be chewed right down to the skin, causing skin bleeding. In a few cases, the attitude of the bird changes from normally quiet to nervous and it jumps at any sudden movement or sound.

Treatment of the Galah syndrome involves removal of damaged feathers, a nutritious diet, and management change. The bird is anesthetized, and broken primary and secondary feather stumps are removed with pliers. Some bleeding may occur but is easily stopped with pressure. The bird is checked 6 weeks later to assess feather regrowth.

Self-mutilation of feathers may sometimes be controlled by adding 2% salt to the diet for a few days (Burr 1982). Daily bathing (misting) with 1 ml chlorhexidine/pt (600 ml) water or 1 ml Nolvason/qt (1200 ml) water may help treat skin infection and eliminate feather mutilation. Spraying with a fine mist promotes feather maintenance and stimulates preening. Providing 8 hours light and 16 hours darkness for 3–4 weeks gives a chance for adequate rest and recovery from stress. The photoperiod is then reversed for the next 3–4 weeks.

Some hand-reared birds require human company, and removal from the owner can elicit the Galah syndrome. They become uninterested in birds of their own kind and even other humans. The first step in correcting a self-mutilating bird is to provide a large enough cage, preferably one with flight space, and adequate nutrition (Burr 1982). Experimental administration of a single intramuscular injection of medroxyprogesterone acetate at 3 mg/100 g body weight can be tried, or megestrol acetate at 1 mg/10 ml drinking water daily until effect (then reduce dose). The observation that many chronic feather pickers (e.g., cockatoos) reduce such behavior when introduced into an aviary suggests that spatial restrictions influence feather picking.

Stress Dermatitis. This condition, an ulcerative dermatitis caused by self-mutilation, occurs chiefly in lovebirds, especially Peach-faced Lovebirds (*Agapornis roseicollis*) and also in pet cockatoos and Budgerigars (Schultz 1981). The shoulder region and the patagial membrane (unior bilateral) are usually affected in birds of any age or sex. Less commonly the inguinal region, the chest (sternal midline), or back is affected. The lovebird is a colony bird, often very spiteful and bullying and therefore probably more prone to psychological insult. The pet cockatoo and Budgerigar can also frequently be exposed to stressful living conditions. Coagulase-positive *Staphylococcus* spp. are often isolated from ulcerative lesions as a secondary contaminant. Treatment includes a mixture of 1.5 ml lincomycin 100 mg/ml injection with 0.45 ml dexamethasone 2 mg/ml injection and 0.05 ml DMSO used alone or in equal combination with vitamin A and vitamin E creams as a topical application (Schultz 1981). Lotagen does not eliminate coagulase-positive staphylocci but appears to aid lesion drying. Sublesional injections of Amoxil 100 mg/ml at 0.05 ml/50 g body weight and Depomedrol 40 mg/ml at 0.025 ml/50 g body weight may be administered. Medroxyprogesterone acetate or megestrol acetate may be used as above.

Scarring and contraction occur during healing, and this area may become torn when the bird attempts to fly, particularly if the lesion was overlying a joint or involved the patagial membrane. Surgical ablation of the affected area is feasible in some situations (especially those in the pectoral region) when skin flexibility can be maintained. Most psittacines ignore surgical wounds other than for normal hygiene (Schultz 1981).

Cockatiel Feather Syndrome. A Cockatiel feather syndrome predominantly affecting lutino, white, and albino Cockatiels (*Nymphicus hollandicus*) occurs, characterized by feather loss, abnormal molt, flank picking, and/or chewing on the wing tips (Fudge 1982). The affected bird will pull out many feathers, self-mutilate, and even draw blood. There are often diarrhea and yellow-tinged urates. Serum lactate dehydrogenase (LDH) and serum glutamic oxaloacetic transaminase (SGOT) are typically elevated. A gram-negative bacterium (coliform, *Pseudomonas* spp.) is usually cultured in large numbers. In most cases, appropriate antibiotics will result in a marked improvement.

Superficial Mycoses. There are over 20 species of fungi belonging to the dermatophytes capable of causing ringworm (syn.: favus, white comb, crête blanche) in birds by invading the keratinized layers of the skin and feathers. The following dermatophytes are among those that have been found on avian hosts: *Microsporum gallinae* (fowl, canary, duck, quail, pigeon, turkey), *M. gypseum* (fowl, canary), *Trichophyton mentagrophytes* (fowl), *T. quinckeanum* (fowl), and *Trichophyton* spp. (unspecified) (robin, European blackbirds) (Eamens 1981). *T. verrucosum* and *T. mentagrophytes* are considered rare on avian hosts, with *M. gallinae* probably the most common.

Fungal infections of the skin and feathers can also be due to *Helminthosporium* spp., which can cause extensive feather loss in psittacines. Rarely other surface-dwelling fungal species are said to cause feather loss, but they may be present only as normal inhabitants of the integument. Ringworm is rare in birds, with the bald-headed species, pigeon, and quail the most commonly affected.

Clinical Signs. Lesions are usually limited to the fleshy or thin-skinned areas of the head and appear as scabs, crusts, or alopecic areas (Eamens 1981). If the lesions are limited to the skin, there may be marked hypertrophy of the epidermis, producing crustlike excretions around the feather follicles similar to those caused by *Candida albicans*. Favus is also known as the honeycomb fungus because of the rough, porous appearance of the scales it produces on affected skin (Arnall and Keymer 1975).

Favic cups can result when inflamed feather follicles become filled with fungal spores and eventually break open at the skin surface. The lesions may extend to the neighboring feathered parts, producing extensive feather loss. As the disease progresses, circular lesions are found on the underlying skin. Birds having combs and wattles are mainly affected (Patgiri 1985).

In poultry, the incubation period of *T. gallinae* is over 3 weeks, and the disease usually persists for 6 months or more in infected birds. Cutaneous mycoses of birds are chronic and spread slowly between birds.

Diagnosis. The diagnosis is mainly based on the clinical signs. Fungal infections sometimes resemble cnemidocoptic mange; therefore direct examination of a skin scraping is necessary. Skin scrapings can be mounted by using 10–20% potassium hydroxide (KOH) solution. The presence of septate hyphal fragments confirms the diagnosis. Cultures should be carried out for further confirmation and identification of the causative dermatophytes. Fungal infections of the integument caused by ingestion of fungal mycelia while preening are sometimes detected by routine fecal culture (Burr 1982). To remove contaminants, the collection site is cleaned first with soap and water and then with alcohol. Clinical material (feathers, scabs) can be placed in a clean envelope and sent to a laboratory for investigation, or they can be placed on a suitable culture medium.

Treatment and Control. The disease is transmissible from bird to bird and, in some cases, bird to man (Madill 1981). Affected birds should be isolated to minimize disease spread. Treatment of birds may prove ineffective. The oral administration of griseofulvin at 125 mg/kg body weight for 3–5 days is suggested, and simultaneously the older remedies may be tried, such as iodine, carbolic acid, mercuric chloride, formalin, and phenyl mercuric nitrate in the form of ointments and lotions (Patgiri 1985). Fungal infections on the feet can be treated twice a day with mycostatin or tinactin cream (Burr 1982). Old litter and nests are a good source of fungal infections in birds. Infected aviaries should be scrubbed with hot soda, detergent solution, or other fungicide such as Halamid at 995 g/kg chloramine (Diseases of Poultry 1965). Proper hygiene and management of housing birds should be maintained to control the infections.

Pseudofavus. Pseudofavus is a nonspecific condition of unknown etiology that affects birds in late summer and early autumn. This disease, which resembles favus, is characterized by thickening of the face skin, extending around the ear orifices to the back of the head. Microscopically there is no evidence of fungal infection. Pseudofavus is not transmissible to other birds and responds quickly to treatment with sulfur or iodine ointment (Diseases of Poultry 1965).

Bacterial Infections of the Avian Integument

Abscesses. Subcutaneous abscesses are often associated with loss of feathers over the affected area. They can arise from infected wounds, damaged feather follicles, blocked sebaceous glands, foreign bodies (e.g., retained mouth parts of ticks), pressure, and friction points. On the scaled part of the leg, abscesses can easily be confused with *Cnemidocoptes* spp. mite lesions.

Ulcers. A cutaneous ulcer is an open infected area on the skin that exposes the underlying tissue. An ulcer is usually slow- or nonhealing in cases where the edges thicken into a rim. Bacteria, especially anaerobes, or other organisms flourish in the tissues but are not necessarily the primary cause. Injuries, burns, foreign bodies, poxviruses, or *Mycobacterium* spp. may start the disease process, and malnutrition and other stresses may predispose the skin to ulcer formation. Tissues with poor blood supplies are commonly affected. The ulcer should be surgically debrided, with or without application of caustics, and an appropriate antibiotic (e.g., chlortetracycline powder in an urea base) applied (Arnall and Keymer 1975). Once the condition begins to resolve, an antibiotic cream can be applied to the area to help maintain a clean wound. To prevent a bird picking the area, an Elizabethan collar may be necessary.

Granulomas. Bacterial granulomas from overwhelming disease processes may appear as little scabs on the mouths of sick parakeets (Rosskopf 1981). Bacterial granulomas involving the cere, beak, or other regions of the integument closely resemble malignant tumors and may require biopsy and histopathology for accurate diagnosis.

Cockatoos may develop feather loss, starting on the legs and gradually spreading over the body. If granulomatous folliculitis is found, it is most likely due to an infectious disorder. Necropsy usually reveals severe degeneration of the skin, myocardial fibers, and adrenal glands.

Skin Infections. Purulent infections occurring in or just under the skin can cause epidermal sloughing. The head is usually affected, but the condition may also be seen in the axillary area of some Sulphur-crested Cockatoos (*Cacatua galerita*) with advanced psittacine beak and feather dystrophy and in the medial aspects of the thigh of Budgerigars (*Melopsittacus undulatus*) (Schultz 1981). The first clinical symptom is drying and crinkling of the epidermis. Treatment with an antibacterial ointment for 5–7 days facilitates skin repair. If the feather follicles have not been damaged, regrowth is normal.

Skin lesions can be associated with many systemic diseases, including those due to *Salmonella* spp., *Escherichia coli*, *Pasteurella* spp., *Yersinia pseudotuberculosis*, *Streptococcus* spp., *Staphylococcus* spp., *Mycobacterium* spp., *Spirochaeta* spp., *Mycoplasma* spp., and *Erysipelothrix* spp. (Arnall and Keymer 1975).

Staphylococcus spp. and *Streptococcus* spp. only occasionally produce purulent lesions in birds; usually dry scabby dermatosis is seen. Wounds most commonly infected are those associated with repeated trauma, especially on the feet (bumblefoot), breast, cere, bastard wing, and eyelids.

Pasteurella spp. (*P. septica, P. avium, P. multocida*) can cause matting of the feathers around the vent, eyes, and beak in combination with systemic infections. In some cases of chronic pasteurellosis, scaly or crusty lesions may develop on the unfeathered parts of the head in combination with signs of systemic illness.

Tuberculosis (*Mycobacterium* spp.) can be associated with the development of wartlike or dry flaking swellings, caseogranulomatous skin lesions, subcutaneous nodules, or raised ulcers of the skin (mainly on the head) in parrots, together with weight loss and other systemic signs (Hughes 1973; Eamens 1981; Hall 1982).

Erysipelothrix insidiosa and *E. rhusiopathiae* occasionally may be associated with accumulation of subcutaneous edema and with skin lesions of the head, together with other systemic signs. Conjunctivitis due to erysipelas has been noted in Budgerigars (Arnall and Keymer 1975).

Viral Infections of the Avian Integument.

Many viral conditions affect the avian integument, namely the various poxviruses, papillomas, and some well-recognized but as yet unconfirmed viral conditions (French molt, psittacine beak, feather dystrophy). Many conditions reported affecting growing feathers may be found to have a viral etiology when further research is conducted.

Duck Viral Hepatitis Virus. This virus often causes the beak of infected ducks to become congested and turn purple.

Papillomas or Warts. Warts occur in birds less frequently than in domestic mammals but are seen in a wide range of bird species (Arnall and Keymer 1975).

Viral Diseases of the Integument

Psittacine Beak and Feather Dystrophy (PBFD).

Psittacine beak and feather dystrophy (syn.: psittacine beak and feather disease syndrome, beak and feather rot, French molt) is characterized by abnormal molts and the development of dystrophic feathers, beaks, and/or claws in many predominantly young psittacines, including Sulphur-crested Cockatoos (*Cacatua galerita*) (Fig. 8.4), Major Mitchell Cockatoos (*Cacatua leadbeateri*), Galahs (*Cacatua roseicapilla*), Little Corellas (*Cacatua sanguinea*), Budgerigars (*Melopsittacus undulatus*), Peach-faced Lovebirds (*Agapornis roseicollis*), Nyasa Lovebirds (*Agapornis lilianae*), Rainbow Lorikeets (*Trichoglossus haematodus*), Eastern Rosellas (*Platycercus eximius*), Western Rosellas (*Platycercus icterotis*), Hooded Parrots (*Psephotus dissimilis*), Mallee Ringnecks (*Barnardius barnardi*), Port Lincoln Parrots (*Barnardius zonarius*), and Red-rumped Grass Parrots (*Psephotus haematodus*). PBFD probably affects many other captive and free-flying psittacines, including Fischer Lovebirds (*Agapornis personata*), Long-billed Corellas (*Cacatua tenuirostris*), Gang-gang Cockatoos (*Callocephalon fim-*

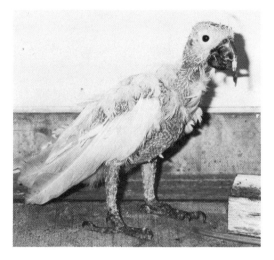

Fig. 8.4. Chronic psittacine beak and feather dystrophy in an immature Sulphur-crested Cockatoo (*Cacatua galerita*). (*From Pass and Perry 1984, by permission*)

briatum), Cockatiels (*Nymphicus hollandicus*), and Eclectus Parrots (*Eclectus roratus*). PBFD is seen in cockatoos more frequently than in the smaller psittacines and has an international distribution. See Altman (1969), Seneviratna (1969), Arnall and Keymer (1975), Perry (1975, 1979, 1981), and Pass and Perry (1984).

Clinical Signs. PBFD may occur as an acute overwhelming disease, with bilaterally symmetrical loss of all actively growing feathers over a few days, followed by death or partial or complete recovery, or it may occur as a chronic, progressive disease. The chronic disease is characterized by repeated replacement of feathers and quills by deformed, twisted, dystrophic quills that fail to mature and are shed prematurely, with death resulting from secondary causes (Fig. 8.5). The gross appearance of chronically affected birds may take several patterns in the early and middle stages of the disease but terminally is similar, probably because of birds succumbing to the disease in different stages in the molt cycle.

The clinical abnormalities of the avian integument are due to a combination of dystrophy and hyperplasia in the epidermis of the feathers, beaks, and claws during the growing phase (Pass and Perry 1984). Subsequent production of hyperkeratosis of the feather sheath and outer layers of the beak and claws then occurs. Powder down feathers are among the first affected because they grow almost continually

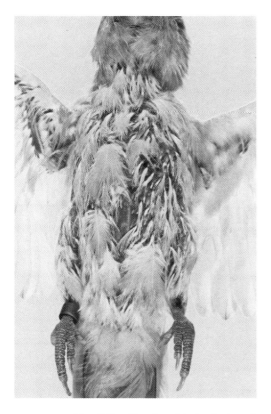

Fig. 8.5. Chronic psittacine beak and feather dystrophy in a Peach-faced Lovebird (*Agapornis roseicollis*), exhibiting replacement of normal feathers by dystrophic feathers and blood quills. (*From Pass and Perry 1984, by permission*)

mild cases birds may lose only one or two tail feathers. "Runners" are birds that are unable to fly due to permanent damage to flight feather follicles. Some Budgerigars and lorikeets affected with the French molt form of PBFD regain the ability to fly, whereas affected cockatoos rarely recover and usually die 6–36 months after infection.

Diagnosis. A characteristic microscopic finding in the dermis of psittacines affected with PBFD is the presence of macrophages containing purple-staining (H. & E. stain) intracytoplasmic inclusion bodies comprised of particles 17–23 nm in diameter, together with the presence of epidermal cells containing similar intracytoplasmic inclusions (Pass and Perry 1984). The particles, which resemble morphologically a densonucleosislike parvovirus, have also been demonstrated in the thymus and bursa of Fabricius of some affected birds. Direct and indirect effects of these particles on affected birds' immune systems may explain their apparent increased susceptibility to other diseases. Pass et al. (1985) have experimentally confirmed the viral cause of PBFD in transmission studies. Other factors, such as hypervitaminosis A and stress, can modify the severity and incidence of the disease. It is known that in birds with French molt the capillaries and red cell membranes in the pulp of growing feathers become fragile, there is a reduced number of circulating red blood cells, and the bone marrow shows evidence of great activity, apparently in an attempt to replace short-lived red blood cells. Deficiencies of vitamin E and/or K aggravate the disease. The mode of transmission of the disease is not yet established, although some evidence suggests that transmission may occur via the egg as well as between nestlings.

Treatment. No reliable cure for affected birds has been found yet, although the following treatments have been tried: (1) prolonged systemic courses of antibiotics (tetracyclines, amoxycillin, tylosin, and lincomycin); (2) topical antifungal and disinfectant rinses in chloramine and captan; (3) topical application of insecticides; (4) hormonal therapy with corticosteriods, thyroxine, and medroxyprogesterone acetate; (5) nutritional supplementation with animal and plant protein, calcium, zinc, vitamins, minerals, and trace elements; and (6) elimination of sunflower seeds and other oily seeds in the diet. Therapeutic efforts should aim at stimulating and supporting the immune system until effective viricidal (assuming the disease has a viral etiology) drugs are available.

Control of ectoparasites, meticulous nest

in normal birds. The lack of powder from these feathers gives the normally gray beaks of Sulphur-crested Cockatoos a glossy black appearance. Overgrowth of the beak is due to hyperkeratosis, failure of the keratinized layers to slough, and degenerative changes within the epidermis that predispose it to split, flake, or crack. Secondary bacterial and fungal invasion of the beak then produces the beak rot seen in some advanced cases.

French molt, which affects the smaller psittacines, especially Budgerigars, is considered to be a form of PBFD. It is characterized by premature molting or breaking off of feathers (often blood quills) beneath or at the skin surface, in a roughly bilateral symmetrical pattern. Primary and secondary flight and tail feathers are usually affected, occasionally covert feathers. In severely affected birds, most feathers are lost before reaching full development, whereas in hygiene and sanitation, interrupting the breeding program, and not breeding from first-year, very old, or affected-offspring-producing pairs may reduce the incidence of PBFD.

Budgerigar Short Tail Disease. This disease, suspected to be viral, commonly affects the feather follicles near the preen gland and the tail of Budgerigars, causing the feathers to grow short, twisted, and otherwise deformed (Fig. 8.6). Similarly affected feather follicles have also been seen in Peach-faced Lovebirds.

The advanced disease is characterized by the appearance of multiple feather quills in a single feather follicle. The disease appears to be contagious between young birds. Rump biters, Budgerigars (usually females) that pluck out feathers from the rumps of other birds, may predispose or hasten spread of the disease. Histologically, there are multiple dermal papillae forming in apparently virus-damaged feather follicles. Apparently once a follicle is damaged,

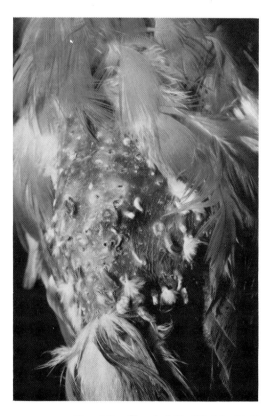

Fig. 8.6. Chronic folliculitis (short tail disease) in a Budgerigar (*Melopsittacus undulatus*) with some secondary self-mutilation.

it continues to grow multiple quills unless excised or destroyed by cautery. This treatment does not stop the slowly progressive disease from extending over other parts of the body, especially the hip area. There is no effective treatment, and control is based on culling rump biters and affected Budgerigars. See Perry and Cooper (1982).

Miscellaneous Conditions

Appendages of the Avian Integument. Wattles, combs, caruncles, and other fleshy protuberances of the head and neck region are richly supplied with blood vessels and are vulnerable to injuries, frostbite, and attack by biting insects. Large hematomas may result from fighting, and in some infections (e.g., pasteurellosis), gangrene of the wattles can occur (Arnall and Keymer 1975).

Ears. The most common lesions involving avian ears are those in pigeons, canaries, and magpies, attributed to poxvirus infections. Occasionally, moist or dry exudate and caseous abscesses are also seen. Treatment involves physical cleansing and application of small amounts of nonoily, antifungal, antibiotic eardrops.

Ticks and neoplasms are rarely found in the external ear canal. Vertigo associated with middle ear infection has been recorded (Small 1969).

Feather Loss Associated with Environmental Stress. Acute loss of tail and/or primary flight feathers from fledgling Budgerigars may occur under heat wave conditions combined with high humidity and overcrowding. Mature fledglings are most likely to be affected. Regrowth of feathers is evident in affected birds before the juvenile molt (Perry 1981).

Stuck-in-the-Molt. This condition, which occurs in psittacines and passerines, is similar to French molt except for the absence of deformed feathers. It is thought to be due to overbreeding or breeding a young bird repeatedly before its molt is completed. The bird's energy reserves are then used for breeding rather than for replacing feathers. Affected birds may exhaust themselves and die if they are kept breeding. The condition can be cured by halting breeding until feather replacement has occurred (Burr 1982).

In canaries, this condition is characterized by cessation of feather shedding or prolonged molt (which normally lasts 8–10 weeks). The disease has been attributed to sudden temperature change, shock during molting, and incorrect diet (Seneviratna 1969). Irregular, artificial photoperiods may predispose stuck-in-the-molt.

Uropygial Gland. This bilobed, holocrine gland (preen gland, oil gland) is situated at the base of the tail and is often associated with a stumpy feather tuft (Lucas and Stettenheim 1972). It is not essential and may be surgically removed if indicated. Ducks, however, have difficulty preening without it and may develop a bedraggled appearance (White 1981).

The organ is commonly affected in Budgerigars, presenting a change in the contour over the tail butt (Madill 1981). The bird will often pick at the area and frequently flick the tail. Impactions may be relieved by gently expressing the gland or flushing it with sterile saline solution. Abscesses may be lanced and dressed and left open to heal.

Vent Gleet. Vent gleet is a condition in which there is inflammation of the cloaca and vent accompanied by a purulent and foul-smelling discharge. Passage of droppings is difficult and causes extreme pain in the parrot. Vent gleet is possibly a venereal disease, and the only known treatment is euthanasia (Burr 1982).

Care of Feathers during Hospitalization. Feathers contaminated with blood and/or feces should be cleaned as soon as the bird is strong enough to tolerate the procedure. The application of oils, ointments, creams, or pastes to feathers should be avoided as these are usually difficult to remove, may initiate self-mutilation, and may interfere with the insulation of the bird.

There must be adequate space available for the bird to turn around without rubbing its tail and wings on the walls of the cage. The position of the perches within the cage should be checked.

It is important to minimize damage to the feathers of birds (e.g., trained falcons) during veterinary examination and treatment (Redig 1981). To help keep the tails in good shape during hospitalization, they should be enclosed in a sheath made of overlapping gummed mailing tape $1\frac{1}{2}$–2 in. (4–5 cm) wide. For greater stability, a piece of X-ray film or balsa wood can be used with the tape. This is especially useful for a bird with a broken leg, as the bird will learn to prop itself with its tail.

For restraining and positioning birds for radiography (and surgery), a piece of thin plywood covered with a velveteen cloth is placed on top of the X-ray cassette. The bird can then be restrained by applying strips of Velcro across the wing tips, legs, beak, neck, etc., with minimal or no feather damage (as might occur with adhesive tape) (Braithwaite 1982).

Repair of Individual Feathers. The art of "imping," as it is known in the sport of falconry, can be applied to the repair of broken feathers (Cooper 1968). This procedure involves removal of the distal portion of the broken feather and the implanation of a corresponding piece of feather from a molted or dead bird. An imping needle made of metal, wood, or synthetic material then glued into the shafts acts to hold the old and new portions together.

Bent or frayed feathers can be improved by immersion of the feather (but not the live tissue) in hot (but not boiling) water for 30 seconds.

References

Altman, R. B. 1969. Conditions involving the integumentary system. In *Diseases of Cage and Aviary Birds,* ed. M. L. Petrak, pp. 243–54. Philadelphia: Lea and Febiger.

Amand, W. 1982. IME 214. *Assoc. Avian Vet. Newsl.* 3(2):35.

Arnall, L., and I. F. Keymer. 1975. *Bird Diseases.* London: Baillière Tindall.

Bird, E. 1982. *Proc. 31st W. Poult. Dis. Conf. 16th Poult. Health Symp.* University of California, Davis.

Braithwaite, T. 1982. IME 232. *Assoc. Avian Vet. Newsl.* 3(2):45.

Burr, E. W. 1982. *Diseases of Parrots.* Neptune City, N.J.: T.F.H. Publications.

Butler, R. 1981. Diseases of non-psittacine birds. In *Refresher Course for Veterinarians on Fauna—Part B,* pp. 473–86. University of Sydney, Post-Graduate Committee in Veterinary Science, Proceedings no. 36. Sydney, Aust.

Cooper, J. E. 1968. The trained falcon in health and disease. *J. Small Anim. Pract.* 9:559–66.

Cooper, J. E., and T. Lloyd. 1974. *Veterinary Aspects of Captive Birds of Prey.* Saul, Gloucestershire, Engl.: Standfast Press.

Diseases of Poultry. 1965. 4th ed. London: British Veterinary Association.

Duncan, I. J. H., and B. O. Hughes. 1973. The effect of population size and density of feather pecking. In *Fourth European Poultry Conference,* pp. 629, 634. Edinburgh: British Poultry Science, Ltd.

Eamens, G. J. 1981. Zoonoses and other human diseases associated with aviary and cage birds. In *Refresher Course for Veterinarians on Aviary and Caged Birds,* pp. 433–60. University of Sydney, Post-Graduate Committee in Veterinary Science, Proceedings no. 55. Sydney, Aust.

Fudge, A. 1982. IME 169. *Assoc. Avian Vet. Newsl.* 3(1):13.

Galvin, C. 1979. The feather picker. *Calif. Vet.* 33(4):12–16.

Gumbs, J. F. 1982. IME 300. Use of synthetic skin during treatment of burned feet. *Assoc. Avian Vet. Newsl.* 3(4):100.

Hall, C. F. 1982. IME 292. Diseases of barnyard game and ornamental fowl. *Assoc. Avian Vet. Newsl.* 3(4):95.

Harrison, G. J. 1982. IME 203. *Assoc. Avian Vet. Newsl.* 3(2):31.

Hughes, B. O. 1973. The effect of implanted gonadal hormones in feather pecking and cannibalism in pullets. *Br. Poult. Sci.* 14(4):341–48.

Hughes, B. O., and I. J. H. Duncan. 1972. The influence of strain and environmental factors upon feather pecking and cannibalism in fowls. *Br. Poult. Sci.* 13(6):525–47.

Humphreys, P. 1978. Ducks (Anseriformes). In *Zoo and Wild Animal Medicine,* ed. M. E. Fowler, pp. 181–210. Philadelphia: W. B. Saunders.

Lucas, A. M., and P. R. Stettenheim. 1972. *Avian Anatomy. Integument. Part 1 and Part 2.* USDA Agricultural Research Service, Agric. Handb. 362.

Madill, D. N. 1981. Avian surgery. In *Refresher Course for Veterinarians on Aviary and Caged Birds,* pp. 197–218. University of Sydney, Post-Graduate Committee in Veterinary Science, Proceedings no. 55. Sydney, Aust.

Pass, D. A., and R. A. Perry. 1984. The pathology of psittacine beak and feather disease. *Aust. Vet. J.* 61(3):69–74.

Pass, D. A., et al. 1985. Personal communication.

Patgiri, G. P. 1985. Unpublished data (College of Veterinary Science, Gauhati, Assam, India).

Peckham, M. C. 1955. Xanthomatosis in chickens. *Am. J. Vet. Res.* 16:580–83.

Perry, R. A. 1975. Beak rot in Sulphur-crested Cockatoos. University of Sydney, Post-Graduate Committee in Veterinary Science, Control and Therapy Article 2, no. 329. Sydney, Aust.

_____. 1979. Beak rot in Sulphur-crested Cockatoos. (Update of Perry [1975]) University of Sydney, Post-Graduate Committee in Veterinary Science, Control and Therapy Article no. 875. Sydney, Aust.

_____. 1981. Beak conditions. In *Refresher Course for Veterinarians on Aviary and Caged Birds,* pp. 73–114. University of Sydney, Post-Graduate Committee in Veterinary Science, Proceedings no. 55. Sydney, Aust.

Perry, R. A., and H. Cooper. 1982. Notes on short tail disease on Budgerigars. University of Sydney, Post-Graduate Committee in Veterinary Science, Control and Therapy Article no. 1385. Sydney, Aust.

Philip, C. J. 1981. Emergencies, shock and post surgical care. In *Refresher Course for Veterinarians on Aviary and Caged Birds,* pp. 256–96. University of Sydney, Post-Graduate Committee in Veterinary Science, Proceedings no. 55. Sydney, Aust.

Redig, P. T. 1981. *Methods for the Delivery of Medical Care to Trained or Captive Raptors.* American Federation of Aviculture, Veterinary Medicine Seminar, San Diego, Calif.

Rosskopf, W. J. 1981. IME 49. *Assoc. Avian Vet. Newsl.* 2(2):14.

Schultz, D. J. 1978. Diseases of parrots. In *Refresher Course for Veterinarians on Fauna,* pp. 223–44. University of Sydney, Post-Graduate Committee in Veterinary Science, Proceedings no. 36. Sydney, Aust.

_____. 1981. The integument, ears, eyes. In *Refresher Course for Veterinarians on Aviary and Caged Birds,* pp. 567–78. University of Sydney, Post-Graduate Committee in Veterinary Science, Proceedings no. 55. Sydney, Aust.

Seneviratna, P. 1969. In *Diseases of Poultry, Including Cage Birds,* 2d. ed., Bristol, Engl.: John Wright and Sons.

Small, E. 1969. Diseases of the organs of special sense. In *Diseases of Cage and Aviary Birds,* ed. M. L. Petrak, p. 354. Philadelphia: Lea and Febiger.

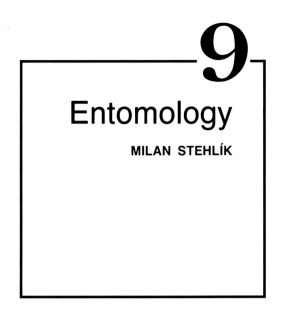

9
Entomology

MILAN STEHLÍK

ARTHROPODS are invertebrates with hard shells (bodies) and pairs of articulated legs. Fleas, lice, and flies have three pairs of legs, while ticks and mites have four pairs (in the larval stage only three pairs are present).

Arthropods can transmit viral, protozoal, and bacterial diseases. They live as parasites mostly on the surface of the host's body; only a few species of ectoparasites inhabit internal organs. Besides causing irritation to the host, these parasites can cause feather damage, anemia, and disease transmission.

Although numerous species of arthropods can infest avian species, only the ones of major importance are discussed in this chapter.

Mites

Sternostoma tracheacolum. *Sternostoma tracheacolum*, the air sac mite, was first described in the trachea of a canary by Lawrence (1948) in South Africa. Small passerines (canaries and finches) are most severely affected, small psittacine birds are rarely affected, and infestation is not known in large psittacines (Mathey 1967; Kummerfeld 1982).

The complete life cycle is spent on the mucous membrane of the respiratory tract; larval, nymphal, and adult stages are found there.

Gouldian Finches (*Poephila gouldiae*) are the passerines most susceptible to this disease.

Clinical Signs. Difficult breathing (dyspnea) through an open beak, coughing, sneezing, clicking sounds, nasal discharge, loss of voice, and a general inability to thrive are seen. Dyspnea is often accompanied by frequent attempts to cough up material from the trachea. Loss of song is also frequently seen in affected passerines.

Aeckerlein (1974) noticed that Gouldian Finches lost feathers primarily around the ear. Clinical signs usually appear several weeks or months after infestation with the parasites. Budgerigars may survive for months after the disease signs appear, but Gouldian Finches usually die within 3 weeks.

The mites penetrate through the trachea into lungs, air sacs, body cavity, and kidneys. Ulceration caused by the mites sucking blood in the air sacs can resemble tumorlike masses (hyperkeratotic tissue) and be accompanied by large amounts of mucus in respiratory passages (Mathey 1967).

Diagnosis. The history, clinical signs, fiber-optic examination of the trachea, tracheal washings, and autopsy aid in making a diagnosis. Postmortem examination may reveal tracheitis, increased slime formation in the respiratory passages, air sacculitis, and black spots (mites) on the mucous membranes. Examination of tracheal washings and exudate under low-power microscope will reveal the mites. Differential diagnosis includes acute bacterial pneumonia, *Syngamus trachea* (gape worm), a pharyngeal form of avian pox, and aspergillosis.

Treatment. Affected birds are placed in a cardboard box or covered cage and 4% malathion powder is dusted into the enclosure for at least 5 minutes. The treatment is repeated once weekly for 4–6 weeks. Recommended for finches (Fringillidae and Estrildidae) is a spot-on treatment in the dorsal shoulder area, using a 2% solution of trichlorphon-1,2-propylenglykol (40–70 mg/kg body weight). Treatment is given on the first, fifth, and ninth days. Supportive therapy may be necessary if the bird is debilitated or harboring a secondary infection. Other effective control measures are treating seed with carbaryl (weekly for 3 weeks) or hanging dichlorvos pest strips near the bird cage (*beware of toxicity*).

Transmission. Transmission is direct from one bird to another, via drinking water and food and from adult birds feeding young. Aeckerlein (1974) recommends hatching of Gouldian Finch eggs only after insecticide treatment and then placing the young with foster Bengalese parents. This isolation technique can also be used to eliminate disease in the species.

Laminosioptes cysticola Vizioli, 1870. Diagnosis of this mite is usually only made postmortem in galliforms and pigeons. Calcified nodules containing these parasites are found in the subcutis, muscle, and lungs. These parasites do not occur in passerines or psittacines (Keymer 1982). Treatment of the disease is unknown.

Cnemidocoptes pilae Lavoipierre and Griffiths, 1951.

The most frequent and most important ectoparasite of small psittacines is scaly face or scaly leg disease caused by *Cnemidocoptes pilae* (family Sarcoptidae). Infestation is commonly found in Budgerigars, other small parakeets, and canaries (Oldham and Beresford-Jones 1954; Kronberger and Haupt 1971; Keymer 1975).

Cnemidocoptes mutans Robin and Lanquetin, 1859.

This is another scaly face/leg mite mange in poultry and canaries (Kummerfeld and Stoye 1981). *Cnemidocoptes jamaicensis* Turk, 1950, causes the same disease in passerines. The disease is widespread, however, and occurs among many different avian species (Kutzer 1964, 1965).

Expertise is required to distinguish between the *Cnemidocoptes* spp.; fortunately the clinical signs and therapy are the same.

Clinical Signs. The disease usually starts from the angle of the beak (Fig. 9.1) and spreads to other areas of the head or body (horn of the beak, cere, eyelids, then the legs and cloaca). Later, in the course of the disease, it may spread to the feathered parts of the body. Overgrown and disfigured beaks are commonly seen as a consequence of dermatitis, along with encrusta-

tion of the cere (hyperkeratosis), nasal obstruction causing respiratory difficulty, lameness of the affected legs and feet, and rarely feather picking. On the feet, a characteristic tassellike appearance (hyperkeratosis) similar to beak infestations is seen in chronic cases. See Blackmore (1963), Kutzer (1964), Richards (1975), and Steiner and Davis (1979).

The mites first penetrate the keratinized layers of epidermis on which they feed, causing cavities in the stratum corneum. During this stage, the first signs of inflammation are seen. Later, affected areas become dry with chalklike, honeycombed encrustations. Budgerigars can be affected as young as 3 months (Freytage and Bendheim 1965).

Transmission. *C. pilae* spends its life cycle (approximately 3 weeks) in the skin of the host; ova, larvae, nymphs, and adult mites can be found on skin examination (Fig. 9.2).

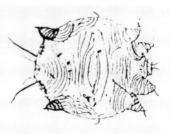

Fig. 9.2. *Cnemidocoptes* spp. mite, which causes scaly leg and scabies of the beak. (× 50) (*Drawing by Elisha W. Burr*)

Adult birds kept separate from other birds sometimes contract the disease, possibly due to a latent nestling infestation. Direct transfer from one bird to another may take place in isolated instances (Zenoble 1982). Inadequate nutrition, metabolic disorders, infectious disease, and poor sanitation are predisposing factors. Experimental transfer of the disease is therefore difficult under good management.

Diagnosis. Clinical diagnosis is made from typical pathological and anatomical changes and the history and condition of the bird. Microscopic diagnosis can be made from parasites recovered from skin scrapings using 10% potassium hydroxide solution. Differential diagnosis includes injury, burns, frostbite, and infectious diseases.

Treatment. Many preparations can be used to treat this disease. Dichlorvos pest strips placed

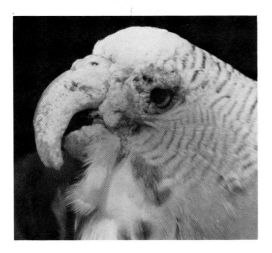

Fig. 9.1. Grossly malformed beak of a Budgerigar (*Melopsittacus undulatus*) with extensive cere and eyelid lesions caused by cnemidocoptic mange. (*Courtesy of Raymond D. Wise, Scottsdale Animal Clinic, Chicago, Ill.*)

around a cage are highly effective in mild cases. Liquid paraffin, petroleum jelly, crotamiton, and mesulphan provide good penetration and dissolution of hyperkeratic tissue when extensive lesions are present; persistent treatment may be necessary to rid the bird of an infestation. Dietary improvement (greens rich in vitamin A) and vitamin and mineral supplements aid in treating the disease. Treatment is usually effective if applied to the affected areas for 3 consecutive days and when necessary repeated in 1 week.

When beak deformities occur, they must be trimmed frequently to allow the bird to eat (Olsen and Dolphin 1978).

Topical treatment alone is usually not recommended because it is messy and the bird may ingest the medicant while preening its feathers. Aerosol therapy in the heavily feathered parts of the body is recommended (Tierney and Baillie 1979). Aerosol treatment can be carried out using a nebulizing apparatus and the following mixture: 20 cc Domoso, 20 cc sterile water, 1 cc Tylan, and 4 cc malathion (95% solution).

Cnemidocoptes laevis. *C. laevis* is the depluming scabies mite that commonly affects parrots (especially macaws) (Altman 1980). Infestation is heaviest during the warmer months of the year. The life cycle is not completely known but probably occurs entirely on the host. Clinical signs include feather pulling, with resulting feather loss, encrustation, and scab formation.

Treatment. Warm soapy water can be used to remove encrustations, followed by topical application of nitrofurazone on the scabby areas (for secondary infections) and application of rotenone or pyrethrin powder. No treatment is entirely effective because the mites often inhabit the feather follicle. Experimental work using the insecticide Ivermectin has produced promising results.

Red or Roost Mite (*Dermanyssus gallinae* De Geer, 1778). The red mite is a temporal, 0.6-mm-long, lively, eight-legged common parasite (Fig. 9.3) that feeds only at night and hides during the day in cracks and cage corners and under droppings (Ebert 1972). This very resistant mite can survive frost and starvation for more than 5 months.

Clinical Signs. Severe infestations can cause anemia, especially in young and debilitated birds. Most frequently affected are canaries, finches, and other small passerines; Budgerigars and other parrots are rather resistant (Keymer 1975).

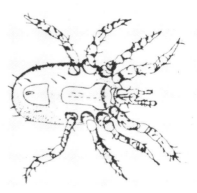

Fig. 9.3. Red or roost mite (*Dermanyssus gallinae*). (× 25) (*Courtesy of the National Pest Control Association*)

Diagnosis. During the daytime, the parasite can be found with the aid of a magnifying glass, embedded in perches, cracks, or corners of a cage. If infestation is suspected and parasites cannot be found, the cage can be covered with a white cloth overnight and examined for mites the following morning. These mites will appear as dark red or black moving spots across the white cloth. During autopsy, mites are occasionally found in the beak cavity, trachea, esophagus, and crop (Hiepe and Ribeck 1982). *Dermanyssus gallinae* can transmit the blood parasites *Plasmodium* spp. and *Lankesterella* spp. and two arboviruses, Japanese B encephalitis and equine encephalitis (Burr 1982).

Life Cycle. The life cycle of the parasite from the egg to six-legged larva to blood-sucking nymph is very rapid (4–9 days, depending upon the environmental temperature). Mite infestation may occur from new introductions into an aviary and from domestic fowl or wild birds.

Treatment. Treatment with common acaricides does not necessarily prevent recurrence of infestations. The use of dichlorvos pest strips will reduce the severity of an infestation. The cage must be cleaned with 5% hot washing soda, the perches burned, and acaricide (malathion, lindane, rotenone) applied to all parts of the cage. Kronberger (1973) recommends repeating the cage cleaning with a water temperature higher than 20°C after 5 days, a temperature of 15–20°C after 7 days, and a temperature lower than 12°C after 20 days.

Northern Mite (*Ornithonyssus sylviarum* Canestrini and Fanzago, 1877). This 0.5-mm-long feather mite spends its entire life cycle on the host. Since these mites prefer to attach themselves to fully grown contour feathers, they are rarely found on young birds (Kummerfeld 1982). Adult forms can survive starvation for only 2–3 weeks.

Adult birds show reluctance to incubate eggs and feed fledglings, resulting in death of young birds (Dodd 1983). Infestation commonly occurs from introduction of new birds into an aviary. Treatment is the same as for red mites.

Harvest Mites (*Trombicula* spp.). These mites are free living as adults, but the larvae (chiggers) are parasitic on birds and mammals.

Clinical Signs. Clinical signs of infestation include localized inflammation, pruritus, and swelling around the point of attachment of the parasite. Nonpruritic edematous swelling of the skin of the legs, ventral abdomen, thorax, and subcutaneous fibrosis is seen in severe cases.

In well-kept aviaries with proper sanitation, the disease is seldom a problem. Infestations usually appear at the start of warm weather. Pass and Jue Sue (1983) described an outbreak in which sixty canaries from various breeders were affected, however, even after strict sanitation was carried out. This indicates the resilience of the parasite.

Treatment. Aviary floors, walls, and nesting sites should be sprayed with a suitable insecticide to prevent infestations (Keymer 1982).

Ticks. Ticks are acarine arthropods. The most frequent tick found on poultry, psittacines, and passerines is *Argas persicus* Oken, 1818 (Fig. 9.4), while *Argas reflexus* Fabricius, 1794, is more commonly found on columbiforms. Both these species belong to the soft or argasic ticks. Hard or ixodic ticks (*Ixodes ricinus* Linnaeus, 1746) are not frequently found in captive birds.

Adult soft ticks lay a large number of eggs, which hatch in relation to temperature (10 days to several months). Larvae molt once or twice into six-legged nymphs and eventually undergo a final molting, forming adults. Individual

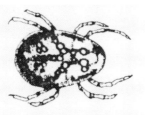

Fig. 9.4. Soft or argasic tick (*Argas persicus*). (×3.5) (*Drawing by Elisha W. Burr*)

stages can survive 6–12 months starvation. Female ticks attach to the bird.

A. persicus and *I. ricinus* transmit *Borrelia anserina* (spirochetosis) and *Aegyptianella pullorum* (aegyptianellosis). *Aegyptianella* spp. commonly affect fowl and rarely passerines and psittacines.

Treatment. The larval and nymph stages of soft ticks hide during the day; therefore birds should be sprayed with suitable acaricides during the night at 2-week intervals (Keymer 1975). This treatment must be followed by thorough sanitation of the surroundings, especially of moist, dark areas.

Adult ticks attached onto birds can be removed by forceps. To prevent breaking off the head of the tick, cover the tick with a piece of cotton soaked in ether or chloroform.

Lice. There are many species of biting lice (order Mallophaga) that appear on wild birds and only rarely attack caged birds. *Amblycera* spp. attack the base of feather quills, sucking vast quantities of blood. *Pectinopygus* sp. (suborder Ischnocera) is a large parasite (2–3 mm) that also infests feathers in psittacines and other bird orders. Companion birds can become infected directly from wild birds if aviaries or cages are placed in the open (Altman 1980).

Life Cycle. Lice spend their whole life cycle on the host, and survive only a short time away from it. Eggs (nits) hatch within 4–8 days into larvae, then molt several times before becoming adults capable of reproducing. The life cycle takes 3–4 weeks. Adults feed on growing feather sheaths and epidermal debris.

Clinical Signs. Clinical signs of louse infestation include poor plumage, pruritus, and frequent vigorous feather chewing (Fig. 9.5). Mouth cavity lesions, ulcerations with subsequent blood loss, and secondary bacterial infection may be seen with oral louse infestation.

Wobeser et al. (1974) described a hemorrhagic ulcerative stomatitis in four White Pelicans (*Pelecanus erythrorhynchos*) caused by the biting louse *Piagetiella peralis* (Mallophaga: Menoponidae).

In the Dvůr Králové n.L. Zoo, Czechoslovakia, newly imported adult White Pelicans (*P. onocrotalus*) from Kenya harbored a large quantity of these parasites in the mouth and pouch but exhibited no clinical signs.

Treatment. A single treatment with Alugan powder is usually enough to successfully treat infestations.

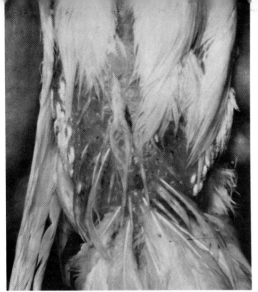

Fig. 9.5. Cockatiel (*Nymphicus hollandicus*) with acute pyoderma of the rump caused by vigorous feathering chewing due to a louse infestation. (*Courtesy of Raymond D. Wise, Scottsdale Animal Clinic, Chicago, Ill.*)

Toxicity is common in birds that frequently preen themselves (due to ingestion of the drug). In these breeds, pyrethrum (0.5–2%) is a more suitable drug because of its few side effects. Bullmore (1983) suggests treating birds by dusting with a 0.5% carbaryl powder (by placing them in a plastaic bag, leaving only the head exposed) once every 7–10 days until infestation is cleared. Mouth infestations may be best treated by hanging a dichlorvos pest strip around the cage after it has been aired for a week to reduce potential toxicity.

Fleas

Clinical Signs. Fleas rarely infest birds, and usually the source of infestation is domestic or wild mammals (Fig. 9.6). Adult fleas suck blood from birds, causing extensive irritation, skin ulceration, and secondary bacterial infections. The larvae feed on the droppings of adult parasites.

Treatment. Ova and pupae are not destroyed by

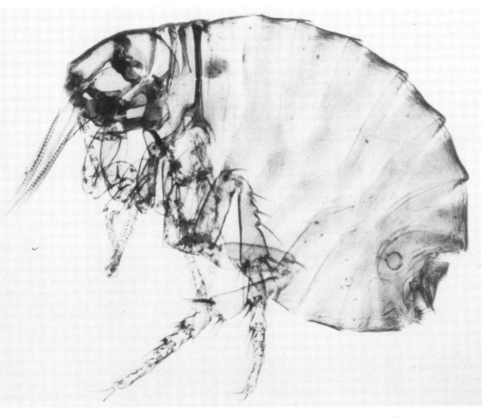

Fig. 9.6. Adult sticktight flea of poultry (*Echidnophaga gallinacea*), which is occasionally found on exotic birds. (*Courtesy of the Department of Agriculture and Fisheries, Veterinary Research Institute, Onderstepoort, Republic of South Africa*)

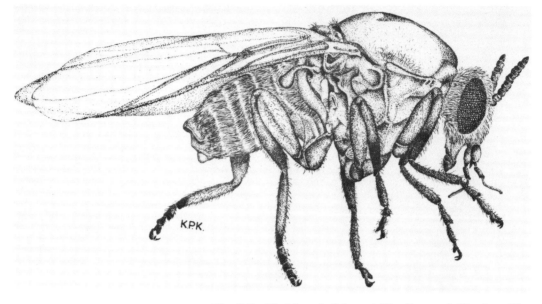

Fig. 9.7.   Blackfly or buffalo gnat (*Simulium* spp.). (*Courtesy of the Department of Agriculture and Fisheries, Veterinary Research Institute, Onderstepoort, Republic of South Africa*)

common acaricides; therefore it is necessary to carry out thorough sanitation of the environment (Boch and Supperer 1977). Treatment is the same as for red mites and is repeated after 3 weeks.

Mosquitoes. Only the females are bloodsuckers. They can cause intense irritation and allergic reactions in birds. *Aedes* spp. and *Culex* spp. can transmit fowl pox virus and *Plasmodium* spp. Control is best achieved by eradication of the vector or removal of birds from affected areas.

Dipterous Flies. Flies are important external parasites of birds because they can transmit blood-borne protozoan infections.

Etiology. Black flies (*Simulium* spp.) (Fig. 9.7) can transmit *Leucocytozoon* spp. and louse flies (*Hippobosca* spp.) (Fig. 9.8) can transmit *Haemoproteus* spp. Larvae or maggots of these two-winged insects can occasionally cause myiasis in birds. Frey and Hinaidy (1978) describe wound myiasis caused by *Lucilia sericapata* Meigen, 1926 in a Short-eared Owl (*Asio flammeus*) as sequel of a wing fracture.

   In Dvůr Králové n.L. Zoo, Czechoslovakia, two White Pelicans (*Pelecanus onocrotalus*) developed myiasis after pinioning.

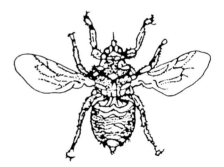

Fig. 9.8.   Louse fly (*Hippobosca* spp.). (*Drawing by Elisha W. Burr*)

Treatment. Larvae found on the yet-unhealed wings were treated effectively with a bath of Neguvon solution. Proper hygiene around wound areas must be carried out to prevent myiasis. Fly control is best achieved by keeping birds in screened areas away from vector sources.

References

Aeckerlein, W. 1974. Luftsackmilben bei Gouldemadinen. *Prakt. Tierarzt* 55:432.
Altman, R. B. 1980. Parasitic diseases in caged birds. In *Current Veterinary Therapy. VI. Small Animal Practice,* ed. R. W. Kirk. Philadelphia: W. B. Saunders.

Blackmore, D. K. 1963. Some observations on *Cnemidocoptes pilae* together with its effect on the Budgerigar (*Melopsittacus undulatus*). *Vet. Rec.* 75:592–95.

Boch, J., and R. Supperer. 1977. *Veterinärmedizinische Parasitologie. 2. Auflange.* Berlin and Hamburg: Paul Parey.

Bullmore, C. C. 1983. Biting louse infestation in a Cockatiel. *Mod. Vet. Pract.* 64:498.

Burr, E. W. 1982. *Diseases of Parrots.* Neptune City, N.J.: T.F.H. Publications.

Dodd, K. 1983. Northern mite (*Ornithonyssus sylviarum*) infestation in canaries. *Vet. Rec.* 113:259.

Ebert, U. 1972. *Vogelkrankheiten.* Hannover: Verlag M. and H. Schaper.

Frey, H., and K. H. Hinaidy. 1978. Fakultative Wundmyiasis bei einer Sujpfohreule – Asio flammeus. *Wien. Tierärztl. Monatsschr.* 65:256–57.

Freytage, U., and U. Bendheim. 1965. Krankheitsbild und Behandlung der Knemidocoptes-Raude des Wellensittichs. *Veterinärmed. Nachr.*, pp. 108–14.

Hiepe, Th., and R. Ribeck. 1982. Lehrbuch der Parasitologie – Rand 4 – Veterinärmedizinische Arachno-Entomologie. Jena: VEB Gustav Fischer Verlag.

Keymer, I. F. 1975. Arthropods. In *Bird Diseases,* ed. L. Arnall and I. F. Keymer. London: Baillière Tindall.

———. 1982. Parasitic diseases. In *Diseases of Cage and Aviary Birds,* ed. M. L. Petrak. Philadelphia: Lea and Febiger.

Kronberger, H. 1973. Haltung von Vogeln – Krankheiten der Vögel. Jena: VEB Gustav Fischer Verlag.

Kronberger, H., and W. Haupt. 1971. Knemidocptesräude bei Wellensittichen. Verhandlungsbericht des XIII. Internationalen Symposiums über die Erkrankungen der Zootiere, Helsinki, pp. 167–72. Berlin: Akademie Verlag.

Kummerfeld, N. 1982. Milben und Federlinge bei Ziervögeln und Tauben. *Prakt. Tierarzt.* 63:36–39.

Kummerfeld, N., and M. Stoye. 1981. Diagnose und Therapie duch die Luftsackmilbe (*Sternostoma tracheacolum*) bei Finken (Fringillidae) und Prachtfinken (Estrildidae) verursachte Acariasis. *Kleintier-Praxis* 27:95–104.

Kutzer, E. 1964. Knemidocoptes Räude bei Ziervogeln. *Wien. Tierärztl. Monatsschr.* 51:36–43.

———. 1965. Ektoparasiten bei Vögeln und ihre Bekämpfung. *Dtsch. Tierärztl. Wochenschr.* 72:15–19.

Lawrence, R. F. 1948. Studies on some parasitic mites from Canada and South Africa. *J. Parasitol.* 34:364–79.

Mathey, N. J. 1967. Respiratory acariasis due to *Sternostoma tracheacolum* in the Budgerigar. *J. Am. Vet. Med. Assoc.* 150:777–80.

Oldham, J. N., and W. P. Beresford-Jones. 1954. Observations on the occurrence of *Cnemidocoptes pilae* Lavoipierre and Griffith, 1951, in Budgerigar and parakeet.

Olsen, D. E., and R. E. Dolphin. 1978. Parasitism in companion birds. *Vet. Med. Small Anim. Clin.* 73:640–44.

Pass, D. A., and L. Jue Sue. 1983. A trombiculid mite infestation of canaries. *Aust. Vet. J.* 60:218–19.

Richards, D. A. 1975. Cnemidocoptes mange in parakeets. *Vet. Med. Small Anim. Clin.* 70:731.

Steiner, C. F., Jr., and R. B. Davis. 1979. Scaly leg and face-mite infestation in a parakeet. *Vet. Med. Small Anim. Clin.* 74:108–14.

Tierney, F., and J. Baillie. 1979. Malathion aerosol for treatment of scaly face mites in caged birds. *Vet. Med. Small Anim. Clin.* 74:69–70.

Wobeser, G., G. R. Johnson, and G. Acompanado. 1974. Stomatitis in a juvenile White Pelican due to *Piagetiella peralis* (Mallophaga:Menoponidae). *J. Wildl. Dis.* 10:135–38.

Zenoble, R. D. 1982. Selected diseases of the head and face in caged birds. *Compend. Contin. Educ. Pract. Vet.* 4:995–1004.

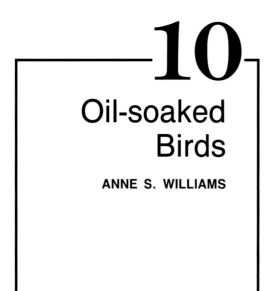

10

Oil-soaked Birds

ANNE S. WILLIAMS

THE DESTRUCTION of wild waterbirds and their aquatic habitat by oil pollution has caused increasing public concern in the last few decades. This interest has led to the development by government and private environmental agencies of detailed emergency plans, delineating procedures for the protection and restoration of habitat threatened by accidental spillage of hazardous substances. Generally these plans also provide guidelines for the capture of oil-contaminated birds and for their transport to centralized facilities where they are cleaned, fed, housed, waterproofed, and conditioned for return to the wild.

Although these rehabilitation centers usually are staffed by wildlife care professionals, the veterinarian also plays a significant role in the care of oil-soaked birds. In large-scale oiled bird rehabilitation efforts, veterinary services are required for clinical and laboratory investigation of disease outbreaks, medical and surgical treatment of injuries, coordination with wildlife disease agencies, and consultation in nutrition, sanitation, and record systems. Veterinarians involved in the emergency treatment of large numbers of oiled birds may wish to consult the International Bird Rescue Research Center's manual *Saving Oiled Seabirds* (second edition; available from the American Petroleum Institute, Washington, D.C.), which provides detailed information on oiled bird rehabilitation.

This chapter is written for the veterinarian in private practice, who occasionally is presented with small numbers of oiled birds or who may be associated with a wildlife care center. Most aspects of oiled bird treatment may be performed by the practitioner, requiring no specialized equipment. The limitation to hospital treatment of oiled birds is that when cleaned they require an intensive period of supervised swimming (to develop waterproofing) before release to the wild. For the majority of waterbird species, this requires transfer to a specialized facility, such as a wildlife care center or zoo, with the requisite pools and staff to complete the process of rehabilitation.

Characteristics of Waterbirds. Waterbirds are a diverse group of birds that utilize a range of aquatic habitat extending from tropical seas to the polar ice, and from open ocean to stream banks and marshland. The group does share a partial or complete dependence on aquatic habitat and thus a vulnerability to oil pollution, either directly through contamination of individual birds and eggs or indirectly through effects on food organisms and habitat. However, the many species of waterbirds exhibit a wide variability in degree of dependence on bodies of water, food habits, size and coloration, reproductive capability, and other adaptations to their aquatic environment. Their variability is further reflected in the differential susceptibility to oil pollution among types of waterbirds and in the varying ease and success with which major groupings of species are rehabilitated and returned to the wild.

A number of species of alcids, loons, and grebes are almost entirely aquatic and move very awkwardly on land, where they come only to breed or molt (Fig. 10.1). Species of surface-feeding ducks, geese, and swans are more nimble on land and alternate periodic use of the water with foraging or idling on shore. Many species rarely alight or swim on the water but are nonetheless dependent on aquatic habitat for food, including the skimmer plowing the surface of the sea with its lower bill for marine orga-

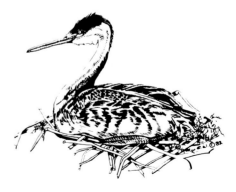

Fig. 10.1. The grebe, an almost entirely aquatic water bird. (*Drawing by Genevieve M. Wilson*)

nisms, the tern plunging into the sea's surface and rising quickly with its prey, and the wading herons and sandpipers foraging in marshes, tide pools, or the surf's edge.

The foods utilized by waterbirds range from the fish, crustaceans, cephalopods, and other marine organisms eaten by the pelagic species to the aquatic tubers, seeds, and grasses eaten by the anseriforms; geese in particular will graze extensively in meadows and fields. The diet of any particular population of waterbirds is not constant but changes periodically according to seasonal or geographic availability of food, age, molt, and reproductive status.

Species Affected by Oil Spills. Not all species of waterbird are equally susceptible to oil spills. The most commonly recorded victims are the alcids (murres, auklets, puffins), bay and sea ducks (eiders, scoters, mergansers), and miscellaneous highly aquatic species (grebes and loons). These species primarily inhabit the open marine and coastal waters, often in large groups, and forage for food by diving and swimming with great maneuverability below the water's surface. The frequency of oil spillage in harbors, shipping lanes, and drilling areas, combined with behaviors that render large numbers of birds susceptible to swimming or surfacing into an oil slick, make this a particularly high-risk group.

Less commonly but still significantly affected are the more aerial and terrestrial species (pelicans, cormorants, gulls, surface-feeding ducks, geese, and swans). These birds are less dependent on strictly aquatic habitat for their livelihood, and in most cases, tend not to congregate in large vulnerable groups on the water's surface.

In some spills, immature and molting birds have been represented in larger proportion than in the local populations; this may represent inexperience or flightlessness. On occasion, terrestrial birds (raptors, passerines, columbiforms) have been contaminated by spilled oil.

Ease of Rehabilitation. Waterbirds also vary in the ease with which they are rehabilitated. The easiest to handle and treat are the surface-feeding ducks, geese, and swans, followed by pelicans, gulls, terns, and coots. These birds readily accept food in captivity, are more easily habituated to proximity with human handlers, and tend to do well in groups. In most cases they are easy to waterproof after cleaning in small troughs or shallow pools, as they are fairly light in relation to their size and are agile on land. Release rates are high with this group.

Intermediate in difficulty are the alcids, the diving bay and sea ducks, and reportedly the Jackass Penguin (Randall et al. 1980). Although these birds are also good feeders in captivity and are gregarious and tolerant of human contact, their care is ultimately more difficult in that they are heavy-bodied birds with dense plumage and many species move poorly on land. Thus their care must include special bedding to prevent the development of keel sores and inflammation of the leg joints and substantial periods of supervised swimming to regain waterproofing.

The hardest group to rehabilitate includes loons and grebes, as well as a few miscellaneous species such as albatrosses and cormorants (Fig. 10.2). These birds tend to resist feeding in captivity and are excitable and highly stressed by crowding and human contact. In this group is included a number of species with very aggressive temperaments, large size, and/or powerful beaks and wings, so that handling is difficult. The grebes and loons, heavy birds that are awkward on land, require deep bedding and long periods of swimming. These and no doubt other factors combine to make release rates lowest for this group.

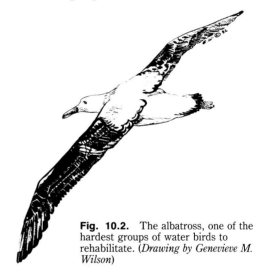

Fig. 10.2. The albatross, one of the hardest groups of water birds to rehabilitate. (*Drawing by Genevieve M. Wilson*)

Effect of Oil on Waterbirds. The effect of oil contamination on waterbirds can be divided into those most attributable to exposure and those due to ingestion. Oil and oil-water mixtures are of sufficiently low surface tension to penetrate the feathers, so that the skin is wetted and chilled and buoyancy is lost. A twofold increase in metabolic rate has been seen in oiled ducks compensating for heat loss in cold water and struggling to keep afloat (Hartung 1967; McEwan and Koelink 1973). Oiled waterbirds often leave the water and stop feeding entirely. Glycogen, fat stores, and the protein of muscle and viscera must then be catabolized for energy. Energy demands at this stage exceed energy production, and hypothermia and exhaustion result.

Oil can gain access to the bird's tissues by inhalation of fumes and aerosols and by cutaneous absorption, but the primary route is through ingestion of oil preened from the plumage. Some highly refined petroleum products (petrol, kerosene, diesel, cutting oils) are toxic on ingestion (Hartung 1966); others, such as certain crude and aged oils, can be consumed in large quantities without overt ill effect, particularly if the bird is in a protected environment (Holmes et al. 1978a). Among the described effects of oil ingestion on a limited number of waterbird species are inhibition of active transport of sodium in the intestine and supraorbital salt gland (Crocker et al. 1975; Miller et al. 1978); interference with glucose and amino acid absorption (Miller et al. 1978); gastrointestinal hemorrhage and renal, hepatic, and pancreatic damage (Hartung 1966; Aldrich 1970); and adrenal hypertrophy and lymphoid regression (Holmes et al. 1978b).

Much of this pathology, particularly the gastrointestinal, adrenal, and lymphoid changes, may be as attributable to generalized stress as to specific effects of ingested oil. Further, when the stresses of captivity (handling, crowding, noise, photoperiod changes, pathogenic organisms) are superimposed on the mechanical and toxic effects of oil, the picture at necropsy reflects chronic stress-mediated conditions, such as emaciation, hepatic and splenic amyloidosis, bacteremia, aspergillosis, and chronic debilitating joint disease (Snyder et al. 1971). Other stresses, such as the increased energy requirements of growth, molt, or reproduction, severe weather conditions, food shortages, and parasites, may also contribute to the cumulative effects of oil on the bird. Thus rapid capture and low-stress supportive treatment in captivity can have a very beneficial effect on the success of a rehabilitation effort.

Treatment of Oil-soaked Birds

Preliminary Examination. When an oiled bird is presented for treatment, its species should be identified, and if possible, its age and sex determined. A field guide to local birds will assist in identification and will also provide information on feeding and characteristics of the species.

Daily Care in Captivity. On a daily basis, the bird should be given a brief examination, which should include weight, cloacal temperature, a check for signs of disease, and a progress check on any injury being treated. The bird's keel should be examined for pressure sores, its leg and wing joints for swelling and heat, its eyes for any ocular pathology, and its droppings for abnormalities. During this period of handling, the bird can be given a tube feeding of fluids, and an emollient cream or lotion should be lightly applied to the feet and legs to keep the skin hydrated. Otherwise, the bird should be disturbed as little as possible.

Caging. For the few days required to treat, clean, and prepare the bird for swimming, it can be kept in any conventional small animal cage or run. The cage must be of sufficient size to allow the bird to stand erect and move freely without damaging feathers on cage bars and must accommodate food and water dishes. Birds of the same species can usually be caged together unless they fight. The room temperature should be kept warm for birds not cleaned, as the plumage cannot provide adequate insulation.

Wild birds stressed by alien sights and noises are best caged in quiet areas, away from other animals and work areas. A visual barrier, such as a towel, should be placed over the front of the cage. Good ventilation is especially important for the heavily oiled bird, as oil fumes can build up to toxic levels in an enclosed space.

With few exceptions, the bird must be provided thick, soft, absorbent bedding to prevent the development of pressure sores along the keel. Bedding may consist of foam padding or plastic-bubble packing material, covered with an abundant layer of cotton sheeting, rags, or towels. A few species (gulls, active alcids, cormorants, surface-feeding ducks) are less prone to keel sores and can be given a thick layer of newspapers covered with cloth to absorb moisture. Many of these "standing species" will perch on a wooden or concrete block placed in the cage, which aids considerably in keeping the plumage clean.

The bedding must be changed several times a day due to the volume and frequency of the bird's droppings. Droppings that are permitted to soil the feathers not only cause the bird to become chilled but also can harden, disrupting feather alignment and removal. Loons and grebes, especially, frequently remain lying in their own droppings and must be checked regularly.

Feeding. Information on the general diet of a particular wild species can be obtained from texts and field guides, but the natural diet is generally impossible to recreate for the captive bird. Even though precise analysis of the nutrient requirements of each wild species is not available, zoos and captive breeding facilities have developed simplified diets that sustain their birds well. For short-term rehabilitation efforts, the dietary needs of these species are simplified even further by dividing them into two groups, fish eaters and grain eaters. (For a discussion of feeding, see Chapter 11.)

Oil Removal

When to Clean. Cleaning is best delayed for 24–48 hours after capture so the bird can be rested, fed, hydrated, and warmed before treatment. The bird is ready for cleaning when the body temperature is normal and when it is active, alert, and defensive and has normal droppings. Exceptions to this rule are in emergency situations, when the oil is suspected or known to be toxic and its continued presence on the plumage may kill the bird. Suspicion of high toxicity should be aroused when lethargy, tremors, ataxia, or unresponsiveness cannot be attributed to hypothermia or when these signs are seen in conjunction with erythematous skin or with ocular epiphora and blepharospasm. The physical properties of the oil can also provide clues, in that the thinner, highly refined, aromatic petroleum products (petrol, kerosene, diesel fuels) tend to be more toxic than aged or tarlike crude oils.

Cleaning Procedure. Cleaning can be accomplished within 20–30 minutes and usually requires only two people, although more help may be needed with very large, strong, or aggressive birds. The following materials and equipment are needed:

1. Sink, basin, or tub large enough to accommodate the bird's body and the workers' hands
2. 10–30 gal (40–120 l) hot water
3. Detergent (Liquid dishwashing detergents are the most satisfactory, but not all are equally effective. Dawn and Lux Liquid Amber, available in the United States, and Joy II, available in Canada, are the agents of choice. Products available in the United Kingdom and reportedly effective include Village, Keynote, Winfield, and Co-op.)
4. Laboratory thermometer for cleaning and rinsing solutions
5. Short hose with shower spray head to attach to the tap
6. Towels or absorbent cloth
7. Dishwashing gloves and aprons, if desired

Just before the cleaning, the bird's eyes should be protected with a bland ophthalmic ointment. It may also be prudent to block the

beak of a very aggressive bird during this extended period of handling. The beak may be taped closed distal to the nares or taped over a small dowel, which will prevent biting without interfering with breathing (see Fig. 4.2).

The wash basin should be approximately three-fourths filled with water 102–110°F (39–43°C). A 1% concentration of detergent should be added to a standard dishwashing basin, which will hold 1.5–2 gal (5–8 l). This concentration is adequate to remove most oils, but detergent can be added in small increments if the oil resists removal. Too high a concentration can inhibit cleaning as badly as too dilute a solution (Berkner et al. 1977).

The bird is held by the wings and its body immersed in the cleaning solution; the solution is then pressed into the feathers with the hands, working with the lay of the feathers (Fig. 10.3). As waterproofing is a function of feather arrangement and integrity, the plumage should not be ruffled or scrubbed during cleaning. When the cleaning solution becomes too dirty to aid cleaning further, the solution must be changed. The head, which cannot be immersed in the detergent solution, can be cleaned with a terrycloth rag.

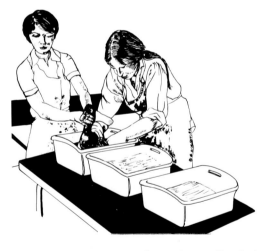

Fig. 10.3. Immersing an oil-soaked bird in cleaning solution. (*Drawing by Genevieve M. Wilson*)

After several baths, when no further oil can be removed and the bird appears clean, it is given a final bath in clear water, then held above an empty basin for rinsing. This is best accomplished by spraying hot water over the wing, starting with a gentle spray for the head and neck and increasing pressure as the breast,

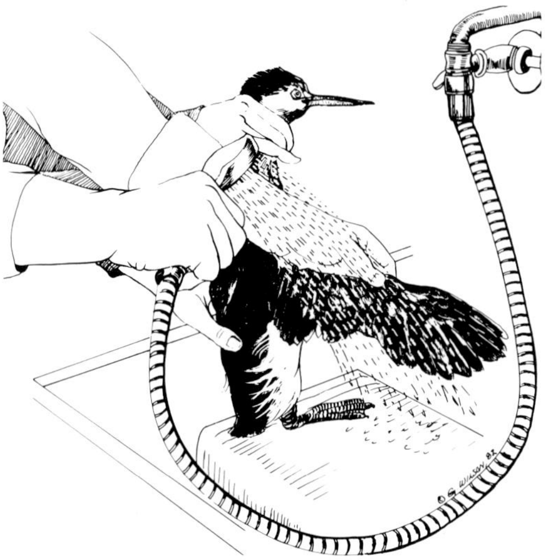

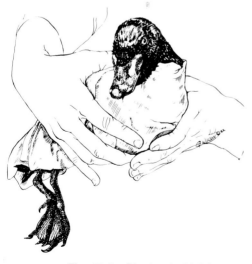

Fig. 10.4. Rinsing the bird with a sprayer. (*Drawing by Genevieve M. Wilson*)

If the bird appears unduly stressed at any point during cleaning, it should be briefly rinsed, blotted dry, and placed in a warm cage to recover. Cleaning can be repeated 24–48 hours later, when the bird has gained condition.

Occasionally a very aged or tarlike oil will not yield satisfactorily to detergent cleaning. In the past, hydrocarbon solvents (kerosene, acetone, chloroform, aliphatic compounds) were used to remove tough oils, but they are not recommended because of health hazards to humans and birds alike. Instead, when oil is impervious to increasing concentrations of an ordinarily effective detergent, cleaning efforts should be halted and the bird briefly rinsed and dried. Once dry, some 24 hours later, the affected areas can be coated with a thin layer of light oil, such as vegetable oil, baby oil, or low-viscosity liquid paraffin (lighter than medical weight). The bird's body heat will aid the light oil's penetration and dissolving of the contaminating oil. Cleaning with detergent can be attempted after 30–45 minutes. This technique delays waterproofing so is only used when absolutely necessary.

back, wings, and tail are rinsed (Fig. 10.4). After a few minutes of rinsing, water should be seen to bead up and run off the plumage, indicating that detergent and oil residues have been removed from the feathers and that the water-repellant physical properties of the feathers are being expressed. Rinsing should be complete within 10–15 minutes, after which the bird is blotted with rags and placed in a cage to dry (Fig. 10.5).

Drying. The rinsed bird is ordinarily dried with radiant or forced-air heat because chilling due to evaporative cooling can be significant when the bird dries at room temperature. The bird is given a tube feeding of fluids before drying, as it may pant and become dehydrated under the dryer. It is then placed in a cage; the bottom of the cage should be covered with rags, and the cage temperature should be 94–104°F (35–40°C).

The bird should be watched for heat or cold stress during drying, although some degree of panting or holding the wings away from the body is not cause for alarm. The cage temperature, however, should be decreased if forceful prolonged panting, prostration, and excessively high cloacal temperature are seen and increased if the bird shivers or registers a below-normal cloacal temperature.

The plumage will dry after 45–60 minutes of forced-air heat. The remaining damp spots under the wings or on the ventral or caudal aspects of the body are dried by exposing these areas to the heat source for a few minutes. After the bird is dry it should be tube-fed fluids once again and offered food.

Waterproofing and Preparation for Release. The last phase of oiled bird rehabilitation consists of restoring the plumage to a waterproof condition. This is best accomplished by providing clean, sheltered pools where the bird can bathe, groom, and preen its feathers into waterproof alignment (Fig. 10.6). Birds that have

Fig. 10.5. Blotting the bird dry with rags. (*Drawing by Genevieve M. Wilson*)

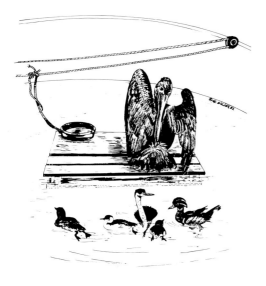

Fig. 10.6. Restoring the plumage to waterproof condition in clean, sheltered pools. (*Drawing by Genevieve M. Wilson*)

been promptly and carefully cleaned may take only a few days to regain water-repellant and buoyant plumage. Time in the water helps prevent the keel sores, cloacal impaction, and joint damage associated with captivity and improves appetite and attitude.

For the majority of waterbird species, the swimming process is best accomplished at a wildlife care center or zoo with pool space to accommodate birds. Until transfer or release in the wild can be effected, the bird should be lightly sprayed with water several times a day to stimulate preening.

An effective method of managing large numbers of birds in a spill situation is to place small groups of birds in pools and allow them to swim until they show signs of waterlogging or chilling. They are then taken out and allowed to preen and dry in warm, sheltered areas, until they are able to swim again. As the plumage improves, birds will spend most of the day in the water without significant wetting.

A pool should be of sufficient depth to stimulate swimming and diving, small enough in diameter to permit easy capture, and easily cleaned (draining or filtering the superficial layer of oil and debris on the water). The partially terrestrial species can be waterproofed in less-elaborate pools. Surface-feeding ducks, geese, coots, gulls, and wading birds will splash and preen sufficiently in low troughs of water or can be wetted with a hose spray periodically. All birds except the wading birds must be tested for waterproofing before being considered for release.

Release. The true test of successful rehabilitation is the rate of survival after release. It is therefore advisable to place permanent bands on released birds to allow individual identification. Some studies have provided evidence that released birds survive poorly (Clarke and Kennedy 1971; Swennen 1977), while other studies are more optimistic (Randall et al. 1980).

To ensure a bird's best chance of survival when returned to the wild, it must not be released until it meets the following criteria:

1. Clean, waterproof plumage that stays dry and beads water even after extended periods of swimming
2. Behavior similar to others of its species
3. Physical capability sufficient for survival in the wild (full use of limbs and eyes, ability to maintain normal body temperature while swimming, weight gain since capture, active, alert attitude)
4. Salt tolerance (in birds released to a saltwater environment)

Birds are best released early in the day, after a good feeding. If possible they should be returned to the area from which they were captured.

References

Aldrich, J. W. 1970. *Review of the Problem of Birds Contaminated by Oil and Their Rehabilitation.* U.S. Fish and Wildlife Service, Resource Publ. 87. Washington, D.C.

Berkner, A. B., D. C. Smith, and A. S. Williams. 1977. Cleaning agents for oiled wildlife. In *Proceedings, 1977 Oil Spill Conference (Prevention, Behavior, Control, Cleanup),* American Petroleum Institute. Washington, D.C.

Clarke, R. B., and R. J. Kennedy. 1971. *How Oiled Seabirds Are Cleaned.* Advisory Committee on Oil Pollution of the Sea, Research Unit on the Rehabilitation of Oiled Seabirds. University of Newcastle Upon Tyne, Engl.

Crocker, A. D., J. Cronshaw, and W. N. Holmes. 1975. The effect of several crude oils and some petroleum distillation fraction on intestinal absorption in ducklings (*Anas platyrhynchos*). *Environ. Physiol. Biochem.* 5:92–106.

Hartung, R. 1966. Toxicity of some oils to waterfowl. *J. Wildl. Manage.* 30(3):564–70.

———. 1967. Energy metabolism in oil-covered ducks. *J. Wildl. Manage.* 31(4):798–804.

Holmes, W. N., J. Cronshaw, and J. Gorsline. 1978a. Some effects of ingested petroleum on seawater-adapted ducks. *Environ. Res.* 17:177–90.

Holmes, W. N., J. Gorsline, and J. Cronshaw. 1978b. Effects of mild cold stress on the survival of seawater-adapted mallard ducks (*Anas platyrhynchos*) maintained on food contaminated with petroleum. *Environ. Res.* 20:425–44.

McEwan, E. H., and A. F. C. Koelink. 1973. The heat production of oiled mallards and scaup. *Can. J. Zool.* 51:27–31.

Miller, D. S., D. B. Peakall, and W. B. Kinter. 1978. Ingestion of crude oil: Sublethal effects in Herring Gull chicks. *Science* 199:315–17.

Randall, R. M., B. M. Randall, and J. Bevan. 1980. Oil pollution and penguins – Is cleaning justified? *Mar. Pollut. Bull.* 11:234–37.

Snyder, S. B., J. G. Fox, and O. A. Soave. 1971. *Mortalities in Waterfowl Following Bunker C Fuel Exposure.* Stanford University, Stanford Medical Center, Division of Laboratory Animal Medicine. Stanford, Calif.

Swennen, C. 1977. *Laboratory Research on Seabirds: Report on a Practical Investigation into the Possibility of Keeping Seabirds for Research Purposes,* Netherlands Institute for Sea Research. Texel, Neth.

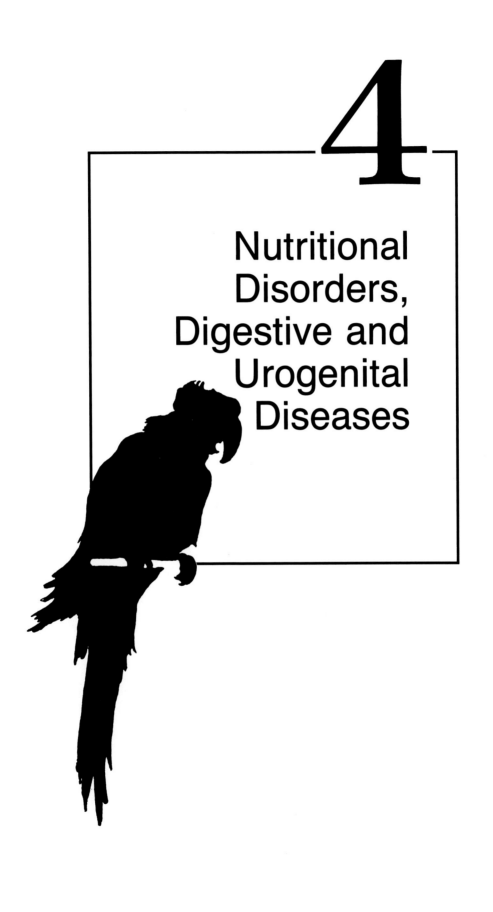

4

Nutritional Disorders, Digestive and Urogenital Diseases

11

Feeding and Nutritional Disorders

ROBERT E. DOLPHIN

IN AVIAN veterinary practice, deficiency diseases are commonly found, affecting all species. Birds in the wild occupy many ecological niches, from the hot, dry, dusty deserts to the tropical rain forests; such diversity in species means differences in nutritional requirements that humans must try to approximate for caged birds.

Controlled studies by nutritionists to determine the exact requirements of different bird species are needed. Most formulas are not yet perfect but have developed a long way in the last 5 years. However, numerous companies still supply mashed and pelleted feeds that are based on quantity rather than quality of nutrients. As a basic rule, most diets should be supplemented with additional foodstuffs.

Deficiencies of one or more indispensable nutrients may lead to signs of disease and death. Deficiencies may be simple or multiple and are more likely to be borderline than marked or absolute. In many deficiency diseases similar general signs are exhibited, such as retarded growth, poor feathering, lethargy, or reproductive failure. Nutritional deficiencies due to poor diet or chronic disease can produce abnormal feather structure if the feathers were actively growing during the period of deficiency or stress. Pinched-off feather bases can result from demands on the body reserves when new feathers are trying to grow, as diversion of nutrients from feather to antibody and defense cell production can cause a feather to die before it has completed growth. Many times a correct diagnosis can be made by obtaining complete information about bird diet and management, in addition to observing the signs of affected birds, and whenever possible, making necropsies. Chronic deficiencies are usually more harmful than acute deficiencies and often much harder to diagnose.

Stress-related conditions such as handling, quarantine, bacterial infections, viruses or parasites, high or low temperature, low humidity, and drug therapy can interfere with the absorption of nutrients or increase the quantity required, causing an adequate diet to become deficient.

Nutritional Requirements. All birds need the following substances: proteins and amino acids, carbohydrates, fats, vitamins, inorganic elements, and water. Different species require different amounts of these substances.

Proteins and Amino Acids. Proteins are composed of approximately twenty nutritionally important amino acids. Ten are essential: arginine, histidine, isoleucine, leucine, lysine, methionine, phenylalanine, threonine, tryptophan, and valine. In the young bird, two amino acids are important, glycine (or serine) and proline; additional amino acids take care of the nitrogen requirement for the synthesis of nonessential amino acids, nucleic acids, and other nitrogenous compounds. In the United States, methionine and lysine are the amino acids likely to be missing in the diet.

Clinical symptoms of lack of protein or essential amino acids include reduction in growth and feed consumption, reproductive problems, and loss of body weight in the adult. Rarely, increases in body fat and feed consumption are seen. Some feather problems can occur with this lack. Feather pulling and poor feather condition have been reported in market-age chickens when the energy level of the feed is increased in relation to the crude protein level.

Excess protein may also have an influence on visceral or articular gout, although other factors are also thought to be involved.

Carbohydrates. There is no deficiency disease attributed to the lack of carbohydrates in the diet. Normal blood sugar levels can be maintained and growth at a normal rate can occur by the substitution of fats for carbohydrates.

Fats. Fats are necessary in the bird's diet as concentrated sources of energy. Two unsaturated fatty acids required by birds, linoleic and arachidonic acid, are important in cell and fatty tissue growth and also as precursors of prostaglandins. In young birds a lack of these fatty acids can result in lack of growth, fatty liver syndrome, and reduced resistance to respiratory infections. In addition, these unsaturated fatty acids are necessary for proper skin condition and feather growth.

Unsaturated fatty acids may be destroyed by oxidation, which forms aldehydes. Aldehydes react with free amino groups in proteins, reducing amino acid availability. The peroxides generated during this oxidation may also destroy the activities of vitamins A, D, and E and water-soluble vitamins such as biotin.

Vitamins. Vitamins are a group of fat-soluble and water-soluble chemicals essential in nutrition. These compounds have no structural or functional relationship to each other. All vitamins, with the exception of vitamin C, are required by birds in minute amounts. Vitamins function as parts of enzymes and act as catalysts in many chemical reactions of the body. Vitamins A, D, and E are the ones most likely to be deficient in a bird's diet.

Vitamin A. Vitamin A is necessary for growth, vision, and epithelial maintenance. Vitamin A deficiencies are probably the most common nutritional disorder seen in practice. They are usually manifested by small, white, necrotic plaques in the mouth and throat.

Vitamin A deficiency is characterized by lethargy, emaciation, and poor plumage. The early signs of a deficiency can appear as a cold or sinus infection. Small, whitish, pus-filled lesions on the roof of the mouth then develop. In chronic cases, the discharges from the eyes and the nose may be so profuse that the eyes are stuck shut. This condition must be differentiated from infectious conditions exhibiting similar lesions. Vitamin A deficiencies, with necrotic mouth lesions, can sometimes be confused with avian pox. Birds exhibiting these signs are treated with either injectible vitamin A and D_3 or vitamin A and D_3 oral preparations. Treatment of choice depends on the severity of the lesions and other management factors. Mouth lesions respond very promptly with vitamin A injections given twice weekly at 1000 IU/100 g body weight. Birds so treated are up and eating within days, whereas avian pox infections may take 4–6 weeks to respond. In severe hypovitaminosis A, the normal absorption of vitamin A from the intestinal tract is interfered with and oral treatment is not successful. Initial treatment must be by injection. In the latter stages of the deficiency, severe ulcerations and secondary infections occur. These must be treated with an antibiotic of choice. Diets should be supplemented with vitamin A on a routine basis.

Vitamin D. Vitamin D is required for a proper use of calcium and phosphorus to form normal bones. It also acts by stimulating the absorption of calcium from the intestinal tract. Vitamin D_3, the form that can be utilized by birds, is produced on the skin through the action of sunlight. It is unlikely, however, that this source is adequate if birds are kept in confinement. Vitamin D_3 deficiencies can also occur from the feeding of stale, high-carbohydrate seed mixtures; unobservable fat necrosis can occur in seed, causing fatty degeneration of the fat-soluble vitamins A, D, and E.

It may take 2 to 3 months or longer for a vitamin D deficiency to develop in the adult bird, but as little as several days in the young bird. Egg production is markedly affected in the older birds, and some may develop a temporary paralysis or loss of leg use. Later on in the disease, the bones, beak, and claws become soft and pliable; in young birds, bowing of the legs occurs. The bones become weak and rubberlike, and birds walk with very obvious effort. Feathering is also poor.

Very high levels of vitamin D_3 (2 million IU or more/lb diet) can cause kidney damage by calcification. In clinical practice, the deficiency is most commonly seen in young raptors because of vitamin D_3 association with calcium and phosphorus levels. Once damage has been done to the bones it is not usually correctable, although further damage can be prevented. Vitamin D_3 should be added to the diet on a routine basis.

Vitamin E. Vitamin E is most important as an antioxidant. It protects the essential fatty acids as well as vitamins A and D_3.

Few or no clinical signs of deficiency are seen in mature birds. In the young, however, nervous symptoms can occur, caused by brain damage and accumulation of fluid under the skin. Muscular dystrophy may also be seen in young birds, associated with a selenium deficiency.

Young birds respond to injections of vitamin E and selenium if the condition is not advanced. When nervous symptoms are present, they often do not respond to treatment.

Vitamin K. Vitamin K is required in the body for production of prothrombin, an important part of the blood clotting mechanism. A bird that lacks vitamin K may bleed to death from a slight injury. This condition occurs in conures and probably also in other species. There is little documentation as to the etiology of the disease. However, an exclusive sunflower seed diet seems to predispose a bird to the condition.

Liver pathology and increased bleeding times are often caused by bacteria, such as

Escherichia coli. Affected birds do not exhibit any condition other than increased bleeding time, and there is no evidence to substantiate other infections or deficiencies. The condition is a separate entity probably involving synthesis in the liver due to lack of essential nutrients. Affected birds respond to vitamin K injections.

Thiamine (vitamin B₁). Thiamine is required by birds for the utilization of carbohydrates. Late in the disease process, deficient birds may "stargaze" because of paralysis of some neck muscles. Treatment must be administered either orally or by injection because when the condition is seen, birds are usually debilitated and refuse to eat.

Riboflavin (vitamin B₂). Riboflavin acts in many enzyme systems of the body and is associated with cell respiration. Deficiencies, however, are usually only seen in the young bird. Lack of riboflavin causes slow growth in the young, and weakness and emaciation in older birds. It is also essential for normal functioning of the nervous system, particularly in growing birds. Appetite remains good, but later in this disease, diarrhea develops. In chronic cases, the wings droop and birds will not walk and are found in a resting position. Severe dermatitis, tissue swelling, and deep fissures in the skin are seen in severe cases. In poultry, this condition is called "curled toe paralysis."

Pantothenic Acid. Pantothenic acid is essential for the metabolism of carbohydrates, proteins, and fats. Clinical symptoms of this deficiency are very similar to a biotin deficiency. Small cracks and fissures may be seen on the skin around the toes and on the bottom of the feet. Severe weakness and unsteadiness can also develop. This condition is rare or nonexistent in companion birds.

Nicotinic Acid (niacin). Nicotinic acid is a part of the enzyme system responsible for carbohydrate, fat, and protein metabolism. A deficiency causes swellings of the hock joint and bowing of the legs. In this deficiency, the Achilles tendon rarely slips away from the condyles, unlike perosis (slipped tendon). Effective supplementation to correct this deficiency is questionable.

Paradoxine (vitamin B₆). Paradoxine is required in amino acid metabolism. There are no reports of paradoxine deficiencies in companion birds.

Biotin. Biotin is necessary for carbon dioxide metabolism. Deficiency symptoms are similar to those for lack of pantothenic acid, making a dif-

ferential diagnosis difficult. In poultry, perosis, ataxia, and skeletal deformities are reported.

If a biotin deficiency is suspected, the presence of uncooked egg white in the diet should be investigated. Raw egg whites contain avidin, which combines with biotin to make it unavailable in the body.

Folic Acid. Folic acid is an enzyme required for amino acid and nucleic acid metabolism and for the formation of nucleo proteins. Folic acid deficiency can produce poor growth, poor feathering, anemia, and perosis. In some avian species, it is required for pigmentation.

Cobalamin (vitamin B₁₂). Vitamin B₁₂ is necessary in nucleic acid synthesis and also in carbohydrate and fat metabolism. Signs of B₁₂ deficiencies are slow growth, decreased feed utilization, perosis, and mortality.

Choline. Choline is involved in body metabolism. This deficiency is also associated with manganese deficiency. The primary clinical symptom is perosis, but in chronic cases, the Achilles tendon slips from its condyle. Once the tendon has slipped, repair is questionable. In some cases, diet supplements and surgery to repair the damage can be tried, but the prognosis is grave.

Vitamin C. In most cases, vitamin C is synthesized in adequate amounts in birds.

Minerals. Collectively minerals enter into many body reactions. Without these essential inorganic elements, life would not be possible. The following inorganic elements are necessary for life: calcium, phosphorus, magnesium, potassium, sodium, chlorine, and the trace elements manganese, iron, copper, zinc, iodine, molybdenum, and selenium. In many cases, two minerals are tied closely together, such as calcium and phosphorus or sodium and chlorine; these will be discussed together.

Calcium and Phosphorus. Calcium is necessary for bone formation, eggshell formation, and blood clotting; and along with sodium and potassium, it is required for normal heartbeat. It also helps in the maintenance of the body's acid-base balance.

Phosphorus is important in the metabolism of carbohydrates and fats. It exists in all living cells, and its salts are also important in the body's acid-base balance, as well as for bone formation. In order for calcium and phosphorus to be utilized properly, there must be an adequate amount of vitamin D in the diet.

A lack of calcium, phosphorus, or vitamin D_3 in growing birds results in rickets. In addition, it is very important that calcium and phosphorus be in the proper ratio in the diet, approximately 1.5:1.

Magnesium. Magnesium is essential, along with calcium and phosphorus, for bone formation. Approximately two-thirds of the magnesium in the body is in the bone. It is also necessary for carbohydrate metabolism and for the action of many enzymes.

Sodium and Chlorine (salt). Sodium is found chiefly in the blood and body fluids. It is important in maintaining the acid-base balance of the body and along with potassium and calcium is necessary for heart activity. A lack of sodium and chlorine in the diet can result in loss of weight and in chickens has been reported to produce cannibalism. A deficiency of chlorine can lead to nervous symptoms.

Excess salt in the diet is toxic. The lethal dose in chickens is approximately 4 g/kg body weight. Younger birds appear to be more susceptible to toxic effects of salt than do older birds.

Potassium. Potassium, in contrast to sodium, is found primarily in the cells of the body rather than in the body fluids. Like sodium, potassium is involved in bone formation and necessary for normal heart activity. Lack of potassium is characterized by overall muscle weakness, poor intestinal tone, and cardiac weakness.

Manganese. Manganese is required for bone formation, growth, and reproduction. Perosis is a condition thought to be caused by a manganese deficiency or a combination of deficiencies of manganese, biotin, choline, and/or other minerals.

In perosis there is an enlargement of the tibial-metatarsal joint. Twisting or bending of the distal end of the tibia and proximal end of the metatarsus occurs and finally, as a result of the twisting, the gastrocnemius tendon slips from its condyles. The slipping of the tendon causes complete crippling in the affected leg. If both legs are affected, the bird usually cannot secure food and water and will die. The condition occurs mainly in young birds. Excess calcium in the diet may prevent the usage of manganese and affect normal bone growth.

Iodine. Iodine is necessary for normal functioning of the thyroid gland. Thyroxine produced by the thyroid gland contains approximately 65% iodine and acts as a regulating agent in body metabolism. When the intake of iodine is restricted, the thyroid tissue enlarges and goiter results.

Iron and Copper. Iron and copper are necessary for hemoglobin formation. In poultry, lack of pigment can result from iron deficiency. When this occurs, a bird is usually also anemic.

Zinc. Zinc is necessary for enzyme activity in the body and possibly other functions that are not well defined. In turkey poults, low levels of zinc can cause extensive feather deformities.

Selenium. Selenium is an important mineral element for muscle toning. Birds deficient in selenium exhibit poor growth and feathering, impaired fat digestion, and pancreas problems. Vitamin E and selenium are synergetic and vital in the young bird to prevent muscle problems.

Water. Without water, life is impossible. It is a solvent and acts as a transport medium for nutrients and products of metabolism, and it enhances cell reaction. Because water evaporates readily, it can remove many calories of heat from the body by vaporization.

Starvation. Starvation is the ultimate nutritional deficiency to occur both in wild and in aviary birds. In the wild, birds that cannot compete for food quickly die off. In caged birds, the condition can occur from a variety of causes. A dominant bird may keep other birds away from the feeding dish, or a bird may have a condition such as face mites that deforms the beak and prevents it from eating. Most important, when birds are sick they often have neither the desire nor the ability to eat and thus die from starvation.

Diets. Exact nutritional requirements for many of the bird species are not known. Therefore quality must be fed to ensure that birds get the proper nutritional requirements. Seeds or food may have to be rotated or fed separately as birds tend to pick what they like and leave the rest.

Bird breeders and aviculturists throughout the world have developed many diet formulas that have worked successfully. They are based on the feed available in that part of the world. The recommended diets that follow are from Muller (1978). (There are, as well, many specialized diets for birds, such as the insectiverous eaters and the fish eaters, that are of specialized interest and probably not of great importance to the average companion bird owner.)

Finches and Canaries. The following mixture is recommended:

2 parts white millet	1 part oat groats
1 part red millet	1 part rape or thistle
2 parts canary seed	seed

A good mineralized grit should always be available, and cuttlebone is desirable. Many finches require animal protein in their diets, especially when feeding young. Finches enjoy green seeding grasses, such as wintergrass (*Poa annua*), chickweed, and most other types found in the garden. Care must be taken to ensure that no insect sprays have been used.

Pigeons and Doves. Some species of rain forest pigeons feed on fruit and must be given an appropriate diet (see the diet for fruit eaters). The majority of species, however, are seed eaters. These range in size from the small Diamond Dove to the larger Wong's Pigeon. All must have a variety of seeds of appropriate size and a good mineralized grit. Grit is especially important, because pigeons swallow their food whole and grind it in the gizzard. The following mixtures are recommended.

For small pigeons and doves:

1 part white millet	1 part yellow millet
1 part canary seed	½ part oat groats
1 part wheat	Mineralized grit and
1 part milo	shellgrit

For larger breeds:

2 parts wheat	1 part whole corn
2 parts milo	1 part white millet
1 part pigeon peas	Mineralized grit and
	shellgrit

Commercial pigeon pellets are available from some feed companies. If the larger species can be induced to eat them, the pellets can provide a balanced diet complete with minerals and vitamins, and they are often medicated against prevalent disease, as well.

Parrots and Cockatoos. There are over 300 species of psittacines, which range in size from the Budgerigar to the Palm Cockatoo and macaws. Most are basically seedeaters, but one group, the lories and lorikeets feed predominantly on nectar, pollen, and fruit. The following mixtures are recommended.

For small parrots (Budgerigar to Red-rumped Parrot):

2 parts white millet	1 part wheat
2 parts canary seed	Mineralized grit and
1 part red or yellow millet	shellgrit
1 part oat groats	Cuttlebone when available

Most smaller parrots appreciate seeding grasses. Care must be taken that no insecticide has been used. Wholemeal bread, crumbled up, is especially good, as it provides extra animal protein and minerals.

For medium parrots (rosella size):

1 part white millet	Green food, fruit (apple, pear, orange), and wholemeal bread
1 part canary seed	
1 part wheat	
1 part oat groats	Mineralized grit and shellgrit (essential)
1 part sunflower seed	
1 part milo	Cuttlebone when available

Many birds enjoy chewing on the leaves and bark of native (*nonpoisonous*) trees. Branches placed in the cage provide birds with something to do and may add minerals to their diet.

For large parrots (cockatoos, macaws, African Gray Parrot):

1 part sunflower seed	1 part whole or cooked corn (or fresh sweet corn)
2 parts wheat	
1 part milo	
1 part oat groats	1 part peanuts (raw)
	Mineralized grit and shellgrit

It is essential that these species have a wide variety of fruits, vegetables, bread, and green branches of nonpoisonous trees. Feather problems are common in larger parrots, as they are prone to boredom; this situation can be partially alleviated by something to chew on.

For lories and lorikeets:

1 cup Heinz dry baby food cereal (high-protein or mixed grain)	2 tablespoons honey, raw sugar, or glucose
	6 drops liquid vitamins for babies
1 cup warm water	
2 tablespoons condensed milk	

Change the food twice daily. In a separate pan offer mixed fruit, apple, pear, grapes, pawpaw (papaya), soaked raisins, tomato, orange, and cantaloupe. Seed should be available (the medium parrot mix). These species also like to chew on bark, leaves, and blossoms of most native (nonpoisonous) trees.

For baby cockatoos and other baby parrots (Baby cockatoos are frequently a problem to veterinarians. The following diet was formulated for them at the San Diego Zoo.):

½ cup Sperry Wheat Hearts or Heinz dry baby food cereal	1 teaspoon corn syrup or honey
	2 fresh egg yolks
⅛ teaspoon salt	Milk or water
½ teaspoon fine cuttlefish bone meal	4 drops vitamin supplement

Mix the dry ingredients; add the syrup and egg yolks and then the milk or water to make a souplike mixture. Boil over low heat 3–5 minutes, stirring gently. Cool until finger warm. Stir in the vitamin supplement. Feed the mixture with a spoon. The baby birds should be fed three to six times daily. The crop is usually visible as a semitransparent bag at the base of the neck so it is possible to determine the amount of food left from the last feeding.

Fruit Eaters. Feed these birds a mixture of fruit, such as diced apple, banana, pear, grapes, pawpaw, cantaloupe, orange, tomato, and raisins. Add a vitamin-mineral mixture and mix well. Very few birds feed exclusively on fruit, and most require some protein in their diet. An insectivorous bird diet should be offered as well as fruit.

Average-sized Waterbirds (500–1500 g). Williams (1984) supplied the following information about feeding and hydration of waterbirds.

Kcal required (2 × basal metabolic rate):

140–200 Kcal/kg body weight/day

Kcal provided by commonly used foodstuffs (metabolizable energy):

Fresh or defrosted smelt: 100 Kcal/100 g
Dry grain feed: 250–300 Kcal/100 g
Tube-feeding mixtures (diluted for passage through tube): 90 Kcal/100 ml

Approximate amounts required:

Fresh or defrosted smelt: 120–200 g/kg body weight/day (equivalent to 8–10 smelt, 15–20 g each)
Dry grain feed: 50–80 g/kg body weight/day
Tube-feeding mixtures (diluted): 160–230 ml/kg body weight/day

Hydration of Waterbirds. Wide, low pans of unsalted drinking water should be provided for all water birds able to use them. Some species, such as pelicans, large herons, and loons, have beaks that make drinking out of water pans difficult, so they may instead require tube feeding of fluids once or twice per day. An occasional bird that persists in sitting in its water pan and becoming chilled will have to be hydrated exclusively by tube. Supplementary tube feedings of fluids are not necessary once a bird is eating or being tube-fed a nutrient mixture regularly. The water content of fish and strained food mixtures is quite high; grain eaters, if their food is presented in water, will be able to ingest sufficient fluids as they eat.

Useful fluids include Gatorade, 2.5% dextrose in half-strength lactated Ringer's solution, a hypotonic solution consisting of 1 level teaspoon salt and 50 ml 50% dextrose/l water, or even tap water. During later phases of rehabilitation, marine and estuarine species are maintained on 2–3% saltwater rather than fresh water or other hypotonic fluids, so as to stimulate and maintain the function of the supraorbital salt gland.

Supportive Therapy. Supportive therapy is designed to keep the debilitated patient alive, often while waiting for laboratory results. The following mixture is suitable for force-feeding as supportive therapy (Schultz 1984):

30% high-protein cereal   30% bread crumbs
25% egg powder   Vitamin supplement
15% skimmed milk powder

To 5 g of this mixture, add:

10 ml 25% sugar solution
1–2 ml vegetable oil

This gives approximately 3 Kcal/g. Using the relationship between existence energy and weight (up to 500 g) at 25°C,

$$\text{Existence energy (Kcal/bird/day)} = \frac{\log W - 1.128}{0.021}$$

where W = weight in grams. The energy requirements and the amount of food are calculated on a daily basis for a given weight. The increased temperature and immobility of a sick bird reduces energy requirements.

Fluid requirements are satisfied by 5% dextrose and 0.9% saline, which provides 154 mmol/l sodium. Other fluids, such as Normosol R, may provide 5 mmol/l potassium but only 140 mmol/l sodium, which may be hypotonic for birds.

Give fluids at 1–2 ml/100 g body weight intramuscularly once or twice daily until skin elasticity over the sternum returns to normal.

References

Muller, Kerry A. 1978. J. S. Stewart Memorial Refresher Course, Taronga Zoo, Mosman, Sydney, N.S.W. Aust.
Schultz, D. J. 1984. Personal communication.
Williams, A. S. 1984. Personal communication.

12

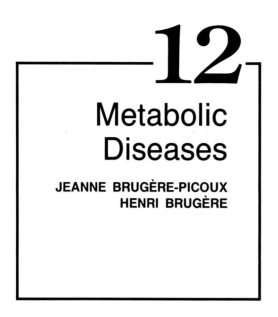

Metabolic Diseases

JEANNE BRUGÈRE-PICOUX
HENRI BRUGÈRE

VETERINARIANS are frequently presented with metabolic disorders in caged birds. A deficiency in one or many indispensable elements (a dietary problem) is the most common cause of metabolic disorders. Imbalances in calcium and phosphorus metabolism can result in bone disorders (rickets, osteomalacia) and in systemic symptoms (as seen in secondary hyperparathyroidism). Excess caloric intake is a cause of obesity, fat deposits, and fatty liver. Some other metabolic disorders can result from an individual predisposition and are more sporadic, such as diabetes mellitus.

Rickets. Rickets is a disease characterized by a failure of mineralization of osteoid matrix in young growing birds. This disease is frequently seen in large or long-legged species, which grow rapidly and need vast amounts of dietary calcium and phosphorus.

Etiology. In caged birds, there are three causes of rickets: deficiency of dietary calcium, deficiency of vitamin D_3, and a severely unbalanced calcium-phosphorus ratio.

Deficiency of dietary calcium occurs when there is not a sufficient supply of calcium in the diet. For example, a common cause of rickets is the absence of a cuttlebone or oyster shell grit (or refusal to use it).

Deficiency of vitamin D_3 can result from insufficient dietary intake or impaired production of provitamin D_3. Most pet birds are kept indoors and do not receive enough direct sun (ultraviolet light) to effect conversion to vitamin D_3. These conditions also reduce the vitamin D secretion of the uropygial gland. Other causes of vitamin D_3 deficiency are impaired intestinal

function (lack of absorption) and diseases of the liver or kidney. In these organs two successive hydroxylations are required to obtain the biologically active form of vitamin D_3. This metabolite stimulates synthesis of a specific calcium-binding protein in the intestinal wall.

The normal calcium-phosphorus ratio is between 1.5:1 and 3:1. Many diets have calcium-phosphorus ratios very different from this optimum, causing disease. An excess of calcium (e.g., from calcium salts as an additive) binds with phosphate ions in the gut lumen and is excreted as $Ca_3(PO_4)_2$, and as a result, deposition of calcium in bone is prevented. An excess of dietary phosphorus ties with calcium ions and is excreted. Some bird foods are rich in phosphorus (seeds given to caged birds, meat given to birds of prey). Diseased animals show a decrease in blood calcium, which can result in secondary hyperparathyroidism.

Clinical Signs. The first signs are softening of the vertebrae, claws, and sternum (which may develop an S shape (Fig. 12.1). Ribs that curve inward and spinal column deformities are also seen. With time, the long bones of the legs may curve and break when manipulated. Af-

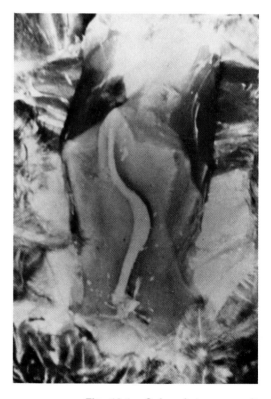

Fig. 12.1. S-shaped sternum resulting from rickets.

fected birds are reluctant to perch, walk, or move their wings. A bird with rickets lacks growth and exhibits a severe weakness of the legs. Birds frequently rest on their hocks and appear to be waiting for death.

Diagnosis. The clinical diagnosis is easy when typical clinical signs as above are presented. At necropsy, bone lesions, structural deformities, and enlarged parathyroid glands can aid diagnosis. Diet evaluation can confirm a dietary origin of the disease.

Therapy. Therapy is possible if the bird is not severely affected. Otherwise euthanasia is indicated.

Treatment includes calcium and vitamin D_3 supplements. For vitamin D_3, cod-liver oil can be placed on seed, vitamin D added daily to the drinking water, or better yet, an oral administration or subcutaneous injection of 500 IU vitamin D_3/30 g body weight given once (Ekperigin and Vohra 1981). For calcium, calcium lactate or gluconate can be given orally, but like vitamin D_3, an injection gives greater efficiency. Calcium gluconate (with or without magnesium or phosphorus) in a 20% or 40% solution (as used for injecting cattle with milk fever) can be given. A dilution of 1 part to 10 or 20 in the drinking water or an injection of a 10–20% solution under the skin of the neck is recommended (Arnall and Keymer 1975).

Treatment must be completed by improvement of the diet, for example, adding cuttlebone, oyster shell grit, fish, and cooked vegetables.

Osteomalacia. Osteomalacia is a disease of adult birds whereas rickets is a disease of young, growing birds. This disease is characterized by mineral loss in the bone when reabsorption exceeds deposition. The osteoid matrix remains, and the bones become soft.

Etiology. The causes of osteomalacia are the same as those of rickets. The disease is frequently associated with prolonged egg laying with an insufficient calcium supply in the diet. Another cause is the lack of grit in the food. Grit in the gizzard is necessary for grinding seeds, and its absence leads to incomplete digestion and absorption of minerals and vitamins. Arnall et al. (1974) reports the occurrence of osteomalacia in old parrots with parathyroid tumors (primary hyperparathyroidism).

Clinical Signs. Signs of the disease are more discrete than rickets. The bones become thin, soft, painful, and fragile and can break sponta-

neously when a bird is handled. Affected birds may appear drowsy, feather-picked, and reluctant to perch, move, or fly. The females lay brittle eggs, or egg production may cease.

Diagnosis. Clinical signs associated with diet evaluation may be sufficient to inform the practitioner: bones are normally formed but soft, painful, and fragile. X-ray examination shows cortice thinning and lowered density. It may also reveal fractures (with minimal callus formation) and kyphosis (deformation of the rachis).

Therapy. When an improvement can be expected, the treatment of osteomalacia is the same as that for rickets. Clinical improvement is often seen after the first week of treatment, but complete recovery needs 3–4 weeks or longer.

Nutritional Secondary Hyperparathyroidism.
Nutritional secondary hyperparathyroidism of caged birds is a common component of rickets and osteomalacia. It appears as a consequence of lowered blood calcium. Bone disorders and other clinical symptoms are seen with the disease.

Etiology. The etiology is the same as that of rickets and osteomalacia. The decrease of blood calcium stimulates the parathyroid glands to release an increased amount of parathormone. This hormone can stimulate calcium reabsorption in the kidney and urinary loss of phosphorus. There is a further leakage of minerals in the bone. The phosphaturia causes polyuria (increased urine volume) and polydipsia (increased water consumption).

Clinical Signs. Clinical signs present a great variability, from clinically inapparent (Arnall et al. 1974) to death. According to the severity, the clinical signs can be as follows: apathy, drowsiness, picked feathers, anorexia, soft stool or diarrhea, polyuria, and polydipsia. Bones can be painful, resulting in difficulty to walk, fly, or perch. The legs and claws may be inflamed and exhibit swollen joints (Fig. 12.2). Claws can be tightly clenched or flexed and twisted over each other (Himmelstein and Bernstein 1978). The most dramatic symptoms are cardiac arrest and death. With or without bone disorders, some birds may exhibit hypocalcemia with functional consequences: muscle spasms, tetany, and cardiac disturbances (Wallach and Flieg 1969; Randell 1981; Altman 1982).

Diagnosis. Diagnosis is difficult except in the most severe cases. Biochemical investiga-

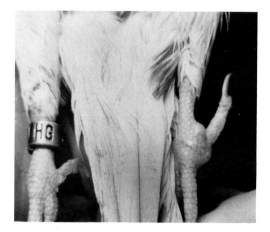

Fig. 12.2. Budgerigar (*Melopsittacus undulatus*) with inflamed and swollen joints due to nutritional secondary hyperparathyroidism. (*Courtesy of Raymond D. Wise, Scottsdale Animal Clinic, Chicago, Ill.*)

tion of the serum (calcium, uric acid, alkaline phosphatase, aspartate aminotransferase) is required for differential diagnosis with liver or kidney dysfunction (Fowler 1978; Blackmore and Cooper 1982).

Therapy. Therapy is symptomatic. Intravenous administration of dilute gluconate solutions is possible in large birds exhibiting tetany. Caution must be taken during infusion by monitoring the heart rate (Halliwell 1979).

Goiter (thyroid dysplasia). Goiter can occur as a result of hypothyroidism caused by iodine deficiency. Some authors consider it very rare (Rosskopf et al. 1982). Others have reported high incidence of this disorder (Blackmore and Cooper 1982). This can be explained by geographical considerations and dietary habit conditions.

Etiology. As in all animals, iodine is required for thyroxin synthesis. A deficiency in the diet can result in decreased secretion of the hormone. Other factors can also stimulate the appearance of thyroid dysfunction (many plants (e.g., soybean) provide goitrogenic principles that inhibit thyroxin synthesis even if iodine is adequately supplied). This disease is unknown in seabirds, which receive large amounts of iodine from the fish in their diet. For caged birds eating only seeds, iodine supply can be insufficient and thyroid dysfunction can appear. Oyster shell grit contains an appreciable amount

of iodine and can prevent the disease (except in Budgerigars). As a consequence of thyroxin deficiency, the thyroid-stimulating hormone from the anterior pituitary is released in increased amounts and the thyroid follicles become hyperplastic.

Clinical Signs. Thyroid hormones stimulate metabolism. Their deficit results in systemic disturbances. Affected birds are lethargic and inactive and exhibit poor condition (dry skin, ragged plumage). They are unable to maintain body temperature when exposed to environmental changes, their blood cholesterol increases, and body weight tends to increase due to the deposition of excess fat. Many birds with fatty tumors and fatty liver have hypothyroidism (Sitbon and Mialhe 1980). The affected birds also show slower heart and respiratory rates and reduced fertility and excrete small, constipated droppings.

Thyroid insufficiency presents a characteristic feature in Budgerigars, in which dystrophy of the glands produces mechanical obstruction of the respiratory and digestive tracts. The weight of the glands is normally 5–40 mg, and when thyroid insufficiency is present, may exceed 300 mg (Schone and Arnold 1980; Blackmore and Cooper 1982). Both lobes of the thyroid gland lie at the thoracic inlet where space is limited; thus an increase in size compresses the trachea, the syrinx, and sometimes the esophagus.

The major clinical signs are labored respiration with squeaking noises. These symptoms are often considered asthmatic or a respiratory infection (chronic respiratory disease). Digestive disturbances, such as regurgitation of food, slow emptying of the crop, and crop dilatation, are also commonly seen. Severe loss of weight (emaciation) ensues (Wise 1980).

Diagnosis. Diagnosis of thyroid disturbance can be made by blood thyroxin evaluation. The normal values vary according to species. Normal ranges for eleven species have been suggested by Rosskopf et al. (1982) in a study where thyroxin was measured in more than fifty species (Table 12.1). Hyperplasia of the gland usually cannot be palpated or seen by X-ray examination. Gastrointestinal disturbances (e.g., slow emptying of the crop) may be revealed, however, after giving a barium meal (Lafeber 1965).

Therapy and Prevention. Goiter can be treated successfully using either iodine or levothyroxine. Iodine can be given by injection to obtain rapid improvement or orally for mild cases

Table 12.1. Suggested ranges for normal thyroxine values (μg/dl) in birds commonly seen in practice

Species	Range of T_1
Blue-and-gold Macaw	1.0–4.0
Yellow-naped Amazon	0.5–1.0
Other amazons	<0.50
Sulphur-crested Cockatoo	0.8–4.4
Red-vented and Goffin's cockatoos	1.0–3.1
Umbrella Cockatoo	0.8–4.2
Budgerigar	2.5–4.4
Cockatiel	0.7–2.4
African Gray Parrot	0.2–2.0
Mynah	0.5–0.9
Lovebird	0.2–1.9

Source: Rosskopf et al. 1982, by permission.

or preventive medicine. Lafeber (1965) recommended daily injections of 20% sodium iodide, 0.01 ml in chronic and 0.02–0.03 ml in acute conditions. Marked improvement may be obtained within 3 days. For oral therapy, Lafeber recommended adding one drop dilute Lugol's solution (2 parts Lugol's solution to 28 parts distilled water) to fresh drinking water.

Steiner and Davis (1979) recommended a solution of 1 ml 7% Lugol's solution in 14 ml water. Every day for 2 weeks, 1 ml diluted iodine solution is diluted in 1 oz drinking water.

The hormone thyroxine is available in thyroid extract or as levothyroxine. The treatment is given orally in the drinking water, the dosage varied according to the bird's drinking habits (Rosskopf et al. 1982).

To prevent recurrence of the disease, the diet may be supplemented with iodine, finely ground oyster shell grit, or cod-liver oil.

Gout. Gout is a metabolic disorder characterized by deposition of urates and uric acid crystals in different tissues or organs. Two forms of gout occur, visceral and articular, depending on the site of urate deposition. Usually they are considered as clinical forms of the same disease; articular gout is regarded as the chronic form and visceral gout as the acute form. Rarely, the two forms have occurred simultaneously in the bird (Hasholt and Petrak 1982; Mehren 1983), although some authors (Sykes 1971; Austic and Cole 1972; Siller 1981) report that the two forms do not occur together. In visceral gout, urate crystals may deposit on the synovial membranes of some joints and tendon sheaths, but there is no tissue reaction as in articular gout. In gout with typical articular lesions, urate deposits on visceral surfaces are not seen. Thus it has been suggested to name the visceral form "visceral urate deposition" to clearly separate it from articular gout.

Etiology. In birds, uric acid is a normal product of nitrogen metabolism. It is the end product of catabolism of purines and of protein in birds, whereas in mammals it is only the end product of purine catabolism. The synthesis of uric acid takes place in the liver and kidney, the precursor being xanthine. The reaction is catalyzed by the enzyme xanthinoxidase, which is slightly different from the xanthinoxidase in mammals (Chin and Quebbemann 1978).

Uric acid is excreted mostly by the kidneys and partly by the gut. In the nephron, it is filtered by the glomerules and secreted in the tubules. An important amount of uric acid is synthesized in cells of kidney tubules. In normal conditions, the average blood concentration of uric acid is 4.5 mg/dl in domestic birds (fowl, duck) (Hasholt and Petrak 1982) and 5.39 mg/dl in female and 5.71 mg/dl in male parakeets (McFarland et al. 1979). Solubility in water is greater for urates in a state of supersaturation because of colloidal components, which allow transport through the tubules and urinary tract (Sykes 1971).

Visceral Urate Deposition. Visceral urate deposition appears as the result of impaired renal function or urinary tract obstruction. Both acute and chronic renal disturbances can lead to visceral gout. There are numerous causes of renal impairment with visceral gout: infectious diseases, mycotoxins, intoxications, water deprivation, high carbohydrate–low protein diets, vitamin-mineral deficiencies, inactivity, decreased water intake, and stress (exposure, shipping) (Halliwell 1978; Siller 1981; Steiner and Davis 1981; Hasholt and Petrak 1982; Julian 1982).

The obstructive form is due to obstruction of the ureters occurring in vitamin A deficiency and excess dietary calcium in the diet (urolithiasis) (Blaxland et al. 1980). Experimental ureter ligation in healthy birds induces visceral gout.

In the nephrotoxic or the obstructive form, there is no correlation between the degree of uricemia and urate deposition. The deposition always occurs in extracellular spaces. Some unknown biochemical factors in the interstitial fluid may be responsible for the urate instability.

Articular Gout. Articular gout is also observed with high uric acid values, but fluctuations are seen. The etiology of articular gout has not been resolved. Several factors are implicated, especially heredity (Peterson et al. 1971) and a protein (meat) diet. It is not the level of the dietary protein that induces the disease, but an imbalance of amino acids causing a greater production of uric acid (Siller 1981).

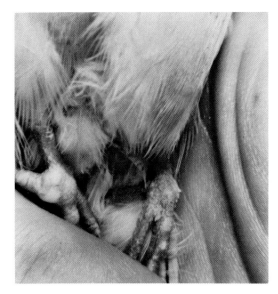

Fig. 12.3. Typical tophi of chronic articular gout. (*Courtesy of Raymond D. Wise, Scottsdale Animal Clinic, Chicago, Ill.*)

Clinical Signs. In visceral urate deposition, clinical signs are not specific. The symptoms account for the poor condition of the bird (anorexia, depression, faintness) and rapid death. Necropsy reveals typical lesions; there is light urate dusting on the surface of the liver and on the pericardium (Plate 1). Such patches may also be seen on the peritoneum and on the kidney (Fig. 12.3). In the nephrotoxic form the kidneys are enlarged, swollen, and discolored (Plate 2). In the obstructive form the ureters appear as thick gray-white cords.

In articular gout, the bird seems in good health in the early stages of the disease and exhibits only local symptoms such as lameness and reluctance to fly or perch. Physical examination shows rigid, swollen, and painful joints (tarsus, heel). As the disease develops, typical tophi with whitish yellow centers can be seen around the joints, ligaments, and tendons and through the subcutaneous and skin tissues. They may disfigure the leg. The hip and shoulder are never involved (Steiner and Davis 1981). At necropsy, incision of joints and synovials shows the thick, whitish masses of urate crystals surrounded by hyperemic tissue reaction.

Diagnosis. Clinical diagnosis of visceral urate deposition is only made on autopsy. Clinical diagnosis of articular gout, on the other hand,

may be obtained when white tophi are seen. For differential diagnosis (e.g., for abscess), material from an incision can be submitted for microscopic examination (needle-shaped or amorphous masses), or a murexide test can be carried out. When using the murexide test, a small amount of deposit is mixed with a drop of nitric acid. After evaporation (with careful heating) and subsequent cooling, one drop of ammonia is added. A red-purple color is indicative of uric acid. The differential diagnosis with arthritis can be established by X-ray examination (Knox 1980). Determination of plasma uric acid can also be carried out (McFarland et al. 1979); however, hyperuricemia can result from other causes and may exist without the presence of gout deposits.

Therapy. Gout in birds is considered incurable.

In articular gout cases, therapy can be attempted to prolong life or alleviate pain. Surgical removal of tophi using either electrocautery (McAffe and Gergis 1981) or silver nitrate (Steiner and Davis 1981) for hemostasis can be done. Hypouricemic drugs used in human medicine (salicylic acid, colchicine) have not proved to be efficient in birds. Allopurinol inhibits xanthinoxidase and uric acid synthesis in birds (Chin and Quebbemann 1978) and may be administered orally at 10–15 mg/kg body weight daily for the rest of the bird's life (Mehren 1983). When medication is stopped, tophi recur.

Glucocorticoids are contraindicated because of increased protein catabolism. Dietary improvement (decreased protein level, especially meat supply; increased vitamin A; access to water) and proper environmental conditions (avoiding cold and other stressors) are recommended.

Obesity and Fatty Liver

Obesity. Obesity is one of the more common metabolic disorders encountered in caged birds, especially in Budgerigars. It is the result of caloric intake higher than body requirements (physical activity, egg production). High-calorie feed (seeds, nuts, eggs, bread) is often converted to fat deposits when feed is supplied ad libitum, tempting birds to overeat constantly. Caged birds are usually sedentary compared with wild birds, and their energy expenditure is insufficient, resulting in fat depositions. In very obese birds, fat deposits localized in the abdomen (Fig. 12.4) and the breast may indicate surgical removal (caution: obesity increases anesthetic risk). To avoid obesity, restriction of a high-calorie diet is necessary.

Fatty Liver. Fatty degeneration of the liver is frequently associated with obesity. Increasing

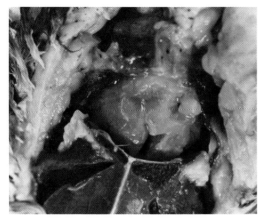

Fig. 12.4. Enlarged liver due to fat infiltration in an obese Galah (*Eolophus roseicapilla*). (*Courtesy of David J. Schultz, Hawthorn, South Australia, Aust.*)

fat content of the hepatocytes is a nonspecific reaction, chiefly in birds where the liver is the site of lipogenesis. Thus numerous factors can result in fatty change: diet, intoxication, infections, environmental conditions, and physiological reactions.

Etiology. The lesion is a common feature of many clinical entities. For example, there are three syndromes with fatty liver known in the fowl: fatty liver and kidney syndrome (FLKS) in the chick (Brugère-Picoux and Brugère 1974), fatty liver syndrome (FLS), and fatty liver hemorrhagic syndrome (FLHS) in laying hens (Haghighi-Rad and Polin 1981). Etiology of these syndromes is not known, but dietary factors are prominent. For example, FLHS can be obtained by force-feeding poultry (as to obtain the *fois gras* in geese or ducks). Estrogens enhance blood lipid concentration, and their administration results in hepatic steatosis in laying hens.

In caged birds, fatty liver is, like obesity, related to an imbalance between diet and energy expenditure. Male Budgerigars are affected more than are females (Minsky and Petrak 1982). Lipidosis, a disease characterized by fatty infiltration of liver and other organs (kidney, spleen, heart), is described in Budgerigars (Minsky and Petrak 1982). The cause is unknown but is similar to the FLKS of the chick associated with biotin deficiency.

Clinical Signs. Clinical signs occurring in birds with fatty liver are apathy, inability to fly, intestinal disorders (constipation or loose droppings), obesity, and abdominal enlargement.

Diagnosis. Diagnosis may be made by abdominal palpation (Davis et al. 1981). Radiography can also be useful (Minsky and Petrak 1982). At necropsy, hepatomegaly and a yellow or yellowish-brown organ color are typical. Atheromatosis and arteriosclerosis are associated with some fatal cases without premonitory signs (Cooper and Pomerance 1982). Similar lesions have been seen in hens; these are related to the cessation of egg production and yolk reabsorption, which allows cholesterol derivatives to enter the bloodstream (Simpson and Harms 1983).

Therapy. Therapy consists of administration of lipotropic substances such as methionine, choline, and vitamin B_{12}.

Diabetes Mellitus. Diabetes mellitus is rarely encountered in birds. Blood glucose regulation is very different in birds and much higher than that of mammals.

Etiology. Normal blood glucose values differ among bird species. After pancreatectomy, blood glucose concentration can reach very high values in meat-eating birds, whereas only a few changes or a decreased concentration occur in seedeating birds after the same operation (Sitbon and Mialhe 1980; Sitbon et al. 1980). There have been some reports of spontaneously occurring diabetes mellitus in birds (Altman and Kirmayer 1976; Douglass 1981).

Clinical Signs. Clinical signs are the same as those in mammals and include polyuria, polydipsia, polyphagia, and glycosuria. Blood glucose can reach very high values (720–1000 mg/dl) (Altman and Kirmayer 1976; Minsky and Petrak 1982).

Diagnosis. According to the few cases reported in birds, glycosuria is the most practical test for diagnosis and adjustment of an insulin therapy. See Chapter 27 for specific tests available for use in birds.

Therapy. Treatment is attempted with valuable birds. Insulin can be given by intramuscular injection, the dose rates established by patient response to treatment. Altman and Kirmayer (1976) obtained successful management of diabetes in a bird with single daily doses of 0.004–0.006 units NPH insulin IM.

Other Metabolic Diseases

Amyloidosis. Amyloidosis, of unknown etiology, consists of shapeless material deposits in liver, spleen, adrenal, and kidney tissues (Plate

3). The parenchyma is often the site of deposit but vasculature may also be affected, especially the iliac bifurcation or renal vessels (Cowan 1968; Speckmann and Luther 1974; Humphreys 1978). This condition occurs mainly in aquatic birds (ducks, swans, flamingos). The disease is more common in older birds suffering from chronic diseases such as tuberculosis. When deposits impair renal function, visceral gout may be an associated lesion.

Hemochromatosis. Hemochromatosis is characterized by an abnormal accumulation of iron, mainly in the liver, with lesser amounts in the heart, kidney, and pancreas. Mynahs are the most commonly affected bird (Lowenstine and Petrak 1980). The causes, nutritional and infectious diseases, are probably as varied as are the causes of hematochromatosis in humans; cirrhosis of the liver with or without ascites is a common finding. Clinical signs are varied but do not affect the body conditions. When ascites is present, the bird shows dyspnea with an abdominal enlargement. No specific treatment is known for the disease.

Capture Myopathy. Capture myopathy (exertional rhabdomyolysis), a disease known in numerous zoo animals, has been described in flamingos (Fowler 1978). It appears after stress (capture or shipping) and consists of leg weakness and inability to stand. Ischemic necrosis of the leg muscles may ensue with increased creatine kinase levels (Schultz 1981). The etiology is unknown, but marked acidosis is possibly a contributing factor. Therapy consists of providing food, rest, and quiet. Selenium and vitamin E administration may be helpful (Rosskopf et al. 1982).

References

Altman, R. B. 1982. Disorders of the skeletal system. In *Diseases of Cage and Aviary Birds*, ed. M. L. Petrak, pp. 282–294. Philadelphia: Lea and Febiger.

Altman, R. B., and A. H. Kirmayer. 1976. Diabetes mellitus in the avian species. *J. Am. Anim. Hosp. Assoc.* 12:531–37.

Arnall, L., and I. F. Keymer. 1975. *Bird Diseases.* London: Baillière Tindall.

Arnall, L., M. A. Kram, H. F. Hintz, H. Evans, and L. Krook. 1974. Nutritional secondary hyperparathyroidism. *Cornell Vet.* 64:37–46.

Austic, R. E., and R. K. Cole. 1972. Impaired renal clearance of uric acid in chickens having hyperuricemia and articular gout. *Am. J. Physiol.* 223:525–30.

Blackmore, D. K., and J. E. Cooper. 1982. Diseases of the endocrine system. In *Diseases of Cage and Aviary Birds,* ed. M. L. Petrak, pp. 478–90. Philadelphia: Lea and Febiger.

Blaxland, J. D., E. D. Borland, W. G. Siller, and D. Martindale. 1980. An investigation of urolithiasis in flocks of laying fowls. *Avian Pathol.* 9:5–19.

Brugère-Picoux, J., and H. Brugère. 1974. A propos de la stéatose hépatique chez les volailles. *Rec. Med. Vet.* 150:1023–30.

Chin, T. Y., and A. J. Quebbemann. 1978. Quantitation of renal uric acid synthesis in the chicken. *Am. J. Physiol.* 234:F446–F451.

Cooper, J. E., and A. Pomerance. 1982. Cardiac lesions in birds of prey. *J. Comp. Pathol.* 92:161–68.

Cowan, D. F. 1968. Avian amyloidosis. *Pathol. Vet.* 5:51–66.

Davis, R. B., C. V. Steiner, and R. L. Toal. 1981. Recognition of abdominal enlargement in the Budgerigar. *Vet. Med. Small Anim. Clin.* 76:220–23.

Douglass, E. M. 1981. Diabetes mellitus in a Toco Toucan. *Mod. Vet. Pract.* 62:293–95.

Ekperigin, H. E., and P. Vohra. 1981. Histopathological and biochemical effects of feeding excess dietary methionine to broiler chicks. *Avian Dis.* 25:82–95.

Fowler, M. E. 1978. Metabolic bone disease. In *Zoo and Wild Animal Medicine,* ed. M. E. Fowler, pp. 55–76. Philadelphia: W. B. Saunders.

——. 1978. Introduction and identification. In *Zoo and Wild Animal Medicine,* ed. M. E. Fowler, pp. 155–63. Philadelphia: W. B. Saunders.

Haghighi-Rad, F., and D. Polin. 1981. The relationship of plasma estradiol and progesterone levels to the fatty-liver hemorrhagic syndrome in laying hens. *Poult. Sci.* 60:2278–83.

Halliwell, W. H. 1978. Toxic and metabolic conditions in birds of prey. In *Zoo and Wild Animal Medicine,* ed. M. E. Fowler, pp. 282–85. Philadelphia: W. B. Saunders.

——. 1979. Diseases of birds of prey. *Vet. Clin. N. Am. Small Anim. Pract.* 9:541–68.

Hasholt, J., and M. L. Petrak. 1982. Gout. In *Diseases of Cage and Aviary Birds,* ed. M. L. Petrak, pp. 639–45. Philadelphia: Lea and Febiger.

Himmelstein, S., and K. Bernstein. 1978. Clinical aspects of nutritional secondary hyperparathyroidism in cage birds. *Vet. Med. Small Anim. Clin.* 73:761–63.

Humphreys, P. 1978. Noninfectious diseases. In *Zoo and Wild Animal Medicine,* ed. M. E. Fowler, pp. 203–4. Philadelphia: W. B. Saunders.

Julian, R. 1982. Water deprivation as a cause of renal disease in chickens. *Avian Pathol.* 11:615–17.

Knox, D. W. 1980. Gout in reptiles and birds, with observations on a comparable syndrome in man. In *Pathology of Zoo Animals,* ed. R. J. Montalic and G. Migaki, pp. 137–41. Washington, D.C.: Smithsonian Institution Press.

Lafeber, T. J. 1965. Thyroid dysplasia in the Budgerigar. *Anim. Hosp.* 1:208–18.

Lowenstine, L. J., and M. L. Petrak. 1980. Iron pigment in the livers of birds. In *Pathology of Zoo Animals,* ed. R. J. Montalic and G. Migaki, pp. 127–35. Washington, D.C.: Smithsonian Institution Press.

McAfee, L. T., and A. L. Gergis. 1981. Gout in a parakeet. *Mod. Vet. Pract.* 62:388–90.

McFarland, D. C., S. G. Henzy, and C. N. Coon. 1979. A micromethod for plasma uric acid determinations in companion birds. *Avian Dis.* 23:772–74.

Mehren, D. G. 1983. Gout. In *Current Veterinary Therapy* VIII, ed. R. W. Kirk, pp. 635–37. Philadelphia: W. B. Saunders.

Minsky, L., and M. L. Petrak. 1982. Diseases of the digestive system. In *Diseases of Cage and Aviary Birds,* ed. M. L. Petrak, pp. 422–48. Philadelphia: Lea and Febiger.

Peterson, D. W., W. H. Hamilton, and A. L. Lilyblade. 1971. Hereditary susceptibility to dietary induction of gout in selected lines of chickens. *J. Nutr.* 101:347–54.

Randell, M. G. 1981. Nutritionally induced hypocalcemic tetany in an amazon parrot. *J. Am. Vet. Med. Assoc.* 179:1277–1378.

Rosskopf, W. J., R. W. Woerpel, G. Rosskopf, and D. Van de Water. 1982. Normal thyroid values for common pet birds. *Vet. Med. Small Anim. Clin.* 77:409–12.

Schone, R., and P. Arnold. 1980. *Der Wellensittich. Heimtier und Patient. Tierärztliche Praxis.* Jena: VEB Gustav Fischer Verlag.

Schultz, D. J. 1981. Disorders of the musculoskeletal system. In *Refresher Course for Veterinarians on Avian and Caged Birds,* pp. 519–33. University of Sydney, Post-Graduate Committee in Veterinary Science, Proceedings no. 55. Sydney, Aust.

Siller, W. G. 1981. Renal pathology of the fowl: A review. *Avian Pathol.* 10:187–262.

Simpson, C. F., and R. H. Harms. 1983. Aortic atherosclerosis in nonlaying hens with fatty-liver syndrome. *Avian Dis.* 27:652–59.

Sitbon, G., and P. Mialhe. 1980. Le pancreas endocrine des oiseaux. *J. Physiol.* (Paris) 76:5–24.

Sitbon, G., F. Laurent, A. Mialhe, E. Krug, H. Karmann, R. Gross, M. T. Strosser, L. Cohen, P. Jean-Marie, C. Koltzer, and P. Mialhe. 1980. Diabetes in birds. *Horm. Metab. Res.* 12:1–9.

Speckmann, G., and J. W. Luther. 1974. Visceral gout and amyloidosis in a Mute Swan (*Cygnus olor*). *Can. Vet. J.* 15:51–53.

Steiner, C. V., and R. B. Davis. 1979. Thyroid hyperplasia in a parakeet (a case report). *Vet. Med. Small Anim. Clin.* 74:739–42.

————. 1981. *Caged Bird Medicine.* Ames: Iowa State University Press.

Sykes, A. H. 1971. Formation and composition of urine. In *Physiology and Biochemistry of the Domestic Fowl,* ed. D. J. Bell and B. M. Freeman, pp. 233–378. London: Academic.

Wallach, J. D., and G. M. Flieg. 1969. Nutritional hyperparathyroidism in captive birds. *J. Am. Vet. Med. Assoc.* 165:1046–51.

Wise, R. D. 1980. Hyperplastic goiter in a Budgerigar. *Vet. Med. Small Anim. Clin.* 75:1013–14.

13

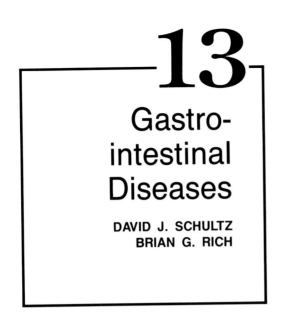

Gastro-intestinal Diseases

DAVID J. SCHULTZ
BRIAN G. RICH

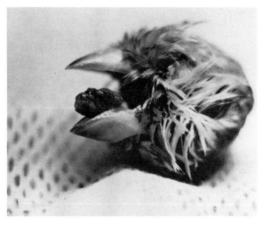

Fig. 13.1. Severe granulomatous glossitis in a Common Canary (*Serinus canarius*), caused by poxvirus.

THE MAIN SYMPTOMS of gastrointestinal tract (GIT) disease are oral discharge/salivation, vomiting/regurgitation, loose feces/dysentery, undigested seed in feces, white-colored feces, and in cases of obstruction, no feces. These may be accompanied by nonspecific signs such as anorexia, depression, ruffled feathers, closed eyes, and head in wing (i.e., the sick bird look, or SBL).

The practitioner is encouraged to investigate the specific signs, utilizing the laboratory. Only clinical symptoms are described in this chapter, as many of the disease conditions are presented elsewhere in the book and many diseases involve other systems as well as the GIT.

Microbiology of the Oral Cavity

Etiology and Clinical Signs. Involvement of the mouth and upper esophagus with gram-negative bacteria, fungi, pox- and herpesvirus, trichomonads (see Chapters 16, 17, and 21), and helminths (see Chapter 22) produces abnormal beak movements and/or oral discharge. Debris is often stuck to the beak. Lesions in the oral cavity may be diphtheritic, granulomatous, or abscessated (Altman 1976) or appear as small necrotic foci (Fig. 13.1).

Diagnosis. Samples can be taken by sterile loop, suction, or biopsy for wet preps and staining.

Bacteria (both gram-positive and gram-negative) can be observed in profusion, but unless they are found in close association with heterophils, it is difficult to ascribe pathogenicity to any one organism. Culture and sensitivity tests for gram-negative bacteria are warranted; however, most bacteria are secondary to another cause (e.g., hypovitaminosis).

Poxvirus can be identified histologically from diphtheritic lesions in the GIT of psittacines (Graham 1978), passerines, and pigeons (Gerlach 1984). Characteristic eosinophilic intracytoplasmic inclusion bodies may be detected in hypertrophied epithelial cells by staining with the Gimenez method (Tripathy and Hanson 1976) (Plate 4). Lesions may extend to the commissures, eyelids, and unfeathered parts of the head and legs, especially in young birds (Fig. 13.2).

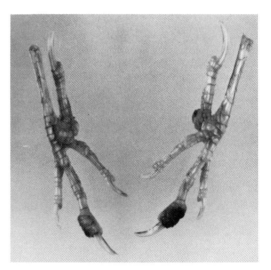

Fig. 13.2. Poxvirus lesions on the feet of a Common Canary (*Serinus canarius*). (*Courtesy of K. E. Harrigan, University of Melbourne Veterinary School, Melbourne, Aust.*)

Treatment. Debridement of focal areas may result in hemorrhage but gives increased efficiency to topical neomycin (2–4 mg) used as a mouthwash. Because of fungal overgrowth, 6,000 IU/100 g nystatin can be incorporated with the antibiotic. Systemic antibiotics can be indicated for severe cases, but immunosuppressive effects should always be considered. Vitamin A injections once or twice weekly are good supportive therapy.

Bacterial cases respond favorably, but viral infections may need additional support in the form of force-feeding. Pox lesions may take 6–8 weeks to disappear.

Control. Discharges and scabs from pox lesions are contagious; therefore hygiene, isolation of affected birds, depopulation to reduce stressors, and removal of insect vectors may effect some control. Vaccination of adult pigeons is generally successful, but the interrelationship between the different pox viridae and their hosts is not completely known at this time.

Microbiology of the Crop, Proventriculus, and Gizzard

Etiology and Clinical Signs. A variety of pathogens similar to those that cause oral lesions also cause lesions further down the GIT, but if the gizzard is affected, the main signs are vomiting/regurgitating movements and undigested seed in the feces. Unusual head movements with vomitus caked over head and neck feathers can indicate esophageal irritation. Feces may not necessarily be affected.

Diagnosis. Crop samples may be obtained for wet preps and staining by suction, using a flexible plastic tube 2–3 mm in diameter. The normal psittacine crop contains squamous epithelial cells with large numbers of gram-positive bacteria in close association with the outside of the cell. Occasional yeasts and gram-negative rods are present. Normally, no inflammatory cells are present. A smear with a large number of bacteria predominantly of one morphological type or with many gram-negative bacteria (in seedeating birds) is abnormal (Campbell 1983). Radiography may aid in differential diagnosis and suggest a GIT problem (Plate 5).

Histopathological examination of the organs may be necessary to determine viral etiology.

Treatment. Treatment is similar to that given for oral lesions except that administration by intubation is preferable. Administration of Buscopan Compositum (4 mg hyoscine-N-butyl bromide plus 500 mg dipyrone/ml) at 0.1 ml/200 g or of Maxalon (metoclopramide hydrochloride at 0.5/100 g may aid in vomition control.

Fluid therapy must be used in the dehydrated patient.

Grit (1- to 3-mm stones, not crushed shell) must be provided for those birds whose stools show undigested seed. In uncomplicated cases this will suffice, but where gizzard pathology is marked, grit cannot be retained.

Microbiology of the Intestines

Etiology and Clinical Signs. Potential pathogens that may be isolated in small numbers from a normal seedeater's stool include *Escherichia coli;* species of *Proteus, Citrobacter, Pseudomonas, Salmonella, Streptococcus,* and *Candida;* and various anaerobes. If these organisms are regarded as significant, the feces will be loose and a fecal Gram stain will show gram-negative bacteria as the predominant organisms. Spores of *Candida* will show developing hyphae. At necropsy, fluid-filled loops of intestine are often revealed (Fig. 13.3).

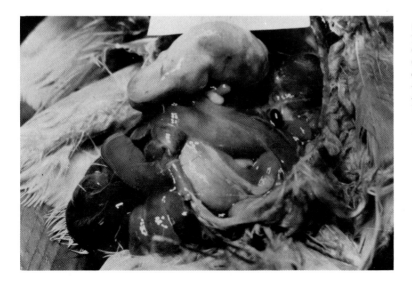

Fig. 13.3. Fluid-filled loops of the intestine of a Crimson-winged Parrot (*Aprosmictus erythropterus*), from which a heavy, pure culture of *Escherichia coli* was isolated.

Chlamydia, herpesvirus, poxvirus, and paramyxovirus can all be isolated from healthy or sick birds so other signs must determine significance (Mustaffa-Babgee et al. 1974). (See Chapters 21 and 22 for a discussion of protozoa and helminths.)

Vomiting and SBL accompany the enteritides, often because of systemic involvement.

Diagnosis. Where the fecal Gram stain has shown gram-negative bacteria as the predominant organism, systemic antibiotics are justified, whether or not the organism is considered primary or secondary. Reduction of these organisms is accompanied by rapid clinical improvement. Inflammatory cells can be identified by staining with Diff-Quik.

Salmonella, viral, chlamydial, or protozoal etiology should be suspected if large numbers of birds are affected.

Culture and sensitivity tests, anaerobes included, are indicated where there are in-contact birds or if the case is unresponsive to antibiotics.

Treatment. Neomycin used orally concurrently with the systemic antibiotics amoxicillin, ticarcillin, chloramphenicol, gentamicin, or metronidazole for anaerobes (see Chapter 29 for a discussion of antibiotic therapy) causes a rapid decline in fecal bacterial numbers. If the stool does not improve in consistency and the fecal Gram stain shows little or no bacteria, then lactobacilli should be force-fed. Whether these bacteria actually colonize the gut is questionable, but their use often coincides with a return to normal flora and an improved stool.

Control. Control of the enteritides depends on adequate quarantine of incoming birds, routine fecal cultures, and cage and floor hygiene. Pet birds must have their cage papers changed daily and perches scrupulously clean, and droppings must be removed frequently from aviary floors. Dirt floors can be turned and lime added, but a bacterial buildup can be expected. Cages with concrete or wire floors offer the best opportunity for consistent cleanliness. Rodents and wild birds are capable of shedding potential pathogens (*Yersinia, Salmonella*) to susceptible aviary flocks. Their control is difficult in open flights.

Oral Cavity Trauma

Clinical Signs and Treatment. Cuts and burns to the tongue occur, especially with young, inquisitive psittacines trying things such as smoking for the first time. Topical antibiotics such as chloramphenicol palmitate at 10–30 mg ad-

ministered every 8 hours to the lesions may help. Healing is rapid.

Cracks in the beak or penetration holes are seen particularly in psittacines because of fighting or their habit of getting into mischief. Splits along the length of the lower bill are most common and do not grow out. Attempts to immobilize the two halves with glue, wire, etc., are not often successful. Most birds seem to handle this situation quite well, once the pain has gone. Penetration wounds eventually grow out. Partial or complete removal of the upper or lower mandible in psittacines, passerines, and ducks occurs frequently. The resilience of affected individuals is remarkable, provided force-feeding and infection control keep the bird alive during the first week postsurgery; then recovery is usually uncomplicated.

Physiological Regurgitation

Clinical Signs. Psittacines, pigeons, and seedeating passerines feed their young by regurgitation, but pet male Budgerigars often carry things too far. They may regurgitate their seed onto any shiny object, toys, ends of the perch, and even their owners. These birds may lose body condition because of the resulting reduced feed intake or develop crop infections due to reingestion of partly fermented seed.

Treatment. Treatment using medroxyprogesterone at 1–2 mg subcutaneously reduces intensity of symptoms for 2–3 weeks. A good appetite and polyuria may follow the administration of this hormone. The bird's weight should be monitored frequently.

Control can sometimes be achieved by removal of target objects; sometimes a complete environmental change is necessary. As a result of imprinting, female mates are often ignored.

Idiopathic Pendulous Crop

Clinical Signs. While a pendulous crop appears in aged geese and fowl, in Budgerigars the condition can be seen as early as 3–4 years of age. Seeds and fluid can be palpated superficially in the crop, even distal to the xiphisternum. Sacculations may occur liberally to the left and right sides. The bacterial content of the crop is often high, with gram-negative rods. Yeasts may also be present. Inflammatory cells are not present, and the feces are usually well formed.

Treatment. Treatment of the gram-negative organisms in the crop does not cure the condition. There is no response to sodium iodide intramuscularly or sodium bicarbonate in the drinking water. Surgical reduction of crop size can be attempted if the bird is strong enough.

Deprivation of feed and water for 4 hours presurgery is necessary to prevent reflux of crop contents.

Crop Impaction.
Fibrous material may be ingested by galliforms allowed to graze long grass, especially after greens deprivation. Pigeons may inadvertently ingest soft nesting material. Threads from cage covers may cause obstructions in the Budgerigar crop region. Feeding tubes are often swallowed by overenthusiastic young psittacines.

Crop calculi have been reported by Beach et al. (1960). The authors have occasionally seen (in psittacines) inspissated necrotic material in the form of calculi, but they did not seem to be associated with any pathology although they probably originated from a previous local inflammation.

Clinical Signs. The main sign is a regurgitating movement, often unproductive. Diagnosis is by palpation.

Treatment. Treatment is surgical if the administration of a vegetable or mineral oil does not shift the obstruction.

Feeding tubes swallowed into the crop do not appear to invoke a violent reaction by the bird. Most can be threaded back out through the mouth, preferably under general anesthetic. Aspiration of refluxed crop contents can endanger life.

Crop Rupture

Etiology. Racing pigeons are often attacked by falcons and goshawks and domestic fowl and ducks by dogs, both with resultant crop rupture. Feeding tubes that damage the juvenile psittacine crop wall predispose to infection, necrosis, and rupture. Trichomonas infections predispose to abscessation in the pigeon and rupture crop walls. The rupture, which is often surrounded by matted feathers, is not always visible.

Treatment. Treatment is surgical. Immobilization with a general anesthetic enables the practitioner to debride the wound, separate the skin and esophageal layers, and suture separately. Inverting layer sutures for the esophagus and continuous mattress sutures for the skin allow good healing, even in contaminated wounds. Small amounts of sugar-rich food may be force-fed 1 hour postsurgery.

Poisons.
See Chapter 32 for a further discussion of toxic conditions.

Plant Poisons. Ingestion of ivy or lily can cause vomiting, but recovery is spontaneous. Other indoor plants can obviously be a danger.

Lead. Lead poisoning has been reported as causing (together with nervous signs) loose feces in psittacines (Woerpel and Rosskopf 1982) and swans (Irwin 1985). Diagnosis is made by confirming lead in a radiograph of the gastrointestinal tract, by monitoring blood lead levels, and by response to chelation therapy.

The disease is treated with intramuscular injections of calcium disodium edetate at 25–50 mg/kg every 8 hours for 5–7 days.

Copper. Copper toxicosis in Canada Geese has been reported as a cause of necrosis and sloughing of the proventricular and gizzard mucosa (Henderson and Winterfield 1975).

Bacterial Toxins. Toxin from *Clostridium botulinum* propagating in stagnant, dirty pond water has been reported by many authors as a cause of diarrhea, nervous signs, and death in waterfowl.

Treatment is accomplished by injection of type C antitoxin, administration of fluids, force-feeding, and removal of the birds from the affected area.

Drug Reactions. Administration of levamisole, both orally and systemically, induces vomiting. Other injectable drugs or their suspending agents (lincomycin, long-acting testosterone, vitamin B complex) can cause vomiting.

Diet Change.
Occasionally a pet bird overindulges in table scraps or spoiled food. A Gram stain of the feces should be carried out, and the food source removed. The feces should regain normal shape within 24 hours.

Diseases of the Liver, Gall Bladder, and Pancreas.
As in mammals, the liver is the hub of metabolism in the bird. It plays the major role in the regulation of carbohydrate, protein, and lipid metabolism. It detoxifies exogenous compounds, eliminates waste compounds, and plays a part in the immune mechanism. Because of the broad spectrum of activity, the liver is involved in many disease processes. The liver has a great reserve, and dysfunction is not always clinically detectable.

The gallbladder is absent in many birds and most psittacines (except cockatoos), and its involvement in disease is not well known. (In the authors' experience, gamma-glutamyl transpeptidase and alkaline phosphatase values are always within the normal considered range.)

Likewise, the avian pancreas is not as well understood, nor as commonly affected, as its mammalian counterpart. While the islet cell secretions control blood glucose levels, the glucagon activity of birds significantly exceeds that of insulin. Nevertheless, glucosuria occurs occasionally in the domestic Budgerigar, usually associated with elevated plasma glucose.

For proper evaluation of these organs the clinician must resort to plasma chemistry (tests are described in detail in Chapter 27).

Liver Diseases

Clinical Signs. Urate color in the normal bird should be white or light cream, depending on the pigments in the diet. Some staining of the urate occurs if the feces are loose. However, liver involvement can be suspected if urate color ranges from mustard yellow to green.

SBL, vomiting, and diarrhea are features of liver disease, to varying degrees.

The liver may be enlarged and palpable behind the xiphisternum (Fig. 13.4). It may be visible through the abdominal wall in the more sparsely feathered passerines. Miliary abscesses may also be visible (e.g., in yersiniosis).

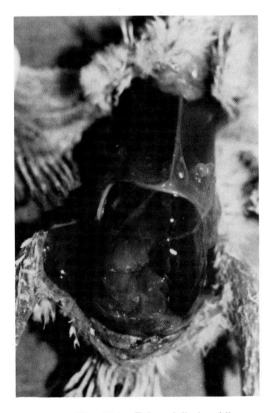

Fig. 13.4. Enlarged displaced liver and hydropericardium caused by papovavirus in a 3-week-old Budgerigar (*Melopsittacus undulatus*) fledgling.

Icterus is not a prominent feature clinically because of the dark skin pigmentation in many species. The white facial skin of the macaw is one exception.

Blood clotting time may be increased, and nonregenerative anemias are common in chronic hepatopathies.

Ascites is commonly present and may cause abdominal enlargement.

Plasma Chemistry. Biochemical evidence to support a diagnosis of liver damage in the bird is (1) lowered plasma albumin (more chronic cases), (2) elevation of aspartate transanimase, and (3) elevation of lactic dehydrogenase.

A liver function test as described in Chapter 27 can be utilized as a prognostic tool.

Etiology

Infectious Disease. A very wide range of microorganisms cause liver pathology in many bird species and account for most cases in practice. The more common causes are the enteric bacteria, yersiniae, chlamydiae, herpes- and papovaviruses, and in game birds, trichomonads and histomonads.

Toxic Disease. Heavy metals (especially lead), insecticides, and mycotoxins from moldy feed cause liver pathology.

Metabolic Disease. Infiltration of fat into the hepatocyte due to energy input exceeding energy output is a common cause of liver failure in pet birds.

Neoplasia. Liver neoplasia is generally the result of metastases from other organs, especially the gonads (Fig. 13.5).

Differential Diagnosis

Bacteria. Bacterial agents often cause hematological change, namely, leucocytosis and heterophilia with left shifts.

Any bacteria seen in the blood film are significant, but it cannot be assumed that fecal gram-negative bacteria are necessarily being shed by the liver.

Chlamydiae. Chlamydiae can be shed in increased numbers from the bowel in clinical cases, and therefore their isolation from the feces is most likely significant. Chlamydial cases invariably evoke a leucocytosis, and the complement fixation test can be performed on plasma. History and epidemiology are also important.

Viruses. Viral involvement is mostly confirmed

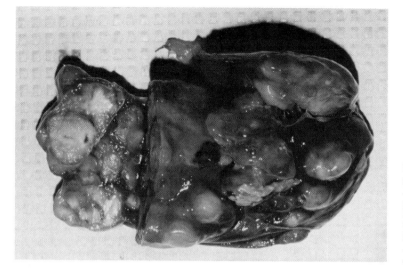

Fig. 13.5. Hepatic granuloma due to *Escherichia coli,* caused by metastasis of a gut infection in an Egyptian Goose (*Alopochen aegyptiacus*). (*Courtesy of V. L. Tham, Hawthorn, South Australia, Aust.*)

at necropsy by histopathology, electron microscopy, or isolation.

Protozoa. Protozoal isolation is mostly made at necropsy although a bird with trichomonads in the esophagus and greenish urate is most likely suffering from hepatic trichomoniasis.

Hematozoa may be detected in the peripheral blood film.

Toxins. Fungal toxins can be isolated from the feed and identified as a cause of hepatitis by a characteristic fibrosis and bile duct proliferation. Samples can be obtained by biopsy; hemorrhage from the liver can be reduced by suturing the cut edges together.

Ascitic fluid, if recoverable, is a modified transudate with minimal inflammatory cells present.

Metabolic Disease. Obese birds are unfit, pant and wheeze, and have luxurious subcutaneous fat deposits, especially over the abdomen. Lipemia is often present, plasma glucose may be elevated, and glucosuria is present.

Neoplasia. Neoplasms in the liver can be identified visually: by palpation in the smaller passerines and by endoscopy, exploratory laparotomy, or at necropsy. Occasionally leukemic cells are seen in peripheral blood smears, the liver being very friable and liable to rupture.

Treatment. Antibiotic therapy is discussed in Chapter 29.

Good supportive therapy consists of maintaining a hydrated, well-fed patient. The quantity of fluid needed can roughly be estimated by the degree of skin elasticity over the sternum

and the amount of fluid being lost. The type of fluid used depends on the plasma sodium and potassium levels. Solutions containing acetate should be avoided because it must be converted to lactate by the liver. Multiple intramuscular injections into the pectoral muscle mass of the standard isotonic solutions used in small animal practice seem to be well tolerated.

Sugar-rich solutions containing the essential amino acids and the vitamin B complex may be force-fed, depending on appetite and weight variations.

Dexamethasone or betamethasone appear to be of benefit in treating mycotoxicoses by limiting fibrosis.

Dieting is a successful way of reducing the obese avian state. Sunflower deprivation, except for a few seeds, causes a healthy weight loss in cockatoos and parrots. For Budgerigars, a reduced feeding time or a given amount (e.g., 1 tsp mixed seeds) is effective in weight control. Whatever system is used, constant monitoring of weight is necessary. Rosskopf (1983) reports that using 5 mg thyroxine dissolved in 100 ml drinking water to treat lipomas in Budgerigars increased the rate of weight loss and the level of fitness.

Control. Infectious disease control depends on hygiene, quarantine, correct stocking rate, and depopulation in the event of an outbreak. Vaccination offers the best hope of control against chlamydiae and herpes- and papovaviruses.

Pancreas Diseases

Clinical Signs. Pancreatic endocrine observations produced polyuria/polydipsia syndrome in psittacines, most commonly in

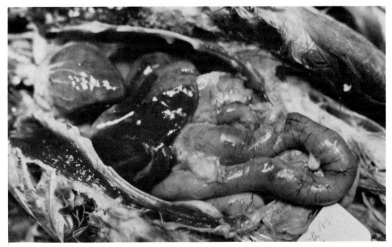

Fig. 13.6. *Escherichia coli* granuloma in a much-reduced pancreas of a Galah (*Eolophus roseicapilla*), revealing no clinical symptoms of pancreatic deficiency.

Budgerigars. The degree of weight loss and dehydration depends on the duration of the disease. Necropsy is often the only means of detecting a pancreas problem (Fig. 13.6).

The vent becomes soiled and the bird kicks at its dirty feathers although the feces maintain normal consistency.

White or pale gray feces are occasionally seen in Budgerigars, usually as a transient condition. A positive starch test using iodine is recorded, but whether this indicates exocrine pancreatic deficiency has yet to be determined.

Biochemistry. Plasma glucose levels can be elevated 3 to 4 times normal. If dehydration is present plasma urea will be elevated. Glucosuria is prominent.

A glucose tolerance (described in Chapter 27) test can be employed.

Etiology. Consistent with the findings of Altman and Kirmayer (1976), the authors have seen hyperglycemia, glucosuria, polydipsia, and polyuria in Budgerigars with normal pancreases but with marked hepatic fat infiltration. The pathogenesis is unclear.

Glandular destruction can be seen in isolated cases of neoplasia or granuloma caused by organisms that have become systemic (*E. coli,* mycobacteria).

Diagnosis. Plasma glucose levels 3 to 4 times normal imply pancreatic gland destruction, and these birds are losing weight while showing marked polyuria/polydipsia. Hematological evidence may suggest an infectious cause.

Plasma glucose elevations that are less marked are more likely to reflect hepatic involvement. These birds are generally obese and polyuric, but weight loss is not as dramatic or as consistent.

Psittacines close to death may exhibit a glucosuria, as can those with renal tubular impairment.

Treatment. Altman and Kirmayer (1976) describe the use of NPH insulin in the Budgerigar with some success.

Dietary control is not a practical means of treatment in the seedeating bird although the obese Budgerigar and cockatoo benefit from a restriction of energy intake.

References

Altman, R. B. 1976. Palatine and lingual abscesses in large psittacine birds. *Annu. Proc. Am. Assoc. Zoo Vet.*

Altman, R. B., and A. H. Kirmayer. 1976. Diabetes mellitus in the avian species. *J. Am. Anim. Hosp. Assoc.* 12(4):531–36.

Beach, J. E., J. S. Wilkinson, and D. G. Harvey. 1960. Calculus in the crop of a Budgerigar. *Vet. Rec.* 72:473.

Campbell, T. W. 1983. Disorders of the avian crop. *Compend. Contin. Educ.* 5(10):813–20.

Gerlach, H. 1984. Virus diseases in pet birds. *Vet. Clin. N. Am. Small Anim. Pract.* 14(2):305.

Graham, Carla L. G. 1978. Pox virus infection in a Spectacled Amazon Parrot (*Amazona albifrons*). *Avian Dis.* 22(2):340–43.

Henderson, B. M., and R. W. Winterfield. 1975. Acute copper toxicosis in the Canada Goose. *Avian Dis.* 19(2):385–87.

Irwin, J. C. 1975. Mortality factors in Whistling Swans at Lake St. Clair, Ontario. *J. Wildl. Dis.* 11:8–12.

Mustaffa-Babgee, A., P. B. Spadrow, and J. L. Samuel. 1974. A pathogenic paramyxovirus from a Budgerigar (*Melopsittacus undulatus*). *Avian Dis.* 18(2):226–30.

Rosskopf, W. J., and R. W. Woerpel. 1983. Remission of lipomatous growths in a hypothyroid Budgerigar in response to L-thyroxine therapy. *Vet. Med. Small Anim. Clin.* 78(9):1415–18.

Tripathy, D. N., and L. E. Hanson. 1976. A smear technique for staining elementary bodies of fowl pox. *Avian Dis.* 20:609–10.

Woerpel, R. W., and W. J. Rosskopf. 1982. Heavy metal intoxication in caged birds: Part 1. *Compend. Contin. Educ.* 4(9):729–38.

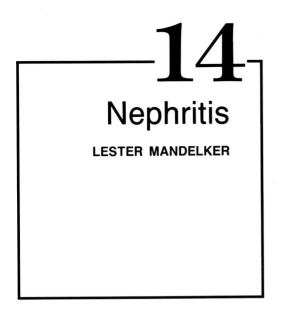

14

Nephritis

LESTER MANDELKER

THE KIDNEYS play an important role in disease processes, elimination of waste products, regulation of acid-base balance, and osmosis. The major diseases of the urinary system are nephritis, tumors and cysts (discussed in Chapter 33), and gout (discussed in Chapter 12). Diabetes and parasites in the urinary system are rare.

Nephritis is a problem for the practitioner because, although it is a common cause of disease in birds, it is often hard to diagnose. The clinical signs (watery droppings, vague symptoms, elevated uric acid levels) are similar to those of many other diseases, and radiographs are helpful but not diagnostic. Blood tests are the most practical method of diagnosing it in birds. Acute nephritis is almost impossible to diagnose antemortem since the course of the disease may be so rapid; the only signs may be lethargy, rapid breathing, and sudden death. Most often the causes are infectious (bacterial, viral) or toxic (e.g., salt poisoning). Chronic nephritis is seen with greater frequency but still can be a diagnostic challenge.

Clinical Signs. Physical findings from birds with chronic nephritis vary, depending on the severity and extent of the disease. The eyes may appear dull but wide open and of normal size. The cere and legs may appear darker in color, swollen, and actually be cyanotic due to circulation impairment. The appearance of extremely dry skin along the feet and legs is evidence of dehydration. Often the bird is ill for several weeks, showing mood change, inappetence, puffiness, and depression. The droppings can vary from a watery, clear fluid to a thick, streaked fluid. The drinking habits may not change or may vary from a slight polydypsia to a decreased water intake. Since most owners don't observe water intake, findings are inconsistent. The extreme polydypsia evident in mammals does not routinely occur in birds with nephritis. The appetite fluctuates, but most often there is a decrease in food intake and little interest in new types of seed, vegetables, and fruit. This reduction in eating results in emaciation.

In advanced cases of nephritis in smaller birds (e.g., passerines), ascites may occur, with the abdomen appearing slightly distended. Unsteadiness on the perch may also be seen.

Diagnosis. Blood uric acid levels are the most consistent and reliable method of confirming renal disease and impairment. In smaller birds (passerines, Budgerigars), levels slightly above 8–10 mg/100 ml are considered suspicious while much higher levels (>15) confirm kidney disease. Blood uric acid levels can be run with various microliter methods, using blood from a microhemacrit tube (obtained from bleeding a toenail). Creatinine is also a reliable indicator of renal integrity. Elevations are associated with primary renal disease and nephritis. Values may decrease in response to diuresis and appropriate medication. Normal range in most birds is .1–.4 mg%. Higher values may occur in psittacines fed on a high-protein diet. Elevated or lowered calcium levels are also highly suggestive of nephritic conditions; levels <5 or >15 mg/100 ml are considered abnormal. A dextrose stick (using blood) will screen out any possibility of diabetes, which can give similar symptoms. With suspect cases a blood glucose test should be taken. Urinalysis is very hard to perform on bird droppings, but occasionally the feces component can be separated from the urates. Results from urine dipsticks usually vary, with false positives for hematuria a common occurrence. Urine glucose determinations are helpful, differentiating normal birds (showing negative to slight positive) from positive birds (a finding that usually indicates diabetes mellitus). Abnormal droppings may also suggest nephritis. A consistently watery-type dropping with or without streaks or urates is typical of renal disease but may also be found in diabetes mellitus and possibly diabetes insipidus. Appropriate testing will help distinguish these from nephritis. The feces color in nephritic birds appears normal. (See Chapter 27 for descriptions of various urinalysis tests.)

A kidney biopsy and/or visualization using fiber-optic endoscopes may be a feasible method of confirming kidney disease. In large birds, intravenous urography has been helpful in defining the location and size of the kidneys, information necessary in determining the presence of primary kidney tumors and other lesions. Avian urography is also useful to determine kidney integrity. Radiographic findings may reveal an increased density and/or renomeglia in advanced cases. This is best viewed on a lateral exposure. The gonads are located at the cranial aspect of the kidney and with seasonal variation can present as a pathological enlargement. Clinical signs and physical examination will help to differentiate the condition. The final differential diagnosis of nephritis relies on blood test analysis. Films are made at 10 seconds (arterial phase), 60 seconds (renal and ureteral phase), and 2 minutes (urethral and cloacal phase) postinjection. The drug of choice of urography is Hypaque at 1.5 mg/g body weight, which calculates to about 3 ml in a 450-g parrot. A large part of a bird's renal blood supply is diluted with splanchnic blood, which causes a considerable dilution of contrast material.

Treatment. The treatment of nephritis consists of symptomatic therapy. Stress is to be avoided; the patient is kept warm, placed on low-protein seed (millet, oats, groats) and given vitamins, especially A and B complex, administered in the drinking water. Antibiotics can be given parentally or orally. Weakened birds should receive extra glucose in the form of honey, and unlimited access to fruits and watery-type vegetables (e.g., lettuce) is recommended. When ascites is present, diuretics may be considered to reduce fluid retention and lower the levels of blood uric acid. Anabolic steroids may also be indicated in the debilitated bird. The administration of sodium bicarbonate at present is questionable, and response to therapy varies greatly. Treatment of nephritis is not specific and often unrewarding. It is important to advise the client of the poor prognosis. Diagnosis and therapy of nephritis should improve as research and advances in avian medicine continue.

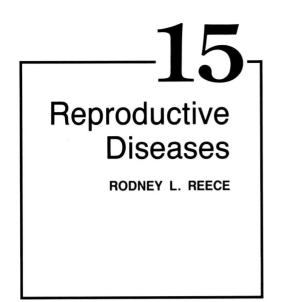

15

Reproductive Diseases

RODNEY L. REECE

DISEASE of the reproductive tract may be restricted to the reproductive tract, originate in the reproductive tract but involve other systems, or be secondary to a disease in some other body system. It is sometimes convenient to consider that diseases of the reproductive tract may be space-occupying lesions, inflammations, and/ or physiological alterations. (For a discussion of surgical techniques, neoplasms, and the structure and function of the reproductive system of birds, see Chapters 23 and 33.)

A diagnosis of a disease of the reproductive tract is usually made on the basis of history, clinical signs, palpation, radiography, and/or laparotomy. The differential diagnosis of the more common clinical signs associated with diseases of the reproductive tract follow.

- Abdominal enlargement may be due to large gonadal tumors, distension of hollow organs (e.g., cystic right oviduct), oviduct impaction (egg binding), or fluid in the abdominal cavity (egg peritonitis). Chronic cardiac insufficiency, hepatopathies, other causes of peritonitis, and other tumors can also cause abdominal enlargement.
- Cessation of egg laying can be due to many factors. The ovary may regress due to the onset of broodiness, stress, or seasonal factors. The infundibulum may fail to engulf the shed oocyte. The oviduct may be obstructed. However, failure to find eggs in the nest does not mean that the bird is not laying eggs.
- Death often results from diseases of the reproductive tract, such as gonadal tumors, egg binding, or salpingitis. A thorough necropsy should indicate the occurrence of any other disease contributing to the death of the bird.

- Depression can be of sudden onset (e.g., with egg retention) or can be long-standing due to gonadal tumors, salpingitis, or peritonitis. Birds are depressed in most diseases, and differential diagnosis is difficult.
- Discharge from the oviduct may be due to salpingitis or vent gleet. Other possibilities are irritation of the vent by external parasites (mites, lice), enteritis, nephritis, or hepatitis.
- Lameness can be caused by the pressure of space-occupying lesions on the sciatic nerve plexus. It is sometimes observed in birds with large gonadal tumors. Other common causes of lameness are foot problems, broken legs, bruising, kidney tumors, and emaciation.
- Loss of libido can be due to, or associated with, degenerative changes and diseases of the testes. It can also occur as a normal phenomenon in birds with a definite breeding season or secondary to other conditions (fear, malnutrition, septicemia, parasitism).
- Prolapse of the cloaca or oviduct is usually associated with straining to pass a retained egg. However, it may be complicated by trauma, cannibalism, and/or hemorrhage. Sequential egg laying complicates the condition and changes it into a life-threatening obstruction.
- Sex changes can occur in response to steroid-sex-hormone-producing tumors. Destruction of the left ovary by disease or surgery leads to hypertrophy of the right gonad, which may develop testicular tissue. Some theca cells of the ovary have the potential to secrete androgens although theca cell tumors generally secrete estrogens. Arrhenoblastomas of the functional ovary are often associated with masculinization due to androgen production (Campbell 1969). Feminization has been reported in some male Budgerigars with various testicular tumors (Beach 1962). Changes in plumage and cere color can be due to a lack of male hormones from a diseased gonad or to an altered state of health (Arnall and Keymer 1975). Some adrenal tumors are probably capable of secreting androgens. Schultz (1981) notes that sex changes of ducks and quail are reported occasionally by aviculturists, but details are lacking. Intersex birds are rare (Arnall and Keymer 1975).
- Straining can be caused by egg retention or protusion of the oviduct. These must be differentiated from other causes of irritation of the cloaca (vent trauma, enteritis, nephritis, pelvic lipoma).
- Vent gleet (cloacitis) is a chronic, foul-smelling, sticky discharge from the vent that soils the ventral feathers. A diphtheritic membrane may be present around the edge of the vent.

The cause is unknown. Male birds can also be affected. Treatment by local application of tetracycline ointments may be of some value. Culling may be considered.

– Weakness can be caused by any long-standing condition, such as gonadal tumors or chronic infections (peritonitis, salpingitis). Other causes of weakness are malnutrition, parasitism, and septicemias.

Hen Birds

Ovary

Oophoritis. Infection of the ovary with *Salmonella pullorum* or other *Salmonella* spp., *Pasteurella multocida, Yersinia pseudotuberculosis, Escherichia coli,* and other bacteria (*Mycobacterium avium, Streptococcus* spp.) produces a congested and distorted ovary. The follicles often contain necrotic debris, fibrin, and cellular infiltrate and are hemorrhaged. Follicular atresia and peritonitis are commonly associated with it.

Oophoritis is usually secondary to systemic disease, and therefore clinical signs in affected birds may be depression, inappetence, wasting, or death.

Antibiotic treatment must be specific for the inciting organism. Control programs for the disease in question should be implemented.

Ovarian Hemorrhage. Hemorrhage from the calyx occasionally occurs at ovulation. If the bird has a defect in its blood clotting mechanisms (e.g., anticoagulant toxicosis from warfarin), it may prove fatal.

The active ovary has an abundant blood supply and is normally congested. Any body trauma may lead to hemorrhage. It is a common finding in birds that have been paretic or recumbent due to some other condition.

Follicular Atresia. Atresia and collapse of the ovarian follicles without ovulation occur in the normal laying cycle of domestic hens. Small yolky follicles become necrotic and are obliterated by connective tissue. Larger follicles may be obliterated or undergo cystic degeneration (Gilbert et al. 1983; Uhrin 1984).

Regression of follicles may be associated with an onset of broodiness or an abrupt cessation of lay due to severe stress. Large follicles then become atretic.

Affected follicles lose their turgidity, but the stigma remains intact. The follicular fluid may be changed in consistency. There may be hemorrhage if the precipitating stress involved trauma or fright.

The only clinical sign associated with significant follicular atresia is a cessation of egg laying. It is only abnormal in birds with long egg-laying cycles, such as domestic hens, or in association with other severe stress. Chronic conditions such as malnutrition and parasitism are usually associated with non–egg laying rather than with an abrupt termination.

Ovarian Tumors. Abdominal adenocarcinomas often have miliary nodules implanted on the serosal surface, particularly in the duodenal loop, the most dependent organ in the peritoneal cavity. The ovary has small nodules on the surface, but there is little follicular activity. Affected birds usually have a fluid-filled abdominal cavity and weight loss. Surgical treatment is not possible. There is some evidence that these tumors originate in the oviduct (Haritani et al. 1984).

The ovary can be involved with lymphoproliferative diseases and hemangiosarcomas. Affected birds usually have signs referrable to involvement of other systems as well as ovarian inactivity.

The ovary can be affected with a mixed cell tumor, teratoma, fibroma/fibrosarcoma, myxofibroma, and hamatoma as well as granulosa cell tumor, theca cell tumor, arrhenoma, or dysgerminoma. The latter may be associated with virilism.

The clinical sign is usually non–egg laying. There may be abdominal enlargement, paresis, respiratory distress, and weight loss if the tumor is large. If the tumor is necrotic there may be lethargy associated with toxemia. Secondary complications of intraabdominal hemorrhage or peritonitis may occur. Histological examination is usually necessary to differentiate these tumors. As biopsy material is obtained by a laparotomy, the affected ovary can be removed at the same time.

Cystic Ovary. This has been recorded in Budgerigars (Beach 1962; Hasholt 1966) and pheasants (Keymer 1980), but there is no reason to suppose that it cannot occur in other species.

The clinical signs are a slowly developing abdominal enlargement with respiratory distress. Egg laying does not occur. There may be a palpable soft abdominal mass.

The ovary of the affected bird may be enlarged, with a mass of thin-walled cysts full of straw-colored fluid. Alternatively there may be a pedunculated cyst. The etiology of this condition is not known.

Removal of excess fluid with a hypodermic needle and syringe may lead to a significant reduction in respiratory distress. Ovariectomy is probably the best long-term treatment.

Right Ovary and/or Oviduct. A right ovary is occasionally reported in diurnal birds of prey, kiwis, corvidae, ducks, a species of swan, and mountain grouse (Koch 1973; King and McLelland 1975; Keymer 1980). It is not clear from these descriptions whether these right ovaries are associated with a functional right oviduct or not. Bilateral ovaries in other species are an abnormality.

If the right ovary is functional but there is no associated oviduct, the ova are shed into the abdominal cavity.

Abdominal Cavity

Abdominal Eggs. Affected birds are also known as internal layers. A fully formed or partially formed egg may be found in the peritoneal cavity. In long-standing cases the egg material may be inspissated.

The presence of an egg free in the abdominal cavity means the ova progressed down the oviduct to a certain point and then either reverse peristalsis or rupture of the oviduct occurred. Oviduct rupture, a sequel to some cases of oviduct impaction, can lead to severe peritonitis.

Affected birds may be found dead without any premonitory signs. Birds with a number of fully formed eggs in the abdominal cavity may exhibit a penguinlike stance. Other birds will have abdominal enlargement. Chronically affected birds may have significant weight loss.

Surgical removal of the abdominal egg via a laparotomy is possible. The success of such a procedure depends on the lack of peritonitis and impaction. The condition can readily recur at the next ovulation, especially if the precipitating factors are still active.

Egg Peritonitis. The presence of egglike material in the abdominal cavity, usually referred to as egg peritonitis, is thought to be due to ectopic ovulation. Recent studies in poultry have shown this material to be fibrin, not egg yolk (Jones and Owens 1981).

Clinical signs in affected birds may be sudden death, depression, abdominal distension, respiratory distress, or weight loss.

In advanced cases peritoneal adhesions are common. This condition is commonly found in association with other problems of the reproductive tract, such as salpingitis, impaction, internal laying, oviduct rupture, and trauma.

Numerous bacterial species have been isolated from this type of lesion, for example, *E. coli, Salmonella* spp., *Proteus* spp., *Klebsiella* spp., *Y. pseudotuberculosis,* and *Pasteurella multocida.* Infection by these organisms may be the cause of this condition or may be secondary to other problems.

In the early stages abdominal irrigation via a laparotomy followed by heavy antibiotic cover may be of some value (Schultz 1981).

(In the course of normal egg laying, occasional ova are shed into the abdominal cavity, but the lipid in these cases is rapidly resorbed [Wood-Gush and Gilbert 1970]. Examination of these birds usually fails to detect the congestion of the peritoneal blood vessels normally associated with egg peritonitis. They are usually bacteriologically sterile. This is a common finding in birds that have been disturbed or handled or are in a recumbent position.)

Leiomyoma of the Mesosalpinx. The free border of the ventral ligament supporting the oviduct is a common place for these tumors, sometimes referred to as "fibroids." They are sharply circumscribed, discrete nodules, with an abundant blood supply. These tumors are composed of variable amounts of interlacing bundles of smooth muscle fibers and fibrocytes; hence they are more correctly called fibroleiomyomas or leiomyofibromas, depending upon the predominant tissue. More invasive tumors are leiomyosarcomas or fibrosarcomas.

The presence of this tumor in the mesosalpinx may interfere with the ability of the infundibulum to engulf shed ova. Internal ovulation could then be a consequence.

These tumors are usually an incidental finding in healthy birds or those that have some other problem. Surgical removal is a possibility, but they do have an abundant blood supply and excision results in impaired mobility.

Large tumors of this type may be presented as space-occupying lesions, with weight loss, abdominal enlargement, and respiratory distress.

Cystic Right Oviduct. In the female birds only the left ovary and oviduct normally develop posthatching. However, vestiges of the right oviduct may persist. These tend to become filled with clear fluid.

If the cyst is large it may act as a space-occupying lesion and thus the bird will have clinical signs of abdominal enlargement and respiratory distress. If the cyst is at the equivalent of the right vagina, obstruction of the left oviduct may occur and the bird may become egg bound. Small cysts are an incidental finding at the necropsy of otherwise healthy birds.

Paracentesis of the cyst with a hypodermic needle and syringe may give some relief. Surgical removal is possible.

Oviduct

Salpingitis. Salpingitis, in severe cases often referred to as "impaction of the oviduct," is a common problem in adult birds. However, it is not restricted to adults and can occur in young birds (Bisgaard and Dam 1980). It is often encountered in association with egg retention or obstruction of the oviduct. Foreign bodies (e.g., wheat grains) in the oviduct can allow infection to become established. Ascending infection can cause salpingitis.

The bacteria most frequently isolated from salpingitis are *E. coli*. Others are also implicated: *Mycoplasma gallisepticum* can cause a salpingitis, as can *Salmonella* spp. and *P. multocida,* but other organ systems are also usually affected in these cases.

The hemagglutinating adenovirus responsible for egg drop syndrome '76 causes an infection of the shell gland with edema and inflammatory cell infiltration (van Eck et al. 1978).

Affected birds show vague symptoms, such as depression and inappetence. There can be significant weight loss in chronic severe affections. No eggs may be laid. Abdominal enlargement can occur as a result of a distended oviduct. There is usually some peritonitis.

Discharge from the vent may be noted. Salpingitis is one of the common causes of vent gleet, a sticky, smelly greenish-white discharge from the oviduct that mats the feathers beneath the vent.

Laparotomy or necropsy will reveal an enlarged oviduct. The wall is usually thin, and there is a fibrinous cast in the lumen. In severe cases of impaction there are concentric rings of coagulated egg material, fibrin, and inflammatory cells.

Antibiotic treatment is of limited value. If there is severe damage to the oviduct, problems will be encountered at the next ovulation so ovariohysterectomy is probably indicated.

Cystic Hyperplasia of the Oviduct. This has been reported in Budgerigars and Japanese Quail.

Affected birds have a dilated oviduct containing mucoid fluid. There may be some association with endocrine disturbances. A cessation of lay, abdominal swelling, and respiratory distress may be noticed in advanced cases. Birds with milder forms may have intermittent mucoid discharges. An accurate diagnosis can only be made after a laparotomy.

Surgical removal of the ovary and oviduct is probably the best method of treatment. If there is an underlying endocrine disorder, temporary remission may be obtained with hormonal therapy.

Cystic Dilation of the Oviduct. Certain strains of infectious bronchitis virus, when given to day-old pullets, can cause damage to the oviduct with resultant hypoplasia and stenosis. This can produce cystic dilation of associated areas of the oviduct (Crinion et al. 1971). When such birds commence ovarian activity they cannot lay eggs so they become affected with internal laying, impaction, and/or salpingitis.

Cystic structures occasionally involve the left infundibulum and may be associated with poor engulfing of shed ova. These are usually discovered as incidental findings or associated with signs of a space-occupying lesion or internal ovulation.

Oviduct Adenoma/Adenocarcinoma. Adenocarcinomas and large nodular adenomas are occasionally observed on the mucosal aspect of the opened oviduct. The serosal surface of the oviduct is commonly involved in metastasized abdominal adenocarcinomas.

An oviduct tumor may predispose to salpingitis. They are more likely to be associated with weight loss and ovarian inactivity rather than with obstruction of the oviduct.

If exploratory laparotomy reveals a single discrete tumor, radical surgery (removal of the ovary and oviduct) may be of value.

Parasites. There are reports of hen eggs containing adult ascarids, presumably carried into the oviduct by reverse peristalsis and subsequently trapped by the descending egg (Hungerford 1969).

Prosthogonimus ovatus and related trematodes inhabit the oviduct and bursa of Fabricius of waterfowl and galliforms. The adult fluke is less than 1 cm long. The life cycle involves an aquatic snail (*Amnicola limosa*) and dragonflies. Birds with heavy infection may have soft-shelled or shell-less eggs, and there may be salpingitis (Kingston 1984). The fluke can be passed in eggs, where it may be mistaken for a hemorrhagic spot (Arundel et al. 1980).

There is no known treatment for parasites. Control is effected by limiting the access of birds to the intermediate host (dragonflies).

Pelvis

Egg Binding. This is a common problem in cage and aviary birds. It is due to obstruction or impaction of the vagina with a fully formed egg. It is brought about by, or associated with, either atony or spasms of the smooth muscles of the oviduct.

The factors associated with egg binding are obesity, oversized eggs, low blood calcium, poor muscle tone, nervousness, variations in temperature, and lack of a suitable nesting place. Birds in poor body condition usually have inactive ovaries.

The clinical signs in affected birds are intermittent bouts of straining and behavior normally associated with egg laying, such as nest seeking. Affected birds often adopt abnormal postures. Paresis can occur. When the bird is examined, an egg is usually palpable just above the pelvic inlet.

If the condition is not treated it can rapidly progress to oviduct and/or cloacal prolapse.

Psittacines with very recent egg binding can be placed in a warmed cage, preferably with infrared irradiation; often the egg is then expelled. Lubrication of the cloacal opening and placing birds over steaming kettles have been tried but with variable success. Gentle manipulation may assist, but this can be easily overdone.

If the egg is accessible in the vagina, the contents can be removed with a hypodermic syringe and needle (Rosskopf and Woerpel 1984). The eggshell may collapse or the fragments can be taken out piecemeal. If the impaction is farther up the oviduct, the egg can only be removed via a laparotomy.

Injection of egg-bound Budgerigars with calcium borogluconate has been associated with rapid expulsion of the egg (Blackmore 1966). Schultz (1981) has used calcium gluconate at 0.5 mg/100 g body weight intramuscularly in psittacines. This tends to confirm that there may be some association of egg binding with low blood calcium and thus decreased muscle contractions.

Oviduct Prolapse. Prolapse of the oviduct can occur in any species. It is usually restricted to birds that are in lay. Birds just coming into lay and overfat birds are more likely to be affected. Birds on suboptimal diets tend not to ovulate. It can be a problem in birds kept in small cages that have not laid an egg for a considerable period of time.

The affected bird may have the distal portion of the oviduct, usually the vagina, prolapsed through the vent. The prolapse is often distended due to the presence of an egg or egg material. Affected birds are often bright and alert and often distress is not apparent. Prolapse of the cloaca is a common complication.

In normal egg laying, the oviduct is partially everted as the egg is passed. The prolapsed oviduct is caused by and/or complicated by straining of the abdominal muscles, rather than by oviduct contractions. It is commonly thought that prolapse is associated with oversized eggs, and although this may well be a factor, Hasholt (1966) and Keymer (1980) found oviduct prolapse associated with deformed, soft-shelled, and shell-less eggs. These findings indicate that there are likely to be problems elsewhere in the reproductive tract, particularly with the shell gland.

Physiological hyperplasia of the oviduct associated with egg laying and flaccidity of cloacal muscles are probably both necessary for a prolapse to occur.

If the prolapse is recent, surgery can be quite successful (Hasholt 1966). If an egg is present in the prolapse, it must be removed. The vagina is opened and the egg removed, the incision closed, and the prolapsed tissue returned to its normal place. A purse-string suture around the cloacal opening helps prevent recurrence. However, the presence of an egg in the prolapsed vagina may not prevent another egg being formed in the shell gland. This can seriously complicate recovery from surgery.

Lipomas and Pelvic Fat. Lipomas are common in large psittacine birds. If lipomas are present in the pelvic area, or if there is a large mass of fat tissue, there may be obstruction to normal egg passage. Hence, the bird may be presented as egg bound.

Birds with lipomas tend to be in good condition with active ovaries.

The cause of the presenting signs must be treated and then a decision made about the offending tumor. They do tend to progress and often become necrotic. Surgical removal is advisable.

Egg Abnormalities. Shell-less eggs occur when the developing egg does not lodge sufficiently long in the shell gland. It may be a spontaneous happening, particularly at the commencement of lay, or it may reflect salpingitis or impaired calcium-phosphorus balance in the bird.

Double-yolked eggs are usually the result of double ovulation, both oocytes entering the infundibulum more or less simultaneously. Yolkless eggs are occasionally produced by normal birds, but if they are regularly produced they may indicate disease of the ovary and/or oviduct.

Eggs occasionally have blood clots in them, probably originating from hemorrhage at ovulation. A developing egg may enclose necrotic debris from a chronic salpingitis. Soft-shelled eggs are usually due to a calcium-phosphorus imbalance. The diet of birds producing such eggs should be investigated. Shell color and yolk color can be influenced by diet as well as by the genetics of the bird.

Unpleasant egg odors can, at times, be derived from feed sources, such as fish meal, rapeseed meal, and other sources of trimethylamine (Fenwick et al. 1981).

Systemic medications given to birds tend to be passed into the egg. Lipotrophic substances (e.g., chlorinated hydrocarbons) are present in the yolk while hydrotrophic substances (e.g., some antibiotics) are present in the egg white. Some medications (e.g., nicarbazin) have an adverse effect on eggshell pigmentation (McClary 1955).

Cock Birds

Orchitis. Granulomas due to infection with a variety of bacteria (*E. coli, Salmonella* spp., *P. multocida*) can occur in the testes of birds. Orchitis can be secondary to foci of infection in adjacent areas, such as phallic prolapse and ulceration in waterfowl or kidney obstruction and infection. It can also be secondary to septicemic conditions.

Affected birds may show signs of generalized infection. Lack of libido is more likely to be noticed than infertility due to interference with spermatozoa.

The causative organism must be identified and treated appropriately. In the event of clinical recovery, subsequent fertility could be poor.

Testicular Atrophy, Degeneration, and Hypoplasia. Testicular atrophy occurs as an annual event in those species with a definite breeding season. Regeneration of spermatogenesis occurs in the next breeding season. The seminiferous tubule cells become distended with fat droplets.

Testicular degeneration is a cessation of spermatogenesis as a consequence of a severe condition such as malnutrition, toxicity, or bacteremia (Figs. 15.1 and 15.2). It is less readily reversible because permanent damage and fibrosis may be present. The predisposing factors must be treated.

The term "testicular hypoplasia" implies that the testes have never developed to their full

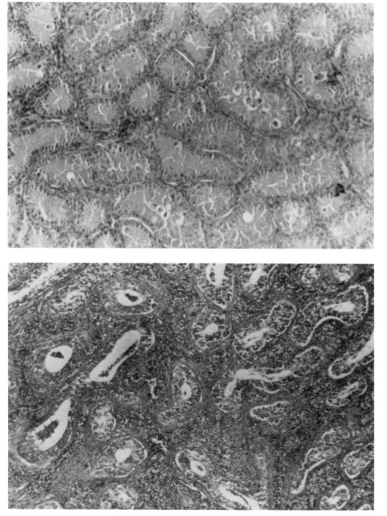

Fig. 15.1. Testes of a 7-week-old Japanese Quail (*Coturnix c. japonica*) with retarded spermatogenesis due to an earlier nutritional problem. Some spermatocytes are present. (H & E)

Fig. 15.2. Testicular degeneration in an adult Emu (*Dromaius novaehollandiae*) with renal abscesses. Note the fibroplasia of the interstitial tissue and lack of normal spermatogenesis in the tubules. (H & E)

potential. Some cases, however, may be merely retardation in attaining full function. A true hypoplasia associated with infertility and impaired libido may be a congenital or heritable condition, and such a bird should not be treated. The breeding history of the parents should be investigated.

It is possible to have congenital absence of portions of the genital tract. Persistent embryonic structures are occasionally found, and these may be cystic.

Testicular Tumors. Unilateral testicular enlargement may be due to a tumor. However, it is common for the left testis to be slightly larger and more caudally placed than the right testis. The testes of sparrows can increase up to a thousandfold during the breeding season (Koch 1973).

Various primary tumors occur in the testes of birds, including Leydig cell tumors, seminomas, and Sertoli cell tumors (the latter tend to metastasize). The testes can also be involved in lymphoproliferative diseases, or they can be affected with fibromas/fibrosarcomas, and teratomas.

If the testes are involved in a lymphoproliferative disease, there will be signs of disease in other systems (splenomegaly, hepatomegaly). Large testicular tumors can act as space-occupying lesions, with paresis, weight loss, and abdominal enlargement. There may be a lack of interest in the general surroundings and a diminution of sexual function and performance. Secondary sex characteristics can revert to an intersex type. In the case of testosterone-producing tumors there may be marked virilism.

If the tumor is single and accessible and the bird in good general health, surgery may be successful (Petrak and Gilmore 1969; Schultz 1981).

Phallic Prolapse. Sexually mature male waterfowl have a large protrusible phallus; the phallus of ratites is smaller. The males of other species of birds have a very small phallus.

The prolapsed phallus may not be readily observed if only a portion of it is involved. As the condition progresses the prolapsed phallus may be subjected to trauma and massive fecal contamination with subsequent ulceration and infection (Fig. 15.3). Birds with severe lesions may be depressed.

The etiology of phallic prolapse is not clear. There may be bacterial infection at the base of the phallus, or it may occur secondary to trauma. A bacterium, *Neisseria* spp., which is antigenically related to but distinct from *N. gonorrhoeae*, has been isolated from phallic ero-

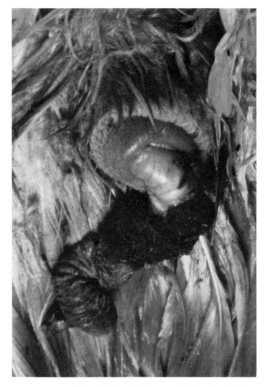

Fig. 15.3. Prolapse of the phallus in a drake with subsequent ulceration and sloughing of necrotic tissue. (*Courtesy of D. Gurney and B. Robinson, Parkville, Victoria, Aust.*)

sions and the oviduct and cloaca of geese (Nalivaiko 1983; Marvan et al. 1983); this may be a sexually transmitted disease.

Birds with a phallic prolapse are rendered infertile. In a breeding flock this may have an adverse effect on flock fertility.

Treatment should be aimed at controlling the infection and ulceration and replacement of the phallus. In early stages topical treatment with a sulfonamide and benzylpenicillin cream may be of value (Marvan et al. 1983). In the likely event that the infection cannot be controlled or the organ replaced, radical surgery is a possibility. In most circumstances the affected bird should probably be euthanized.

Flock Reproductive Diseases. Most flock reproductive diseases, whether infectious, nutritional, or behavioral, can be prevented. The reason these diseases occur is usually related to a management decision, often based on economic considerations. Therefore, advice from the veterinarian to the owner should cover treatment (how to overcome the effects of the disease), control (how to minimize the effects), and prevention (how to ensure the disease does not recur).

Parameters of Reproduction. The parameters determining a flock's reproductive performance are the production of eggs, the fertility of the eggs laid, the hatchability of the fertile eggs, the survival of the progeny to an age of independent existence and their attainment of successful sexual maturity. In many aviary-type situations the only parameter available is the number of fledglings that leave the nest.

Defining the Disease. In order to solve a flock reproductive disease it is useful to identify which of the above parameters are involved. This cannot always be done by a veterinarian remaining in a clinic or laboratory. At least one visit, and probably more, to the flock may be required. A multidisciplinary approach is appropriate for these types of investigations.

The records of the flock's reproductive performance must be examined. In many cases the owner can supply accurate and meaningful records that are of immense value in the ensuing investigation. Records of previous performance can act as a comparison for the present disease state and may possibly highlight which parameters are involved. Sometimes, however, the records are not made available or may be vague, inaccurate, invested, or even deliberately falsified. It is also important to determine what the owner expects from the flock; the expectations may be quite unrealistic and the flock may be performing satisfactorily. Investigations of such cases often lead to wasted time and considerable frustration.

The other major problem encountered with investigations of flock diseases is related to sampling. What do the birds presented for clinical and/or necropsy examination represent? In any apparently normal flock, a small number of birds may be affected with a variety of diseases and conditions. It is common for these birds to be presented by the owner when requesting investigation of a flock disease because they are "sick." Such specimens are of little value, as they usually do not represent the flock disease. Owners must be advised to present birds that are relevant to the problem under investigation. Of course, if the flock is visited by the investigator, the specimens can be collected personally. Such visits also provide an opportunity to look at the flock management, arrangement of nests, population dynamics, and feeding and housing.

Objectives of Investigations. The objectives of investigations of a flock reproductive disease are the following:

− To define the disease in terms of its effects
− To suggest the likely pathogenesis and most probable etiology
− To advise the most suitable treatments to alleviate the disease (nursing, management alterations, medications)
− To assess the response to treatment
− To advise appropriate control and prevention methods

In assessing the response to treatment, it is necessary to know the reproductive potential of the type of bird in the flock. In seasonal breeders, recovery from a disease may not be associated with a return to normal reproductive performance until the following year. However, when a flock improves after treatment it should be determined if the treatment was responsible for the recovery; the flock might have recovered anyway or the benefits of nursing and altered management might have outweighed a negligible (or even deleterious) effect of medications. On the other hand, when a flock fails to respond positively to treatment the diagnosis might have been wrong. The medication might have been inappropriate (wrong drug, ineffective dose rate, too-short treatment period), a new disease might be causing the current problem, or advice might not have been followed. Medications with toxic effects can sometimes compound the problem. Seasonal breeders and birds that lay eggs in definite clutch periods tend to be difficult to assess.

Causes of Flock Reproductive Diseases. Any disease is usually manifest in a variety of ways, either on an individual or on a flock basis. For example, the presence of a predator outside an aviary of passerines or psittacines may be sufficient to lead to the death of some birds (whose eggs and hatchings subsequently die), cause others to abandon their nests and their hatchings or incubating eggs, and not affect still others. A disease such as riboflavin deficiency leads to a reduction in the number of eggs laid and also results in lowered hatchability and poor survival of the chicks (Davis et al. 1938). This variety of symptoms and reactions must be borne in mind when reading the following sections. The information provided is by no means exhaustive but should serve as a general guide.

Poor Egg Production. A reduction in the number of eggs may be due to (1) fewer eggs laid, (2) some eggs not counted (i.e., laid elsewhere), or (3) eggs laid not present (stolen, eaten, broken, shell-less). Fewer eggs on a flock basis may be due to a combination of birds not laying eggs, some birds laying fewer eggs, and still other birds laying satisfactorily. Careful inspection of the owner's records, nests, birds, and aviary should reveal any evidence of (2) or (3).

A lack of eggs laid may be due to ovarian inactivity attributed to the following factors:

1. The bird is unable to lay because the ovary is nonfunctional.
   a. What is thought to be a female bird may be a male.
   b. The ovary may be involved with a neoplasm or teratoma.
   c. The bird may have been castrated.
   d. The bird may be too young or too old.
2. The bird is unwilling to lay because of inappropriate or adverse stimuli exerting an effect via the hypothalmic-pituitary axis.
   a. The nesting places and nesting material may be unsuitable.
   b. The birds may not have been successfully paired.
   c. It may be the wrong season for breeding.
3. The bird is not in a suitable state to lay eggs.
   a. The bird may be suffering primary malnutrition; that is, the diet is unbalanced or deficient, particularly in water, energy, protein, vitamin A, vitamin B, calcium, and/or phosphorus.
   b. The bird may be affected with secondary malnutrition; that is, suitable feed is provided but not utilized (e.g., because of shortage of feeder space accentuating peck-order problems; feeders inaccessible or blocked; blindness, weakness or deformities; beak problems; feed available but in an inappropriate form; or a neurological disorder that interferes with feed uptake).
   c. The bird may be affected with a generalized condition, such as parasitism, chronic toxicities (pyrrolidine alkaloids or aflatoxins), obesity, infectious disease (trichomoniasis, pox, respiratory disease complex), or large space-occupying lesions (neoplasms).

Atresia of the ovary is usually a physiological response induced by severe stress such as water and feed restriction, fright (fire, flood, predators, nearby construction work), or pyrexia and septicemia (velogenic Newcastle disease, avian influenza, chlamydiosis, pasteurellosis, yersiniosis or paratyphoid).

A reduction in the rate of lay, either by reducing the total number of eggs in a clutch or by increasing the interval between eggs laid, is usually due to any of the above factors occurring less dramatically.

In some cases the ovary may be functional but no eggs may be laid, either due to the failure of the infundibulum to engulf the shed oocyte (which can happen with severe disturbance) or due to a blockage of the oviduct. These problems usually occur in individual birds and are not normally a flock problem.

Low Fertility. A reduction in the fertility of the eggs is a difficult parameter to measure, as it must be differentiated from fertile eggs that are not incubated. It may be due to male and/or female factors and in any individual may be an absolute infertility or a reduced fertility.

Male factors (the males must be present and effective) follow:

1. The male shows a lack of libido (little or no interest in the female).
   a. There may be a lack of testosterone because the bird is too young or too old, there are estrogen-producing neoplasms, or there are severe pathological conditions in the testes.
   b. There may be neurophysiological distress due to overcrowding, excessive disturbances, or fighting.
2. The male shows an inability to mate (interested in the female but unable to copulate).
   a. There may be neurological disturbances, such as cerebellar hypoplasia or neurotoxicities due to pesticides, nitrofurans, dimetridazole, dinitolmide, or lead (Reece and Hooper 1984).
   b. There may be anatomical problems, such as debilitating conditions and general weakness or physical infirmities (broken legs or claws).
   c. The perches may be unsuitable for copulation.
   d. The female may be unreceptive (because it is the wrong season or the birds are incorrectly paired) or physically unable to be copulated with (because of a uropygial gland tumor, for example).
3. Copulation occurs but is not successful.
   a. Spermatogenesis may be suppressed by the specific action of a toxin, such as copper fungicides (Shivanandappa et al. 1983) or 2-amino-5-nitrothiazole (Hudson and Pino 1952).
   b. There may be testicular hypoplasia, degeneration, or atrophy, either congenital/genetic or acquired following septicemia or malnutrition.
   c. There may be an inherent infertility.

Some of the factors mentioned above can also be applied to hen birds. Any factor that reduces the number of eggs laid is also likely to reduce the fertility of the hen bird.

Low Hatchability. The term "low hatchability" usually refers to a combination of infertility, poor incubation, death of embryos in the eggs, and/or failure of the chicks to pip. Although there is some overlap between these, these sections are presented – and should be considered – separately.

Infertility. See the previous section on low hatchability.

Poor Incubation. Unincubated fertile eggs can be differentiated from infertile eggs. The former have a blastoderm.

Some hen birds lay fertile eggs but fail to set. This may be due to neurological-behavioral defects, lack of suitable nests, or disturbance or abandonment of nests by the birds. Occasionally aviary birds lay more or less continuously like a domestic hen but fail to become broody.

It is possible to use surrogate birds to incubate eggs laid by other birds. These may be of the same species (e.g., altricial birds such as pigeons) or of different species (e.g., precocial birds such as the domestic hen, which can incubate duck, quail, or turkey eggs).

Mechanical incubators should be used according to the manufacturer's directions, accepted practices, and/or practical experience.

Death of Embryos in the Eggs. The developing embryo is a suitable bacterial culture medium. Under ideal conditions, however, bacterial growth is not a significant problem. The inherent resistance of the embryo can be overcome by the following factors:

1. Infection may occur prior to the egg being fully formed. Mycoplasmas in the left abdominal air sac are able to infect the oocyte as it enters the infundibulum. *Mycoplasma iowea* causes embryo mortality in turkeys (McClenaghan et al. 1981), as does *M. gallisepticum* in chickens (Yoder and Hofstad 1965).
2. The natural protection of the egg may be bypassed by cracks or by mechanical damage to the cuticle, such as from scrubbing.
3. The bacterial challenge may be overwhelming. This is usually caused by bad nest design (leading to dirty eggs), by adult birds contaminating eggs with fecal material and therefore *Salmonella* spp., *E. coli, Pseudomonas* spp., etc., or by human-assisted contamination (washing eggs in an ineffective detergent).

The original isolation of fowl adenovirus was from chick embryos (Yates and Fry 1957);

whether infected prelay or postlay was not known. Leukosis virus is also transmitted to the descending egg (Burmester et al. 1955).

Death of embryos in the eggs can also be caused by a cessation in incubation (power failure or birds abandoning nests).

Poor viability of embryos is due in part to occasional monstrosities and other congenital problems. More important, nutritional deficiencies (particularly riboflavin; biotin; pantothenic and folic acids; vitamins B_{12}, D_3, and E; zinc; and manganese) of the hen bird often are associated with reduced viability of the embryos. It has also been shown that, in chickens at least, the relative number of embryos that survive can also be related to the time since insemination of the hen (van Drimmelen 1951).

Failure to Pip. Any factor that reduces the viability of the embryo will reduce its chances of pipping successfully. Therefore, this will include congenital defects, respiratory disease (mycoplasmosis), and yolk sac infections. If the shell is too hard (due to low humidity) and/or too thick, the embryo may not be able to pip. In nests the eggs are usually on their sides and the birds roll them around frequently, whereas in artificial incubators the eggs may not be rolled and are sometimes placed upside down, so the embryos adhere to the shell membranes and are not able to move.

Survival of Hatchings. Altricial bird hatchings are dependent on their parents for warmth, protection, and nourishment. Some birds are poor parents, which may be related to their age, presence of other birds, nest disturbances, and neurological disorders and other diseases. The parental care necessary for the successful rearing of the progeny may not be provided, so some or all may die.

In precocial birds, the environment must be suitable for the survival of the young birds; warmth, shelter, and suitable feed and water are necessary. It has been shown that the viability of chicks is related to the age of the hens laying the eggs and is probably dependent on egg size (McNaughton et al. 1978). Young birds are highly susceptible to cold stress. A delay in placement after hatching can significantly increase chick mortality (Fanguy et al. 1980). Mortality can also be substantial if inappropriate feed is made available for birds (e.g., quail chicks cannot handle turkey breeder pellets).

Many infectious diseases can cause significant early losses. In some cases these may be directly linked to the parent stock (trichomoniasis in pigeons and Budgerigars, mycoplasmosis), while in other cases the link is more tenuous (salmonellosis, colibacillosis). Other diseases are enzootic in the population, and therefore infection of the young birds is likely to occur (parasitism, pox, Pacheco's disease, pigeon herpesvirus, chlamydiosis, yersiniosis).

Attainment of Successful Sexual Maturity. In leukosis infection of domestic fowl, total egg production of progeny of infected hens is less than that of noninfected hens (Gavora et al. 1980). In other situations congenital or genetic defects, such as cerebellar degeneration of chickens (Markson et al. 1959) and related conditions in psittacines, may render the progeny infertile, thus limiting or preventing carryover of that trait into succeeding generations.

References

Arnall, L., and I. F. Keymer. 1975. Surgery. In *Bird Diseases*, ed. L. Arnall and I. F. Keymer, pp. 401–40. London: Baillière Tindall.

Arundel, J. H., J. L. Kingston, and P. J. Kerr. 1980. *Prosthogonimus pellucidus* in domestic poultry. *Aust. Vet. J.* 56:460.

Beach, J. E. 1962. Diseases of Budgerigars and other cage birds: A survey of post-mortem findings. Part II. *Vet. Rec.* 74:63–68.

Bisgaard, M., and A. Dam. 1980. Salpingitis of poultry. I. Prevalence, bacteriology and possible pathogenesis in broilers. *Nord. Vet. Med.* 32:361–68.

Blackmore, D. K. 1966. The clinical approach to tumours in cage birds. I. The pathology and incidence of neoplasia in cage birds. *J. Small Anim. Pract.* 7:217–23.

Burmester, B. R., R. F. Gentry, and N. F. Waters. 1955. The presence of the virus of visceral lymphomatosis in embryonated eggs of normal appearing hens. *Poult. Sci.* 34:609–17.

Campbell, J. G. 1969. Tumours of epithelial tissues. In *Tumours of the Fowl*, ed. J. G. Campbell. London: William Heinemann Medical Books.

Crinion, R. A. P., R. A. Ball, and M. S. Hofstad. 1971. Pathogenesis of oviduct lesions in immature chickens following exposure to infectious bronchitis virus at one day old. *Avian Dis.* 15:32–48.

Davis, H. J., L. C. Norris, and G. F. Heuser. 1938. Further evidence on the amount of vitamin G required for reproduction in poultry. *Poult. Sci.* 17:87–93.

Fanguy, R. C., L. K. Misra, K. V. Vo, C. C. Blohowick, and W. F. Kruger. 1980. Effect of delayed placement on mortality and growth performance of commercial broilers. *Poult. Sci.* 59:1215–20.

Fenwick, G. R., C. L. Curl, A. W. Pearson, and E. J. Butler. 1981. Production of egg taint by fish meal. *Vet. Rec.* 109:292.

Gavora, J. S., J. L. Spencer, R. S. Gowe, and D. L. Harris. 1980. Lymphoid leukosis virus infection: Effects on production and mortality and consequences in selection for high egg production. *Poult. Sci.* 59:2165–78.

Gilbert, A. B., M. M. Perry, D. Waddington, and M. A. Hardie. 1983. Role of atresia in establishing the follicular hierarchy in the ovary of the domestic hen (*Gallus domesticus*). *J. Reprod. Fert.* 69:221–27.

Haritani, M., H. Kajigaya, T. Akashi, M. Kamemura, N. Tanahara, M. Umeda, M. Sugiyama, M. Isoda, and C. Kato. 1984. A study on the origin of adenocarcinoma in fowls using immunohistological technique. *Avian Dis.* 28:1130–34.

Hasholt, J. 1966. Diseases of the female reproductive organs of pet birds. *J. Small Anim. Pract.* 7:313–20.

Hudson, C. B., and J. A. Pino. 1952. Physiological disturbance of the reproductive system in White Leghorn cockerels following the feeding of Enheptin. *Poult. Sci.* 31:1017–22.

Hungerford, T. G. 1969. *Diseases of Poultry, Including Cage Birds and Pigeons.* 4th ed. Sydney, Aust.: Angus and Robertson.

Jones, H. G. R., and D. M. Owens. 1981. Reproductive tract lesions of the laying fowl with particular reference to bacterial infection. *Vet. Rec.* 108:36–37.

Keymer, I. F. 1980. Disorders of the avian female reproductive system. *Avian Pathol.* 9:405–19.

King, A. S., and J. McLelland. 1975. *Outlines of Avian Anatomy.* London: Baillière Tindall.

Kingston, N. 1984. Trematodes. In *Diseases of Poultry*, 8th ed., ed. M. S. Hofstad, H. J. Barnes, B. W. Colnek, W. M. Reid, and H. W. Yoder, Jr., pp. 668–90. Ames: Iowa State University Press.

Koch, T. 1973. *Anatomy of the Chicken and Domestic Birds*, ed. and trans. B. H. Skold and L. DeVries. Ames: Iowa State University Press.

McClary, C. F. 1955. The restriction of ooporphyrin deposition on egg shells by drug feeding. *Poult. Sci.* 34:1164–65.

McClenaghan, M., J. M. Bradbury, and J. N. Howse. 1981. Embryo mortality associated with avian mycoplasma serotype 1. *Vet. Rec.* 108:459–60.

McNaughton, J. L., J. W. Deaton, F. N. Reece, and R. L. Haynes. 1978. Effect of age of parents and hatching egg weight on broiler chick mortality. *Poult. Sci.* 57:38–44.

Markson, L. M., R. B. A. Carnaghan, and G. B. Young. 1959. Familial cerebellar degeneration and atrophy: A sex-linked disease affecting Light Sussex pullets. *J. Comp. Pathol.* 69:223–30.

Marvan, F., E. Vernerova, and M. Lavickova. 1983. Inflammation of the copulatory organs in geese from the spermatogenesis and therapy point of view. *Biol. Chem. Vet. (Praha)* 19:355–62.

Nalivaiko, L. I. 1983. A disease of the genital organs of geese caused by species of *Neisseria. Veterinariia (Moskva)* 10:60–61.

Petrak, M. L., and C. E. Gilmore. 1969. Neoplasms. In *Diseases of Cage and Aviary Birds*, ed. M. L. Petrak. Philadelphia: Lea and Febiger.

Reece, R. L., and P. T. Hooper. 1984. Toxicity in utility pigeons caused by the coccidiostat dinitolmide (3,5-dinitro-ortho-toluamide). *Aust. Vet. J.* 61:259–60.

Rosskopf, W. J., and R. W. Woerpel. 1984. Egg binding in caged and aviary birds. *Vet. Med. Small Anim. Clin.* 79:437.

Schivanandappa, T., M. K. Krishnakumari, and S. K. Majumder. 1983. Testicular atrophy in *Gallus domesticus* fed acute doses of copper fungicides. *Poult. Sci.* 62:405–8.

Schultz, D. J. 1981. Reproductive system. In *Refresher*

Course for Veterinarians on Aviary and Caged Birds, pp. 584–89. University of Sydney, Post-Graduate Committee in Veterinary Science, Proceedings no. 55. Sydney, Aust.

Uhrin, V. 1984. Follicle atresia in the growing ovary of fowl. *Vet. Med. (Praha)* 29(3):181–88.

van Drimmelen, G. C. 1951. Artificial insemination of birds by the intraperitoneal route: A study in sex physiology of pigeons and fowls with reports upon a modified technique of semen collection, a new technique of insemination, and observations on the spermatozoa in the genital organs of the fowl hen. *Onderstepoort J. Vet. Res.* (Suppl. no. 1):1–212.

van Eck, J. H. H., L. Elenbaas, P. Wensvoort, and B. Kouwenhoven. 1978. Histopathological changes in the oviduct of hens producing shell-less eggs associated with precipitins to adenovirus. *Avian Pathol.* 7:279–87.

Wood-Gush, D. G. M., and A. B. Gilbert. 1970. The rate of egg loss through internal laying. *Br. Poult. Sci.* 11:161–63.

Yates, V. J., and E. F. Fry. 1957. Observations on a chicken embryo lethal orphan (CELO) virus. *Am. J. Vet. Res.* 18:657–60.

Yoder, H. W., Jr., and M. S. Hofstad. 1965. Evaluation of tylosin in preventing egg transmission of *Mycoplasma gallisepticum* in chickens. *Avian Dis.* 9:291–301.

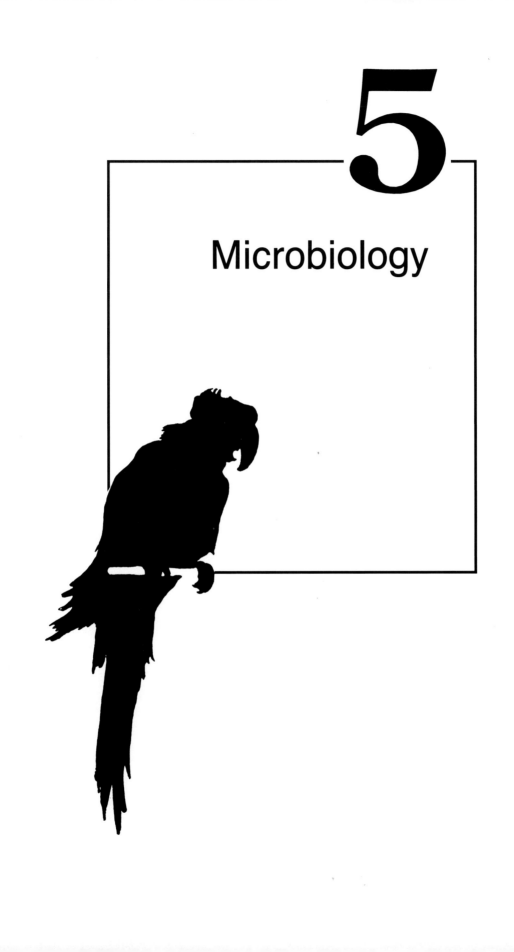

5

Microbiology

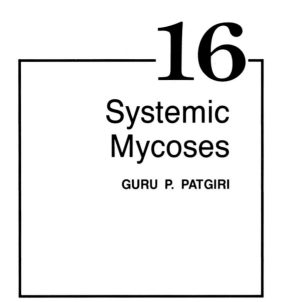

16

Systemic Mycoses

GURU P. PATGIRI

FUNGAL INFECTIONS were among the first diseases of birds to be discovered. Aspergillosis was observed in the air sac of a wild scaup duck (*Aythya marila*) as early as 1813 and in a captive flamingo in 1833. Since then, numerous reports of fungal infections in various species of birds have appeared (Fowler 1978). In recent years fungal infections in free-living as well as captive birds have been reported.

The vast majority of fungi and their spores are ubiquitous, existing as saprophytes in the environment and as parasites of plants, mammals, and birds. Fungi require suitable nutrients, temperature, humidity, and protection from direct light for their growth. These requirements are provided by warm-blooded birds and other animals. Fungi are aerobic, gaining their oxygen requirement from the air and the body of the host. Fortunately only a few species of fungi are known to be pathogenic to birds. Most fungi are soil inhabiting and noncontagious; only a few are highly contagious and passed from animal to animal with or without resorting to a soil-inhabiting phase. Birds acquire infection from soil, decaying keratinized animal tissue, and dung. Free-living wild birds are less likely to acquire fungal infections because they are devoid of predisposing factors, such as poor sanitation, capture, change in food habits, malnutrition, and other physiological stress problems that can affect caged birds (Arnall and Keymer 1975). Another problem of caged birds is that continuous and indiscriminate use of antibiotics favors the establishment of mycotic infections.

Two groups of mycoses can be recognized: the superficial (dermatophytes), which are almost always contagious, and the systemic, in which the contagion plays only a minor role.

The superficial fungi are described in Chapter 8.

Aspergillosis. In avian species, aspergillosis (syn.: brooder pneumonia, pseudotuberculosis, bronchomycosis, cytomycosis, chick fever) is commonly caused by *Aspergillus fumigatus.* Aspergillosis has been described in a variety of captive and free-living birds, being particularly common in penguins, waterfowl, flamingos, and recently captured wild birds (Burr 1981). Newly imported birds are at high risk if they have been subjected to adverse management conditions. Stress factors include capture, transport, dietary change, trauma, surgery, and debilitating conditions. In free-flying psittacines and passerines, aspergillosis can be influenced by prevailing weather and climate (Jungerman and Schwartzman 1972; Burr 1981).

The disease is mainly contracted by inhalation of spores or hyphal fragments. Ingestion of a large number of spores may also lead to the disease. Contaminated seeds, chaff, hay, and straw and other dirty materials are a good source of the disease. *A. fumigatus* exists as a saprophyte but can also live as a parasite. Other species of *Aspergillus,* notably *A. flavus, A. nidulans,* and *A. terreus,* have also been isolated from captive and wild birds (Keymer 1969) (see also Chapter 32).

Debilitated, weak, and overcrowded birds are most prone to infection. The nestlings and older birds therefore are the first to contract the disease. *Aspergillus* spp. can also attack fresh and incubating eggs by penetrating through the pores of the shell, killing the embryo (O'Meara and Witter 1971).

Clinical Signs. Aspergillosis is an acute or chronic infection usually affecting the respiratory tract and occasionally the peritoneum and abdominal organs. Affected birds exhibit gasping, labored and rapid breathing, anorexia, and emaciation. Difficulty in mucus movement in the trachea results in gurgling sounds. In later stages of infection, diarrhea, ataxia, and other nervous symptoms develop. The disease is usually fatal within a few days in young birds. However, death may follow without showing any characteristic clinical changes. In adult psittacines and some other species, the disease course may progress for weeks.

Fungal mycelia penetrate the bronchial walls and parenchyma, where they multiply and branch. Combining with tissue exudates, they tend to block air passages and fill the air sacs. Radiating hyphae often form a nodule (plaque) over which a capsule is formed. These are seen by the naked eye as yellow, green, or bluish plaques in the lung, air sacs, and other organs. The consistency of the plaques may be spongy, soft, or hard. Plaques are frequently loosely attached to the organs; only occasionally are firm adhesions seen. Extensive plaque formation may result in severe tissue changes in affected organs (pleurisy, cirrhosis). Abscess formation and peritonitis are seen with abdominal adhesions.

Diagnosis. Suggestive diagnosis of aspergillosis in birds is made by the detection of plaques in the lung, air sacs, and other organs. The demonstration of septate hyphae can be made directly by examining crushed plaques in 10–20% potassium hydroxide (KOH). Confirmation of a fungal infection is made by culturing fungi on a suitable medium. Sabouraud's dextrose agar containing antibiotics is commonly used for fungal isolation. Histological examination of tissue sections should be carried out to identify aspergillus hyphae as well as to demonstrate tissue damage.

Treatment and Control. Captive birds can occasionally be treated by using fungicides in the feed or by injection. Injection consists of a mixture of amphotericin B at 1 mg/kg body weight to treat the primary infection and chloramphenicol at 75 mg/kg body weight to combat secondary bacterial infections; 100,000 IU nystatin is given once daily subcutaneously to combat secondary fungal infections. The total volume should not exceed 3 ml/kg body weight.

Birds showing diarrhea and vomiting should be administered 5% dextrose, four doses daily, at the rate of 4% body weight, to maintain hydration. Recent studies using miconazole indicate its effectiveness in treating fungal infection, but dosage rates have not been formulated.

When an outbreak occurs, all litter from a contaminated cage should be removed and a suitable disinfectant or fungicide sprayed over the area. Feed and water utensils should also be properly cleaned to avoid mold accumulation. Old feed should be discarded and potassium iodine placed in the drinking water. Incubators must be cleaned and disinfected between hatches and eggs candled before incubation to remove infertile or dead embryos. Birds living in a planted aviary free from loose litter and debris are least likely to contract the disease. To prevent disease occurrence, attention should be given to a high standard of nutrition and the proper hygiene and housing of cage and aviary birds.

Candidiasis. Candidiasis (syn.: moniliasis, oidiomycosis, crop mycosis, sour crop, thrush, muguet, soor, levurosis) is caused by the yeast *Candida albicans*. Like many bacteria, yeasts are ubiquitous in nature and live as commensals in the skin, mouth, and alimentary tracts of warm-blooded animals and birds. Candidiasis has been reported from a variety of bird species, including turkeys, chickens, pigeons, geese, pheasants, parrots, quails, ruffed grouse, herring gulls, partridges, and jackdaws (Austwick 1968). Some factors (prolonged antibiotic therapy, feeding a high level of carbohydrates, vitamin deficiencies) predispose birds to infection. The disease is commonly contracted by ingestion of *C. albicans* in the feed and water. Outbreaks of candidiasis have been reported, but most commonly infections occur in individual birds.

Clinical Signs. The initial clinical sign of candidiasis in birds is unthriftiness and listlessness. Young birds are most susceptible to the disease. The disease is characterized by the formation of necrotic pseudomembranous patches over the mucosa of tongue, pharynx, and crop. These patches of dead epithelial tissues can be easily scraped off the mucous membranes. The mucosae are often thickened, raised, corrugated, and white and look like terry cloth (Fig. 16.1). Advanced candidiasis in ratites (emus,

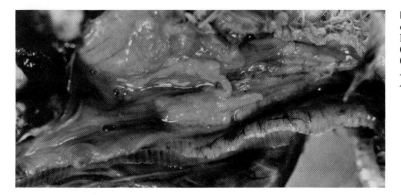

Fig. 16.1. Candidial esophagitis in a young, hand-reared Little Corella (*Cacatua sanguinea*). (*Courtesy of David J. Schultz, Hawthorn, South Australia, Aust.*)

rheas, cassowaries, ostriches) is associated with the development of a yellowish pseudomembrane on the oral muscosa, extensive necrosis of the upper beak with concurrent beak deformity, poor growth, unthrifty appearance, and listlessness (Dolensek and Bruning 1978). Candidiasis may result in beak deformities (especially in adult parrots and soft-bills) (Fig. 16.2), frequently secondary to impaction with soft mushy foods (Burmeister et al. 1972). These lesions give rise to mechanical impairment, causing difficulty in swallowing and breathing. Eating and maintenance of appetite are difficult, and some affected birds regurgitate their food. A mouth-rot-like syndrome may eventually develop and destroy the tongue, leading to fatal starvation (Fig. 16.3). Characteristic lesions may also be present in the proventriculus and intestine of infected birds. Occasionally the disease is found around the commissures of the mouth and on the feather follicles of the head, back, and underside.

Diagnosis. Commonly, characteristic lesions are observed in the mouth of an infected bird. Without laboratory procedures, the crustlike lesions may be difficult to differentiate from bacterial and parasitic infections. Initial diagnosis of a fungal infection can be made by using a wet crush mount. For this, a scraping of deep tissue from the lesion is made and treated with 10–20% KOH. Diagnosis is easily made by plating a piece of necrotic tissue on Sabouraud's dextrose agar containing antibiotics. The site where material is removed is treated with 2% iodine to reduce surface contaminants. The presence of yeastlike cells and occasional budding indicates a *Candida* infection. Histological examination of the affected tissue may be warranted for positive diagnosis.

Treatment and Control. Cage and aviary birds can be treated effectively with nystatin at 10,000 IU/kg body weight twice a day in the feed or drinking water. This should be followed by diet supplementation with an adequate quantity of vitamins A and B and reducing the carbohydrate level of the feed. Amphotericin B lotion may be used for feather infections. Amphotericin B at 1 mg/day orally, griseofulvin at 125 mg/kg body weight orally once a day, and 5-fluorocystosine at 100 mg/kg body weight orally twice a day are other effective treatments.

Unsanitary housing, overcrowding, dirty utensils, and litter are all factors that contribute to an outbreak. All footwear should be disinfected before visiting an infected flock to prevent spread of the disease. Isolation and quarantine of new stock and of suspected or known

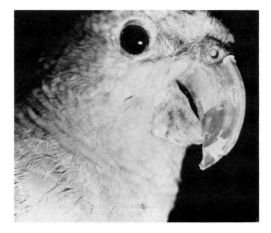

Fig. 16.2. Orange-winged Amazon Parrot (*Amazona amazonica*) with candidiasis. The growth plate of the lower mandible has been damaged, resulting in disfiguration and hyperplastic tissue growth. (*Courtesy of Walter J. Rosskopf, Jr., Hawthorne, Calif.*)

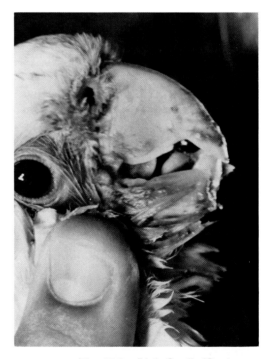

Fig. 16.3. Little Corella (*Cacatua sanguinea*) with candidiasis. Oral discharge adhering to the beak was the first clinical sign of the disease. (*Courtesy of David J. Schultz, Hawthorn, South Australia, Aust.*)

infected birds should always be practiced. The spraying of 2–5% formic acid at the rate of 20 ml/100 g food minimizes mortality.

Mucormycosis. Mucormycosis (syn.: phycomycosis, zygomycosis) is rare among birds but may occur secondarily to malnutrition and other debilitating diseases. Prolonged antibiotic therapy predisposes birds to infection. The most common species involved is *Absidia corymbifera* (Burr 1972). The disease has been reported in African Gray Parrots, horned owls, flamingos, and penguins.

Clinical Signs. Mucormycotic infections may exhibit lesions confined to the lung, air sacs, kidney, and myocardium or may follow a disseminated form. Sometimes exudative and granulomatous lesions are observed in the tongue. The thickened growth on the tongue may occlude the oral cavity and thus starve the bird.

Diagnosis. Diagnosis can be made by a wet crush mount of the affected tissue in a 10–20% solution of KOH. A piece of granulomatous tissue is placed on suitable mycological media for fungal identification (Fig. 16.4). The presence of nonseptate mycelia in the mount confirms the diagnosis. Histological examination of affected tissue should be carried out for positive diagnosis and determination of tissue damage.

Treatment. There is no effective treatment or control for mucormycosis in birds. Amphotericin B may be tried since the drug was found effective in suppressing the development of phy-

comycosis in experimental animals. It is advisable to practice good hygiene and supply adequate nutrition to prevent recurrence.

Gizzard Malfunction Syndrome. Fungal mycelia of several species have been found penetrating the koilin layer, the epithelium, and even the muscle in a small number of Australian parrots and finches. Diagnosis, if possible, depends on finding fungal elements in feces. Treatment of a gizzard fungal condition may best be attempted by a systemic fungicide, such as amphotericin at 0.075 mg/100 g body weight intravenously once a day for 4 days. Nystatin and amphotericin are poorly absorbed from the seedeater's gut; therefore adequate penetration into the deeper layers of the gut or gizzard is difficult and outbreaks may recur.

Toxicoses. Aflatoxicosis (T-2 toxin) may be caused by *Fusarium tricinctum,* which is commonly found in moldy feed (Burmeister 1971; Burmeister et al. 1972). Other causes of aflatoxicosis are discussed in Chapter 32.

Clinical Signs. Small concentrations of T-2 toxin (4–16 μg/g) in the feed of broiler chickens caused dose-related lesions in the mouth of birds (Wyatt et al. 1972). The gross lesions appeared as raised yellowish white areas and microscopically as a fibrous surface layer with intermediate layers (invaginations) filled with rods and cocci and a heavy infiltration of the underlying tissue with granular leucocytes. Mouth secretion of affected birds may contain greatly increased numbers of bacteria, including *Staphylococcus epidermidis* and *E. coli,* which often prove

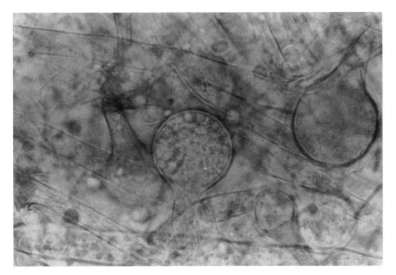

Fig. 16.4. Conidia and conidial spores of the fungus *Absidia corymbifera* isolated from tissue taken from the buccal cavity of an African Gray Parrot (*Psittacus erithacus*). (*From Burr et al. 1982, by permission*)

avirulent when inoculated into scarified tissue of control birds (Wyatt et al. 1972). In experimental birds, T-2 toxin in small concentrations caused a relative decrease in the weight of the spleen and the bursa of Fabricius and a relative increase in the weight of the pancreas and crop (Wyatt et al. 1973a). T-2 toxin has also been found to cause abnormal wing positioning, hysteroid seizures, and impaired righting reflex in young chickens (Wyatt et al. 1973a). Other investigators found T-2 toxin caused dose-related abnormal feathering in chickens, characterized by sparse, short feathers protruding at odd angles, missing feathers, and altered feather shape (Wyatt et al. 1973b). Aflatoxins may also produce a palpable liver with or without ascites.

Diagnosis. Serum albumin levels are usually low. Abdominocentesis may exhibit a straw-colored fluid with minimal cellular content if hepatomegaly is present (Fig. 16.5) (Schultz 1984). Histological examination of the liver must be used to differentiate between a fibrotic fat-infiltrated liver and the hepatocyte necrosis with bile duct proliferation caused by aflatoxin. Liver biopsy is feasible, even in Budgerigars, as the fibrotic liver bleeds minimally and the edges can be effectively sutured together. Removal of ascitic fluid makes a bird more comfortable before surgery, as well as a better surgical risk.

Treatment. Treatment of aflatoxicosis involves low-dose steroids, such as dexamethasone at 0.1 mg/100 g body weight once a day for 3 days. Supportive therapy includes vitamin B complex and a reduction of sunflower seeds. Control may be difficult to achieve if the source of toxin cannot be traced. Most seeds produce an abundance of fungi when damp for any length of time, so cage floors must be kept clean since psittacines and other bird orders readily seek out germinating seeds on aviary floors.

References

Arnall, L., and I. F. Keymer. 1975. *Bird Diseases.* London: Baillière Tindall.
Austwick, P. K. C. 1968. Mycotic infections. *Symp. Zool. Soc. Lond.* 24:249–71.
Burmeister, H. R. 1971. T-2 toxin production by *Fusarium tricinctum* on solid substrate. *Appl. Microbiol.* 21:739–42.
Burmeister, H. R., J. J. Ellis, and C. W. Hesseltine. 1972. Survey for fusaria that elaborate T-2 toxin. *Appl. Microbiol.* 23:1165–66.
Burr, E. W. 1981. Enzootic aspergillosis in wild Red-vented Cockatoos in the Philippines. *Mycopathologia* 73:21–23.

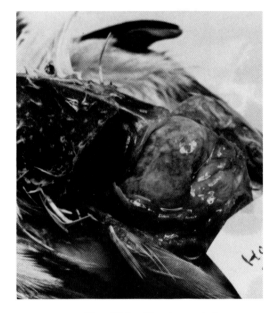

Fig. 16.5. Hepatomegaly in a Budgerigar (*Melopsittacus undulatus*) due to aflatoxicosis. (*Courtesy of David J. Schultz, Hawthorn, South Australia, Aust.*)

Burr, E. W., F. W. Huckzermeyer, and B. v. d. Made. 1982. Mucormycosis in a parrot. *Mod. Vet. Pract.* 63:961–62.
Dolensek, E., and D. Bruning. 1978. Ratites (Struthioniformes, Rheiformes and Casuariiformes). In *Zoo and Wild Animal Medicine,* ed. M. E. Fowler, pp. 165–80. Philadelphia: W. B. Saunders.
Fowler, M. E. 1978. Special Medicine: Birds. In *Zoo and Wild Animal Medicine,* ed. M. E. Fowler, pp. 323–34. Philadelphia: W. B. Saunders.
Jungerman, P. F., and R. M. Schwartzman. 1972. *Veterinary Medical Mycology.* Philadelphia: Lea and Febiger.
Keymer, I. F. 1969. Mycoses. In *Diseases of Cage and Aviary Birds,* ed. M. L. Petrak, pp. 453–58. Philadelphia: Lea and Febiger.
O'Meara, D. C., and J. Witter. 1971. Aspergillosis. In *Infectious and Parasitic Diseases of Wild Birds,* ed. J. N. Davis, R. C. Anderson, L. Kerstad, and D. O. Trainer. Ames: Iowa State University Press.
Schultz, D. J. 1984. Unpublished data.
Wyatt, R. D., P. B. Hamilton, and H. R. Burmeister. 1973a. The effects of T-2 toxin in broiler chickens. *Poult. Sci.* 52:1853–59.
Wyatt, R. D., W. M. Colwell, P. B. Hamilton, and H. R. Burmeister. 1973b. Neural disturbances in chickens caused by dietary T-2 toxin. *Appl. Microbiol.* 26:757–61.
Wyatt, R. D., B. A. Weeks, P. B. Hamilton, and H. R. Burmeister. 1972. Severe oral lesions in chickens caused by ingestion of dietary fusaritoxin T. *Appl. Microbiol.* 24(2):251–57.

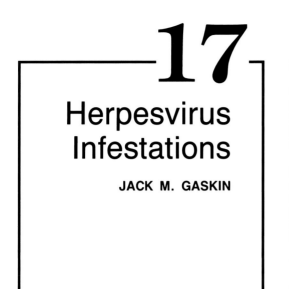

17

Herpesvirus
Infestations

JACK M. GASKIN

ALTHOUGH herpesviruses are known to be pathogens for domestic poultry and account for diseases such as infectious laryngotracheitis, duck virus enteritis, and Marek's disease, few herpesvirus infections of exotic and caged birds have been described. This may reflect inadequate research and documentation rather than an actual lack of such infections since many outbreaks of disease in caged birds are not thoroughly investigated. Herpesvirus infections have been described in raptors, parrots, pigeons, cranes, and cormorants. In psittacines, three distinct herpesvirus infections have been reported. Pacheco's disease is best known, but there are descriptions of an infectious laryngotracheitislike herpesvirus that affects amazon parrots and of a herpesvirus of Budgerigars that is harbored predominantly in the feathers and may cause decreased hatchability of eggs (Gerlach 1984).

Because there is such a vast array of avian species, it is often difficult to assess the pathogenicity of a herpesvirus of one species for birds of another species without experimental inoculations. For example, infectious laryngotracheitis is principally a disease of chickens but has been reported in pheasants and peafowl; turkeys can be experimentally infected when young but are refractory as adults, and quail, guinea fowl, and nongalliform birds resist infection. In another example, pigeon herpesvirus (PHV) is experimentally pathogenic for some parrots and causes a disease very similar to Pacheco's disease, a naturally occurring herpesvirus infection of psittacines. Whenever different avian species are housed in close proximity, the possibility exists for exchange of viruses and the development of disease.

Etiology. Herpesviruses are medium-sized viruses (70–150 nm in diameter) that contain deoxyribonucleic acid (DNA) as genetic material. Since they are surrounded by a lipoprotein envelope, they usually are readily destroyed by the effects of sunlight, drying, and disinfectants with surface-active properties.

Generally, herpesviruses that affect one species of birds may cause disease in other species in that taxonomic order but do not affect species in other orders. A dramatic exception is pigeon herpesvirus, which may cause naturally occurring fatal infections in raptors (owls, hawks, falcons) that eat infected pigeons.

Transmission. Herpesviruses are noted for their ability to cause latent infections in birds that survive the initial encounter with them. A latent infection is one in which the infected bird shows no clinical evidence of infection but may periodically shed virus during times of stress. Latently infected birds are often referred to as carriers since they serve as a source of infection for disease outbreaks. They are responsible for initiating disease in other susceptible birds but usually show no illness themselves.

In several mammalian herpesvirus infections, latently infected animals have been demonstrated to maintain virus in a noninfectious state in nerve ganglion cells. In times of stress, the virus infection is reactivated, and infectious virus moves down nerve trunks from the ganglion cells to be shed in small quantities in secretions and excretions of the carrier animal. Susceptible animals that encounter the virus become sick, shed large quantities of virus, and thereby amplify the possibility that other susceptibles will become exposed. This same phenomenon has been demonstrated in duck virus enteritis (duck plague) and undoubtedly occurs in other avian herpesvirus infections.

Since PHV primarily causes fatal infections in squabs less than 6 months of age, it is likely that adult pigeons that are asymptomatic carriers of the virus may initiate infections through regurgitation feeding. Introduction of PHV via carrier birds to pigeon lofts that have never been exposed to the infection may cause mortality in adult as well as young pigeons.

In Pacheco's disease, latently infected carriers initiate infection, and acutely ill birds shed large quantities of virus in pharyngeal secretions and in droppings. Contamination of food and water with infective droppings probably accounts for the rapid transmission to susceptible cage mates. Contact and aerosol transmission undoubtedly also occur. Many outbreaks of Pacheco's disease occur during cold weather; thus cold stress seems to be a major factor in initiat-

ing virus shedding by carrier birds. Other outbreaks have accompanied the introduction of
new birds into an aviary. Under these circumstances, the stressing factor is socialization and
the establishment of a pecking order.

Clinical Signs. Pigeons affected with PHV develop an illness characterized by listlessness, loss of appetite, dyspnea, and ocular and
nasal discharge. The disease causes a mortality
rate of up to 50% and is most severe in birds
less than 6 months of age. Examination of the
organs of dead squabs may reveal pale foci on
the livers and spleens (focal necrosis) as well as
diphtheritic laryngitis and esophagitis.

Another herpesvirus infection of pigeons
has recently been described from the Middle
East. Pigeon herpes encephalomyelitis virus
(PHEV) was recovered from pigeons that consistently showed nervous signs a few days prior
to death. Depression, inappetence, and inability
to fly was followed by paresis and/or paralysis of
the extremities. Head tremor, circling movements, torticollis, and greenish diarrhea were
also observed. The morbidity rate was over 50%
in some flocks, with death occurring in over
90% of the affected birds. PHEV was noted to
differ from PHV in that it produces smaller lesions on the chorioallantoic membranes of experimentally inoculated embryonated hen's
eggs. PHEV is also more rapidly fatal to the
embryos and causes primarily nervous rather
than respiratory signs in affected pigeons. Necropsy findings in PHEV infections include visceral congestion and microscopic lesions
(neuronal degeneration and multifocal gliosis) in
the central nervous system. Although the signs
and lesions of PHV and PHEV differ, no serological studies have been done to determine if
they are different herpesviruses or merely
pathogenic variants of the same virus.

With Pacheco's disease the signs of illness
vary to some degree with the species of psittacine affected. Smaller psittacines (lovebirds,
parakeets, *Pionus* spp.), amazons, and cockatoos
often die acutely after showing minimal signs of
illness. They continue to eat and drink and may
be obviously weak and listless for only a matter
of hours prior to death. Some larger psittacines,
especially macaws, may become visibly ill, exhibiting lethargy, regurgitation, and diarrhea
with a distinctive orange coloration. These birds
may also show increased thirst, and some may
recover. The course of Pacheco's disease may be
as short as 5 days or as long as several weeks.
Usually it is an acute, rapidly fatal infection.

Sudden deaths in a group of psittacines are
suggestive of Pacheco's disease, but a specific
diagnosis often requires laboratory assistance.

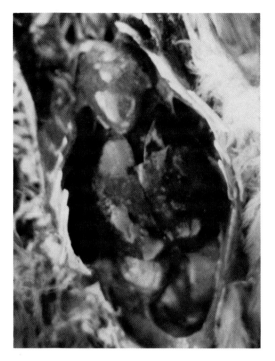

Fig. 17.1. Severe liver lesions
exhibiting focal necrosis in a Monk
Parakeet dead of Pacheco's disease.

Mottling (due to focal necrosis) may be observed on the livers and spleens of dead birds
(Fig. 17.1), but birds that have died abruptly
may exhibit no gross lesions. Histopathologic
recognition of viral intranuclear inclusions in
liver lesions, electron microscopic examination
of liver lesions for direct visualization of the herpesvirus (Figs. 17.2 and 17.3), or recovery of
virus from organ suspensions in fertile hen's
eggs or chick embryo cell cultures are laboratory methods to confirm the diagnosis.

Epidemiology. The propensity of herpesviruses
to produce latent infections in some birds
that survive exposure makes their epidemiology
particularly intriguing. The carrier birds may
show no signs of disease yet shed virus under
various stressing influences, thereby exposing
other susceptible birds and resulting in a disease
outbreak. The ramifications of this virus-host interaction is the same for all avian herpesviruses
but is best illustrated by Pacheco's disease.

Although Pacheco's disease was first
described in psittacines from Brazil and is usually associated with species of Central and
South American origin, psittacine varieties from
around the world are susceptible. Presently it is

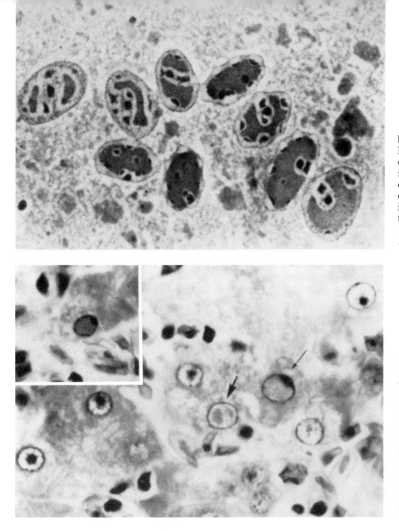

Fig. 17.2. Chick embryo kidney cells containing eosinophilic intranuclear inclusion bodies characteristic of Pacheco's disease 48 hours after inoculation with parrot tissue suspension. (H & E. ×700) (*From Randall et al. 1979, by permission*)

Fig. 17.3. Section of a parrot liver with eosinophilic intranuclear inclusion bodies in the hepatocytes characteristic of Pacheco's disease. Visible are a rare halo (*large arrow*) and beading of chromatin (*small arrow*). (H & E. ×700) Inset: Solid basophilically staining intranuclear inclusion body in hepatocyte. (×1200) (*From Randall et al. 1979, by permission*)

not known whether psittacines of Pacific or Afro-Asian distribution have their own herpesvirus infections caused by viruses serologically different from South American strains, but diseases similar to Pacheco's disease have been reported in native birds in Africa and New Zealand. It also is not resolved whether more than one serotype of Pacheco's herpesvirus occurs in the western hemisphere. In limited studies only one serotype has been recognized so far.

Outbreaks of Pacheco's disease in the United States have usually occurred between November and February. Because of the reversal of seasons in the northern and southern hemispheres, young susceptible birds are captured during the summer months in South America and shipped to the northern hemisphere, where it is winter. The stress of shipping, accompanied by abrupt changes in climatic conditions, results in virus shedding by carrier birds. Spread of infection is potentiated under conditions of crowding at quarantine stations and import holding facilities where Pacheco's disease is most devastating.

Considerable variation occurs among psittacine species with regard to the severity of the disease. Most amazon parrots (*Amazona* spp.) are highly susceptible, and 100% mortality is not unusual. African Gray Parrots (*Psittacus erithacus*), Senegal Parrots (*Poicephalus senegalus*), Monk Parakeets (*Myiopsitta monachus*), lovebirds (*Agapornis* spp.), macaws (*Ara* spp.), cockatoos (*Cacatua* spp.), Cockatiels (*Nymphicus hollandicus*), parakeets (e.g., Canary-winged, *Brotogeris;* Red-rumped, *Psephotus*), and Budgerigars (*Melopsittacus undulatus*) are also highly susceptible.

Among conures there is a great variation in susceptibility. Orange-winged or Half-Moon Conures (*Aratinga canicularis*) suffer losses approaching 100% while White-eyed Conures (*A. leucophthalmus*), Maroon-bellied Conures (*Pyrrhura frontalis*), and others are less severely affected. Some species of conures show little or no mortality while other psittacines in contact with them are dying in large numbers. The Patagonian Conure (*Cyanoliseus patagonus*) and the Nanday Conure (*Nandayus nenday*), for example, are seldom affected by Pacheco's disease. Nevertheless, there are some reports that implicate these species as possible sources of introduction of the disease.

Control. Although there are commercial vaccines for certain herpesviral diseases of domestic poultry (Marek's disease, infectious laryngotracheitis, duck virus enteritis), no vaccines are available for the known herpesvirus infections of caged and aviary birds. Since the different herpesviruses are serologically distinct, vaccination with the products designed for poultry would be of little value for aviary birds.

Research has indicated that vaccination against Pacheco's disease is feasible. Inactivated vaccines with adjuvants have been effective under experimental conditions and would be safe for all psittacine species. Whether they would be effective in protecting birds under the rigorously stressful conditions encountered in the import trade has not yet been resolved. Commercially useful vaccines against herpesviruses of domestic poultry are of the modified live virus type. A modified live vaccine for Pacheco's disease is being sought by a number of research groups and would provide ease in protecting birds since one administration might be effective. Because of the varying susceptibilities of different psittacine species, however, such a vaccine would require extensive testing to assure that it was safe for all varieties. In addition, if future research indicates that there is more than one serotype of Pacheco's disease virus, multivalent vaccines would be necessary to ensure protection.

Without the benefit of vaccines, the aviculturist must rely on strict sanitation and good husbandry procedures to prevent or control herpesviral infections. Stressful conditions such as overcrowding must be avoided. Food and water containers should be covered to minimize fecal contamination. Daily washing and disinfection of dishes should be done, with care taken to return them to the cages from which they came. Since healthy carrier birds may introduce disease, new birds should be acquired from trusted sources only and quarantined 2–4 weeks before introduction to an established aviary. This acclimation period helps ensure that the new bird is not incubating disease and permits a gradual adjustment to the stressful conditions of a new environment. With Pacheco's disease, avoiding contact of susceptible species with possible carrier species like the Patagonian and certain other South American conures is a wise precaution.

In situations where the introduction of Pacheco's disease might be especially devastating,

yet new birds of questionable history must be introduced to an aviary, an inexpensive susceptible bird such as a Cockatiel may be used as a sentinel. The healthy sentinel bird must be housed so that it has direct exposure to the new birds, and this exposure should last for at least 1 month. With compatible species, the sentinel can be kept in the same cage; under other circumstances, the respective cages can be placed closely together and seed and water dishes interchanged on a daily basis. If the sentinel dies, laboratory confirmation of the cause of death is necessary to determine that Pacheco's disease was actually involved. The dead sentinel should be refrigerated and presented to the laboratory while still fresh.

Faced with a disease outbreak of possible herpesviral origin, the aviculturist should redouble sanitation efforts and immediately isolate exposed birds. Caging birds individually or in separate small groups can minimize disease spread and mortality. Since laboratory diagnosis may require up to several weeks, it is unwise to await laboratory confirmation before taking action.

To minimize the spread of an outbreak of Pacheco's disease, some aviculturists have recommended the incorporation of chlorhexidine into the drinking water. The disinfectant is diluted according to the manufacturer's directions and should not be used for prolonged periods (>10 days) to avoid possible toxic effects. Chlorhexidine solution given orally with vitamins, minerals, and glucose may increase the survivability of sick birds. It is administered several times a day in small quantities directly into the crop.

When the outbreak has run its course, the owner must decide what to do with the remaining birds. Some survivors may never have been exposed, while others may have recovered. Since the possibility exists that surviving birds may become carriers, care should be taken to house survivors according to species and to eliminate contact between previously exposed and newly introduced birds.

Herpesviruses are serious pathogens for avian species. Undoubtedly many herpesvirus infections of caged and aviary birds have yet to be discovered. Cooperation between aviculturists and avian disease specialists will provide the increased knowledge needed to understand and control these infections.

References

Gerlach, H. 1984. Virus diseases of pet birds. *Vet. Clin. N. Am. Small Anim. Pract.* 14:299–315.

Randall, C. J., et al. 1979. Herpesvirus infection resembling Pacheco's disease in amazon parrots. *Avian Pathol.* 8:229–38.

18

Velogenic Viscerotropic Newcastle Disease

MURRAY E. FOWLER

NEWCASTLE DISEASE (ND) is a highly contagious virus disease of birds. Four major strains of the virus (classified as a paramyxovirus) affect poultry and nondomestic birds. Velogenic viscerotropic Newcastle disease (VVND), the most virulent form, causes high morbidity and mortality in poultry (Hanson 1978), psittacines (Clubb 1984), raptors (Zuydam 1952; Chu et al. 1976), waterfowl (Cavill 1980), and other orders of birds (Mathey and Olsen 1974; Pearson and McCann 1975; Cavill 1980, 1982).

World trade in nondomestic birds has caused great alarm in the domestic poultry industry for fear that VVND (syn.: fowl pest, avian pest, avian distemper, Asiatic Newcastle disease, avian pneumoencephalitis) might be introduced into domestic flocks. These fears are reasonable; epidemics originating from nondomestic birds have cost millions of dollars to control.

Detailed histories of outbreaks throughout the world may be found in literature reviews (Hanson 1978; Cavill 1980). The avian practitioner needs to understand the epidemiology of this infection, the clinical manifestations, and how the disease may be diagnosed and controlled.

Etiology. The origin of this virus is unknown. Original isolations were made almost simultaneously in 1926 in England, Java, and Korea. Since then, VVND virus has been isolated from birds in many countries of the world.

Epidemiology

Transmission. VVND virus is spread primarily by aerosols (Hanson 1976, 1978; Clubb et al. 1980; Clubb 1984). During the incubative and clinical stages, the virus is released into the air during normal breathing. This may begin within 2 days following exposure to the virus. Dense populations of birds in confined areas are at significant risk. The virus may continue to be shed by aerosolation for several days, constituting a ready source of infection for other birds. Although sneezing and coughing occur in birds with ND, neither is necessary for expulsion of the virus from the respiratory tract of infected birds. The virus is also shed in the feces, contaminating food, water, and bedding during the acute phase of the disease (Luthgen 1975; Hanson 1978).

Infection is spread to other facilities either by virus particles adhering to the shoes and clothing of people moving from one place to another or by the transporting of birds during the incubation period. Numerous small outbreaks have occurred in the United States from a single distributor (Pearson and McCann 1975).

Lentogenic strains of ND virus have been isolated from wild migratory passerines and waterfowl in the United States (Pearson and McCann 1975). When ND virus is isolated from a cloacal swab, the strain must be typed to establish whether or not VVND virus is present.

Hosts. VVND has been reported in one or more species of eighteen of the twenty-six orders of birds. It has been recorded in most of the families of the order Psittaciformes (Cavill 1980). There is, however, variation in the susceptibility among species and even from one outbreak to another. Insufficient data are available to provide precise lists of sensitive and resistant species. Some work indicates that African psittacines may be more resistant than others (Luthgen 1975).

Passerines seem to be more resistant, but two mynahs (*Gracula religiosa* and *Acridotheres* sp.), Java Sparrows (*Padda oryzivora*), and canaries (*Serinus canarius*) have experienced mortality when exposed to VVND virus.

Reservoirs. A number of theories have been published attempting to explain the origin of the virus and how it is maintained in various regions of the world. No conclusive evidence supports any of the theories. As is common in many virus infections, there is likely a species of bird that is minimally infected with a given ND virus strain. In an evolutionary sense, this reservoir species evolved with the virus, adjusting to the extent that the virus did not destroy its host population and the host did not totally overpower the virus. This is the "nidus concept of disease" of Pavlovsky (1966). There is a possibility that the VVND virus is a mutant, sufficiently virulent to cause mortality in previously resistant species.

Hanson (1976) postulates that VVND virus is harbored by many tropical birds in Africa, Asia, and South America. With the advent of heavy world trade in tropical species and more intensified chicken production, conditions favored the distribution and perpetuation of the infection.

The carrier state has been recognized. Amazon parrots have been known to shed virus for a full year after undergoing experimental infection (Cavill 1980). Other species, such as the Indian Hill Mynah, Budgerigar, and some conures also shed virus for long periods following infection.

Clinical Signs. Newcastle disease is rarely suspected at the onset of an illness in a bird. There are no pathognomonic signs or lesions. Other viral, bacterial, or fungal diseases may mimic ND; thus an outbreak in a flock usually has ample time to infect cage mates before a diagnosis is made. Normal husbandry practices allow spread of the virus to other birds cared for along with sick birds. When a pattern of high mortality in recently acquired birds is recognized, concern for ND arises.

The incubation period for VVND in psittacines is 3–16 days (Cavill 1980). In young birds, especially, the only sign may be a peracute disease unresponsive to antibiotic therapy and with high mortality. The degree of severity of the signs noted may be dependent on the age of the bird, virulence of the virus strain, virus dosage, species of bird infected, and high ambient temperatures. In resistant birds, anorexia and depression are early signs and the course of the disease may be quite prolonged.

In more susceptible birds, the following signs may be noted: yellowish or hemorrhagic diarrhea, coughing, sneezing, and dyspnea. The virus is pantropic, and various visceral organ system malfunctions can occur.

The central nervous system (CNS) is commonly affected, resulting in a bird that is ataxic, incoordinated, or hyperexcitable. Other CNS signs include torticollis, opisthotonus, tremors, nodding, jerking of the head, and bilateral paralysis of the limbs. Neurologic signs may persist following recovery from the primary disease. Nervous system manifestations may occur in the absence of respiratory or digestive system signs.

Diagnosis. If ND is suspected on the basis of a history of recent acquisition, high mortality, and/or CNS involvement, appropriate governmental agencies should be notified. In the United States, this is the United States Department of Agriculture, Animal Disease Eradica-

tion Branch. They conduct appropriate necropsies and submit tissues to laboratories equipped to deal with ND virus isolation and identification.

Necropsy. As with clinical signs, the lesions noted in an individual bird are of little help in establishing a diagnosis, especially in nondomestics. A composite list of lesions observed in psittacines include petechial hemorrhages of the serosa of the proventriculus, intestines, pericardium, and air sacs (Hanson 1978; Clubb et al. 1980; Cavill 1982). Petechiae may also be noted on the mucosa of the trachea. Other lesions seen are airsaculitis, hepatomegaly, and splenomegaly. These lesions are also characteristic of chlamydiosis. Gross lesions in the CNS are minimal.

Histopathologic studies are not rewarding in ND. There may be hyperemia, hemorrhage, and a general inflammatory response of the serosa and mucosa of visceral organs. Hemorrhage may also be noted in the trachea, pericardium, lungs, and air sacs. Lesions in the brain consist of multifocal, nonsuppurative meningoencephalitis, particularly of the cerebellum. There may also be gliosis and mononuclear perivascular cuffing. None of these lesions are pathognomonic for ND (Hanson 1978; Clubb et al. 1980; Clubb 1984).

Laboratory Procedures. In live birds, the virus is isolated from cloacal or pharyngeal swabs. At necropsy, samples from the brain, lung, colon, spleen, or trachea may be used to inoculate the allantoic chamber of embryonated chicken eggs. If the embryo dies after 2–5 days, both hemagglutination and hemagglutination inhibition tests are performed. If these tests are positive, specific pathogen-free chickens are inoculated with material from the infected eggs for pathotyping (Clubb 1984).

Control. The obvious control is to prevent exposure of cage birds to carrier birds or those in the incubative stage of the disease. In the United States this is effectively carried out by official quarantine and testing in government-operated facilities.

Unfortunately, birds are smuggled into most countries and sold at reduced prices. Diagnosis is frequently delayed because owners are reluctant to have anyone know where they acquired a bird that became sick within a few days of purchase.

ND is population dependent (Hanson 1976; Hanson et al. 1978). If an outbreak is suspected, immediate isolation of sick birds is crucial. If a flock can be segregated into isolation pens on the same premises, the rate of spread will be decreased.

Disinfection. Government regulations dictate clean-up and disinfection procedures. VVND virus is sensitive to a number of disinfectants. The official disinfectant of the USDA is orthophenyl phenol (Wright 1974).

Infected and exposed cage birds are killed. The vaccination programs so important in commercial poultry operations are not an option for control of VVND in cage birds.

The keys to prevention and control:

1. Purchasing birds through reputable firms
2. Proper quarantine and testing prior to introduction of newly purchased birds into a resident flock
3. Proper sanitation and periodic disinfection of feeders, waterers, and handling equipment
4. If infection does occur, early isolation and depopulation of infected birds and dispersing others to minimize exposure

References

Cavill, J. P. 1980. Newcastle disease in aviary and pet birds. *Vet. Rev.* 25(7):6–9.

———. 1982. Virus diseases. *Diseases of Cage and Aviary Birds,* 2d ed., ed. M. L. Petrak. Philadelphia: Lea and Febiger.

Chu, H. P., E. W. Trow, A. G. Greenwood, A. R. Jennings, and I. F. Keymer. 1976. Isolation of Newcastle disease virus from birds of prey. *Avian Pathol.* 5:227–33.

Clubb, S. L. 1984. Velogenic viscerotropic Newcastle disease. In *Zoo and Wild Animal Medicine,* 2d ed., ed. M. E. Fowler. Philadelphia: W. B. Saunders.

Clubb, S. L., B. M. Levine, and D. L. Graham. 1980. An outbreak of viscerotropic velogenic Newcastle disease in pet birds. *Annu. Proc. Am. Assoc. Zoo Vet.,* pp. 105–9.

Hanson, R. P. 1976. Avian reservoirs of Newcastle disease. In *Wildlife Diseases,* ed. L. A. Page, pp. 185–95. New York: Plenum.

———. 1978. Newcastle disease. In *Diseases of Poultry,* 7th ed., ed. M. S. Hofstad, pp. 513–35. Ames: Iowa State University Press.

Luthgen, W. 1975. Newcastle disease in psittacines. In *Report on Proceedings 20th World Veterinary Congress,* p. 2265. Geneva: World Veterinary Association.

Pavlovsky, E. N. 1966. *Natural Nidality of Transmissable Diseases.* Translated by N. D. Levine. Urbana: University of Illinois Press.

Mathey, W. J., and D. E. Olsen. 1974. A Newcastle disease virus from newly imported birds: Pathogenicity and persistence. *J. Am. Vet. Med. Assoc.* 165:740.

Pearson, G. L., and M. K. McCann. 1975. The role of indigenous wild, semidomestic, and exotic birds in the epizootiology of velogenic viscerotropic Newcastle disease in southern California, 1972–1973. *J. Am. Vet. Med. Assoc.* 167:610–14.

Wright, H. S. 1974. Virucidal activity of commercial disinfectants against velogenic viscerotropic Newcastle disease virus. *Avian Dis.* 18:526–30.

Zuydam, D. M. 1952. Isolation of Newcastle disease virus from the osprey and the parakeet. *J. Am. Vet. Med. Assoc.* 120:88–89.

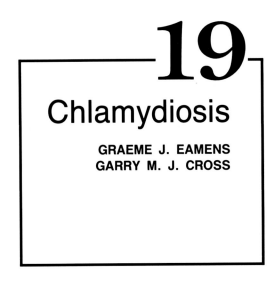

19

Chlamydiosis

GRAEME J. EAMENS
GARRY M. J. CROSS

Etiology. Chlamydiosis (formerly termed "psittacosis" in psittacine birds and humans and "ornithosis" in nonpsittacine birds) is the term commonly used to describe generalized infections in mammals and birds caused by *Chlamydia psittaci*.

Avian chlamydiosis occurs worldwide, and the majority of cases exist as latent, inapparent infections. The most commonly affected cage and aviary birds are the psittacines (parrots, parakeets, Budgerigars, macaws, cockatoos, Cockatiels, lories, lorikeets, lovebirds) as well as all types of pigeons and doves. Occasional clinical disease occurs in pheasants, partridges, ducks, hummingbirds, magpies, tits, thrushes, finches, canaries, and cardinals.

Developmental Cycle of *C. psittaci*. *C. psittaci* exists in two forms during its intracellular developmental cycle: a small 300-nm-diameter elementary body with an electron-dense nuclear region and a larger 800- to 1200-nm-diameter initial body (the reticulate body) with a less-dense nuclear region.

The elementary body is a highly infectious, stable, extracellular transport form that becomes phagocytosed to become an intracytoplasmic elementary body in a membrane-bound phagosome. At this site, the elementary body undergoes cellular rearrangement to form the larger initial body, which has a lower infectivity. The initial body undergoes binary fission several times, and the products condense to form new elementary bodies, the developmental cycle taking 24–28 hours. Both forms stain well with Macchiavello, Castaneda, Gimenez, or Giemsa stains but poorly with Gram stain.

Transmission. Transmission occurs by inhalation or ingestion of chlamydiae contained in the feces, nasal secretions, or lacrimal secretions of infected birds. Most transmission probably occurs in the nest, by direct transfer of infected crop milk to the young nestling.

Chlamydiae can remain infective for several months in dried feces, and contamination of eggshells by feces in nesting birds is a source of nestling infection. In addition, vertical transmission is known to occur in psittacines, ducks, seagulls, and chickens. Aerosols of fecal dust are a frequent source of infection for birds of all ages.

Mechanical transfer by nest mites and lice has been reported in poultry. Ticks and fleas may also transfer chlamydiae mechanically.

In the absence of stress, infections remain either latent or associated with only mild transient signs. In the unstressed nestling, such signs will disappear by the time the young birds are able to fly. However, the chlamydiae can persist in the spleen and kidneys until the next breeding season, when they may infect the new generation of young birds. Clinically normal birds may be carriers and shedders. Overt clinical disease is induced by stress, and affected birds excrete chlamydiae in large numbers in their feces and lacrimal and nasal secretions.

Predisposing Factors. Stress caused by a low plane of nutrition, a change of diet, fluctuating temperature, overcrowding, prolonged transportation (particularly with little food or water), racing, handling, and nesting may all contribute to convert latent to active infections and result in increased shedding of chlamydiae.

Young birds are particularly susceptible. Birds kept intensively in large numbers and bred collectively are most vulnerable to serious outbreaks of clinical disease. Parent birds that are stressed by nesting may become mild clinical cases, thus exposing their young to high numbers of infectious organisms.

Clinical Signs. Clinical disease may be peracute, acute, subacute, or chronic in nature. Several or all forms can be seen in any given outbreak of chlamydiosis.

The incubation period varies from 5 to 98 days in psittacines. In pigeons, an incubation period of 7–14 days is common, while experimental infections in turkeys may have an incubation period as short as 2 days. The incubation period depends on the virulence of the agent, the susceptibility and stressing of the host, and the route of exposure.

Signs of clinical disease may vary and are not specific, as the outward appearance of affected birds is similar to that seen in other systemic diseases.

The peracute form results in sudden death or death within a short time without marked premonitory signs. This form has been reported in small psittacines, Australian King Parrots, rice birds, finches, canaries, and pigeons.

In the acute form, common signs are ruffled feathers, depression, decreased appetite, greenish or grayish diarrhea, and a soiled vent. Weight loss and emaciation often occur. Blepharitis, conjunctivitis, and a serous or seropurulent oculonasal discharge are frequently seen. Due to weakness and listlessness, flight is inhibited. Breathing may become labored and even rattling in nature. Birds often tend to shiver or huddle together and show drooping wings. Progress of the disease may be over 1–2 weeks, followed by prostration, convulsions, and death. Alternatively there may be sudden death or a slow recovery with retarded growth. Occasionally, cases show staggering and paralysis. Markedly decreased egg production occurs. In various species the diarrhea may differ, feces becoming yellowish, rust-colored, or blood-tinged.

The subacute form has a protracted course with a variety of clinical signs that may disappear and then reappear after a few days. Growth is retarded, and some birds may become cachectic.

The chronic form is characterized by severe pectoral muscle wasting, leg and wing weakness, fluffing of the feathers, and lack of feathering around the eyes from previous bouts of conjunctivitis and blepharitis.

The signs of disease may be influenced by age. Some birds, usually adults, may suffer only conjunctivitis and blepharitis. Among pigeons, young birds often show most of the signs of the acute form whereas adults may suffer sudden death or symptoms may be limited to a uni- or bilateral conjunctivitis and rhinitis (with accompanying serous or seropurulent oculonasal discharge, swollen eyelids, and cloudy corneas), respiratory disturbances, and sometimes diarrhea.

Specimens for Laboratory Examination.

If chlamydiosis is suspected, care must be taken to avoid infection of laboratory staff and others who may be handling the birds, cages, or feed utensils or who may come in contact with discharges, feathers, or dust from the birds.

The suspect birds should be handled with gloves. Birds submitted to a laboratory should be euthanized in a sealed container, and all subsequent laboratory handling of the carcasses should be performed in a biological safety cabinet.

Diagnosis.

A presumptive diagnosis may be made on the basis of clinical signs, typical gross lesions, and the demonstration of chlamydial elementary and initial bodies in stained impression smears of liver, spleen, air sacs, or conjunctival scrapings. Definitive diagnosis depends on the isolation and identification of *C. psittaci* from typically diseased birds. Culturing of specimens from live birds is unreliable.

At necropsy, lesions are basically similar in all avian species. Variations are caused by factors such as route of exposure, length of illness, virulence of agent, and host susceptibility.

Common necropsy findings include the following:

1. Fibrinous or fibrinopurulent airsacculitis and peritonitis, and often similar pericarditis and perihepatitis
2. Splenomegaly in psittacines, not regularly seen in pigeons (The spleen may vary from congested to pale and may show subcapsular hemorrhage or focal granulomas. Splenic enlargement may be so severe that rupture and sudden death occur.)
3. Hepatomegaly (The liver may vary in appearance from pulpy to mottled or show evidence of focal necrosis/granuloma formation.)
4. Pulmonary congestion
5. Catarrhal enteritis

None of these lesions is sufficiently characteristic to give a conclusive diagnosis. Species of *Mycoplasma, Salmonella,* and *Pasteurella, Escherichia coli,* and other infectious agents may cause similar lesions or may occur concurrently with chlamydiosis. However, the presence of fibrinous or fibrinopurulent exudates on various serosal surfaces as well as enlarged, congested somatic organs is sufficient to initiate the following further confirmatory tests:

1. Staining of impression smears for elementary bodies and initial bodies (Fig. 19.1) (Liver, spleen, air sac, or conjunctival scraping smears may be stained by Giemsa, Macchiavello, Gimenez, Castaneda, or modified Ziehl-Neelsen methods.)
2. Isolation of chlamydiae from liver, spleen, air sacs (may be frozen) via (a) yolk sac inoculation into embryonated chicken eggs, (b) intraperitoneal inoculation into chlamydia-free mice, or (c) inoculation into tissue culture, where the presence of intracytoplasmic inclusions may be demonstrated by fluorescent antibody technique
3. Histopathology (for the liver, lung, spleen, heart, or kidney)

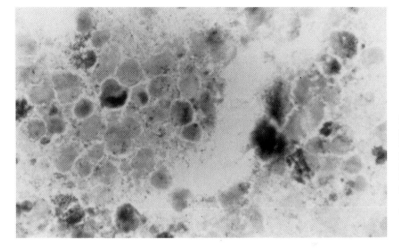

Fig. 19.1. Gimenez staining of an air sac impression smear from a psittacine. Chlamydial elementary and initial bodies are evident in the smear. (*Courtesy of D. K. Windsor, Jr., and J. E. Grimes, Texas A&M University, College Station, Tex.*)

4. Bacteriology (for alternate diagnosis for the liver, spleen, heart, or intestine)

Control Procedures. Infected birds should be removed and treated or destroyed, and all carcasses either disinfected using a phenolic (e.g., 5% Lysol) or iodophor compound or forwarded to a veterinary laboratory. Confirmation of the diagnosis is important when other birds and humans are at risk.

Any bird or specimen suspected of being infected must be regarded as dangerous. Clinicians handling sick birds should take precautions (masks, gloves) because of the risks, particularly of aerosol inhalation of large numbers of infective particles. All necropsy examinations, tissue collection, smearing, or cultural procedures should be carried out in a biological safety cabinet, and all carcasses should be disinfected with phenolics or iodophors prior to any examination.

Increased awareness of the disease and its early recognition and treatment will assist in disease control. In outbreaks with considerable numbers of clinical cases and mortalities, depopulation must be considered.

According to the United Kingdom Public Health Laboratory Service (1976), infected premises should be disinfected with iodophors (cages), 5% formalin (surfaces), and phenolics (wastes). Alternatively 1% formaldehyde solution (3% formalin) is satisfactory for daily rinsing and disinfection of floors and weekly cleaning and disinfection of cages (Wachendorfer 1973).

If the infected premises can be made airtight, formaldehyde gas fumigation (after preliminary cleaning to remove organic matter) is ideal. However, formaldehyde fumigation is rendered ineffective if the relative humidity and temperature are too low. During fumigation, a relative humidity of over 70% and a temperature of over 18°C enable efficient disinfection.

Formaldehyde gas can be generated in four ways:

1. By adding formalin to a shallow layer of potassium permanganate, which results in a violent exothermic reaction with a rapid release of gas. A metal bucket or earthenware container with sides 3 times the depth of the chemicals should be used and placed 1–3 m from any inflammable material. To ensure good gas distribution, 600 ml formalin is poured onto 400–500 g potassium permanganate/30 m³, using no more than one container for every 30 m³. For buildings in excess of 360 m³, the above amount of chemicals per 30 m³ is halved.
2. By heating paraformaldehyde flakes or granules (320 g paraformaldehyde flakes/30 m³) 180°C in a thermostatically controlled electric frying pan, hot plate, or deep fryer (set at 200°C).
3. By boiling formalin in a kettle with an automatic cutout at the rate of 500 ml formalin + 1000 ml water/30 m³ air space.
4. By dispersing formalin as an aerosol (200 ml formalin/30 m³, diluted 1:1 with water if humidity is low) using a mechanical generator. This method is suitable for buildings that cannot be made completely airtight.

Treatment. Sick birds should be well isolated and kept uncrowded and warm in freshly cleaned holding cages. Cages should be kept clean throughout treatment. A combination of parenteral and oral medication is recommended. Monitoring the hemogram of sick birds aids in the treatment (Table 19.1).

Table 19.1. Typical hemogram of chlamydiosis

Leukocytosis
   Persists 5–14 days, depending on species, even
   with correct therapy. Leukocytosis of bacterial
   septicemia usually falls rapidly with correct antibiotic therapy. Leukocytosis of egg-yolk peritonitis
   may mimic leukocytosis of chlamydiosis.
Left-shift
   Increased heterophil count, often with meta-
   myeloctyes and band heterophils (the latter two
   usually rare). Bands and metamyelocytes usually
   disappear rapidly with correct therapy.
Low PCV
   Stabilizes with therapy (e.g., doxycycline) or continues to fall until death ensues without (or with
   incorrect) therapy. Occasional acute case treated
   on day 1 or 2 does not show a low PCV (very rare).
Moderate to marked polychromasia (in regenerative
   anemia)
Moderate to marked anisocytosis (in regenerative anemia)
Elevated SGOT (SAAT), LDH, AP, creatinine, uric
   acid, BUN (in septicemia)
Glucose and/or calcium may be decreased

   Source: Drs. R. W. Woerpel and W. J. Rosskopf,
Jr., and Tech. M. Monahan-Brennan, Animal Medical
Centre of Lawndale, Hawthorne, Calif.

For sick parrots, especially those that refuse to eat, suggested treatment is intramuscular injections of oxytetracycline (100 mg/ml) at 1 mg/10–30 g body weight either daily for 5 days or every second day for a total of six to eight injections (Schultz 1978). For small psittacines, intramuscular injections of oxytetracycline at 1 mg/20–30 mg body weight is suggested, but injected volumes must be small (e.g., 0.05 ml), taking care to avoid the subpectoral venous sinuses (Hungerford 1969; Olsen and Dolphin 1978).

Recommended oral treatment either for sick birds or for prophylaxis is by feed medication for a period of at least 45 days for parrots and other large psittacines and at least 30 days for small psittacines and other birds (Wachendorfer 1973). Schultz (1978) also suggests that intramuscular oxytetracycline at 1 mg/10 g daily for 3 days, followed by another course after 3 days, is useful in prophylaxis, but handling of birds is to be avoided. For parrots and other large psittacines, chlortetracycline at 0.44% in cooked mash (antibiotic added daily), at 0.5% in pellets (antibiotic stable for 6 months), or at 0.5% to any hulled seed they like is used successfully in treatment and prophylaxis (FAO/WHO 1967; Arnstein et al. 1968; Hungerford 1969; Wachendorfer 1973). For small psittacines, chlortetracycline at 0.05% in impregnated hulled millet is successful in treatment and prophylaxis (FAO/WHO 1967; Wachendorfer

1973). The antibiotic in the medicated seed is stable for 6 months if stored at 10–27°C in tightly closed plastic or glass containers kept in a dark place. Direct oral dosing may be an alternative with small numbers of birds, but care must be taken that the drug is actually swallowed.

For nectar-feeding psittacines (lories, lorikeets), chlortetracycline at 0.05% should be used in a liquid diet (1/6 honey, 1/6 canned food, 4/6 water) for 45 days (Arnstein et al. 1969).

For pigeons, the following oral medications have been recommended for treatment and prophylaxis: chlortetracycline at 0.5% in pellets or at 50–80 mg/bird/day in drinking water (Wachendorfer 1973), chlortetracycline at 0.89% in hen scratch (milo/corn/wheat/kafir) (Arnstein et al. 1964), and chlortetracycline at 0.4–1.0% in a palatable grain (Hungerford 1969). All oral medications for pigeons should be maintained daily for at least 30 days.

For canaries and finches, chlortetracycline at 0.05% in palatable medicated seed for 30 days is suggested (Wachendorfer 1973).

Unless a constant therapeutic level of antibiotic can be maintained in blood (>1 μg/ml) for a sufficiently long time, elimination of chlamydiae may not occur (Wachendorfer 1973). Long-term in-feed medication with tetracyclines has been criticized because of the risk of derangement of the intestinal flora, and supplementary treatment with multivitamins daily in the drinking water is recommended to prevent deaths during chemotherapy (Wachendorfer 1973).

For oral treatment, chlortetracycline is preferred to oxytetracycline because of the latter's greater tendency to chelate copper, iron, and calcium and the subsequent poorer intestinal absorption. Tetracyclines are reported to be anti-vitamin B in activity. Plastic or glass feeding vessels are recommended for medicated feed, as vessels lined with iron, copper, or zinc have a deleterious effect on tetracyclines. Treated birds should be kept under observation for 1 month after cessation of treatment before being transferred back to their usual quarters. If there is any evidence of recurrence of the infection, they should be returned to the treatment cages and retreated.

Tetracycline medication of drinking water is contraindicated in cage birds because such medication is unpredictable and unlikely to achieve therapeutic blood levels (Wachendorfer 1973). For example, a Budgerigar weighing an average 45–50 g eats daily an average of 14–15% of its body weight (range 12–22%) (Universities Federation for Animal Welfare 1967; Wachendorfer 1973). However, it drinks only 2–3 ml water daily, which is only 4–6% of its body weight. Generally all healthy birds eat 15–20% of their body weight in feed daily, but the larger psittacines drink less than 2% of their body weight daily. Therefore, water medications require at least 3 times the concentration of feed medication, and this level would be unpalatable for small psittacines and almost syruplike for large psittacines. Also, water intake in many small, healthy birds may be negligible.

Because of such problems, strict veterinary supervision of treatment programs is advisable (Keymer 1973; Wachendorfer 1973).

Prevention. Stress must be avoided in transport, housing, environment (especially cold), feed, water, crowding, and the mixing of birds (bullying). Recently captured wild birds such as psittacines should be avoided, and when possible, birds should be bought directly from breeders with known healthy stock. Effective quarantine of all incoming stock and the maintenance of all birds under sanitary conditions at all times are important prevention measures.

References

Arnstein, P., D. H. Cohen, and K. F. Meyer. 1964. Medication of pigeons with chlortetracycline in feed. *J. Am. Vet. Med. Assoc.* 145:921.

Arnstein, P., B. Eddie, and K. F. Meyer. 1968. Control of psittacosis by group chemotherapy of infected parrots. *Am. J. Vet. Res.* 29:2213.

Arnstein, P., W. G. Buchanan, B. Eddie, and K. F. Meyer. 1969. Chlortetracycline chemotherapy for nectar-feeding psittacine birds. *J. Am. Vet. Med. Assoc.* 154:190.

Epidemiological Research Laboratory of the Public Health Laboratory Service, United Kingdom and Ireland. 1976. Outbreak of Psittacosis. *Br. Med. J.* 2:1017.

FAO/WHO. 1967. *Medicated Feed for Psittacosis Control in Budgerigars and Parrots.* Joint FAO/WHO Expert Committee on Zoonoses Third Report, Annex 10. Rome: FAO.

Hungerford, T. G. 1969. Cage birds. In *Diseases of Poultry, Including Cage Birds and Pigeons,* 4th ed., ed. T. G. Hungerford, pp. 566, 592. Sydney, Aust.: Angus and Robertson.

Keymer, I. F. 1973. Psittacosis. *Vet. Rec.* 93:654.

Olsen, D. E., and R. E. Dolphin. 1978. Administering therapeutic agents to cage birds. *Vet. Med.* 73:1045.

Schultz, D. J. 1978. Diseases of parrots. In *Refresher Course for Veterinarians on Fauna,* p. 224. University of Sydney, Post Graduate Committee in Veterinary Science, Proceedings no. 36. Sydney, Aust.

Universities Federation for Animal Welfare. 1967. Section IV: Birds, poikilotherms and invertebrates. In *The UFAW Handbook on the Care and Management of Laboratory Animals.* Edinburgh: E. and S. Livingstone/UFAW.

Wachendorfer, J. G. 1973. Epidemiology and control of psittacosis. *J. Am. Vet. Med. Assoc.* 162:298.

6

Parasitology

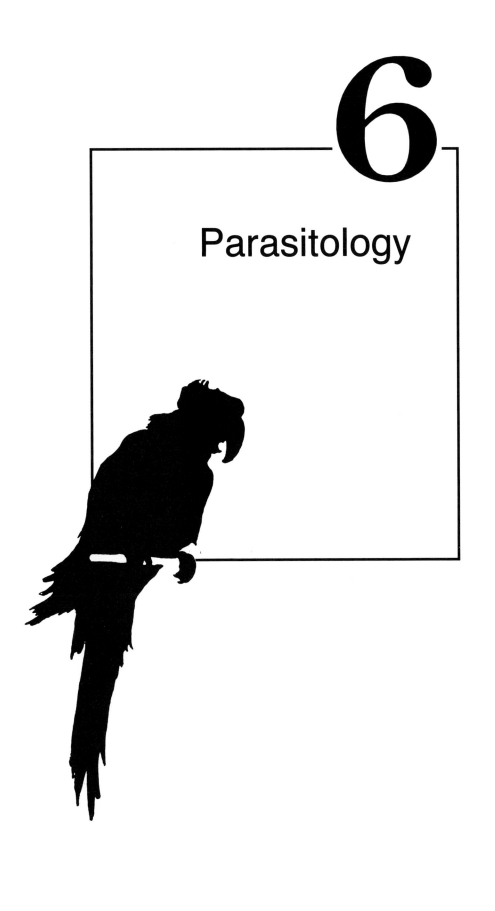

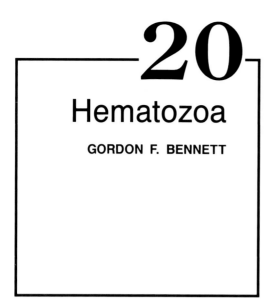

20

Hematozoa

GORDON F. BENNETT

THE PRESENCE of parasites in the peripheral circulation of birds was first demonstrated by Danilewsky in 1885, when he described *Trypanosoma avium* from the little owl *Athene noctuae.* Sir Ronald Ross, using chickens, first described an avian *Plasmodium* (under the generic name of *Proteosoma*) life cycle and established the protocols for the study of all insect-borne diseases (Ross 1898, 1899). Since then, nearly 4000 species of birds (approximately 50% of the known species) have been examined for blood parasites. At present 200 species of *Haemoproteus,* 96 species and varieties of *Leucocytozoon,* 75 species and varieties of *Plasmodium,* 86 species and varieties of *Trypanosoma,* and a large number of the embryonic stages of filarioid nematodes (under the designation *Microfilaria*) have been described (Bennett et al. 1982).

For a considerable period of time, blood parasitologists used a one host–one parasite philosophy, particularly among parasites described from birds. It is possible that many of the species described will prove to be synonyms as little attempt has been made to determine their life cycles, modes of transmission, and cross-infectivities. Experimental evidence suggests that the haemoproteids and leucocytozoids are host family, not host species, specific. The avian malaria parasites of the genus *Plasmodium,* on the other hand, have a much broader host range, with many species infecting a wide range of avian species from a variety of avian families. The relative ease of transmitting *Plasmodium* via blood inoculation has greatly assisted studies of this genus, with the result that this group has received the most critical attention. The Trypanosomatidae pose a difficult problem, as the species are highly pleiomorphic and few life cycle studies have been conducted; there is little information on the host specificity, cross-infectivity, and mode of transmission for most species. The microfilaria also pose a unique problem in that specific identification is only possible on the basis of the adult worms. Compounding the problem is the fact that the genus *Microfilaria* has been erected, on the basis of the embryonic worms only, to contain many of the species. However, it is probable that many of these will prove to be synonyms when the embryos are associated with their parents. Parasites of the genera *Atoxoplasma, Babesia, Haemogregarina, Hepatozoon, Lankesterella, Nuttallia,* and *Toxoplasma* are rarely encountered except in a few avian families and species. The taxonomy and relationships of these groups is poorly known, and little consensus among various authorities can be found. Veterinarians should be scientifically precise in their reports and identifications of parasitic infections. Overgeneralizations, imprecision in identification, and identifications based on symptoms alone lead only to confusion. If the causal agent of disease is unclear or unknown, especially in such exotic fields as blood parasites, it is better to obtain the opinion of an expert than to hazard a guess. Incorrect guesses are perpetuated in the literature, contributing to erroneous diagnoses.

Parasite Diagnosis. Avian hematozoa can only be identified with certainty from stained thin-film preparations. Thin films can be made from blood drawn from the brachial vein/artery in small birds and from the femoral vein/artery in larger birds. Blood smears made by clipping toes are not recommended as abundant contaminants can lead to diagnostic error. Thin smears made from tissue imprints are also useful. Specific identification of avian blood parasites should be confirmed by sending the material to specialists in the field, such as those at the International Reference Centre for Avian Haematozoa, Memorial University of Newfoundland, St. John's, Newfoundland, Canada.

Parasite Control. From the veterinary point of view, avian blood parasites are of both academic and economic interest. There is no question that some species of blood parasites can contribute to severe economic loss in the poultry industry. On the other hand, some blood parasites occur in a high percentage of individuals but apparently cause little harm. The practicing veterinarian, therefore, must be able to distinguish those of economic importance. In particular the veterinarian must know the life cycle and mode of transmission to provide adequate control measures. This is of primary importance for birds in zoological gardens where a number of species are in close proximity, many of them exotic to the geographic locality. Such proximity provides opportunity for the transmission of disease or parasites to display species that would not normally come in contact with such pathogens. Frequently species involved have had no previous contact with the pathogens and thus are highly susceptible to infection. Manwell and Rossi (1975), Peirce (1969), Peirce and Bevan (1977), Poelma and Zwart (1972), and numerous other parasitologists have all recorded the remarkably high prevalence of blood parasites in birds imported from various countries to zoological gardens. If possible, therefore, it should be determined whether a blood parasite infection was contracted locally or at the bird's point of origin. If locally, in the case of pathogenic blood parasites, some form of control measures must be instituted. If at the point of origin, it is equally important to know whether the blood parasites can or cannot be transmitted by local vectors. While most blood parasites have little clinical effect on their natural hosts, entry into an aberrant host can cause severe problems and mortality, as has been frequently recorded with respect to avian *Plasmodium* species in penguins (Stoskopf and Beier 1979). Therefore, all newly acquired birds should be checked for hematozoan infections prior to introduction into a display aviary.

The Avian Hematozoa

Genus *Haemoproteus*
(Apicomplexa:Haemoproteidae)

Synopsis. The genus *Haemoproteus* is the largest and most commonly encountered blood parasite group, containing nearly 200 species and varieties (Bennett et al. 1982) in over 1700 species of birds representing 110 families. However, on close examination many of these species will probably prove to be synonyms. Aragao (1907) and Adie (1915) demonstrated that *Haemoproteus columbae* was transmitted from pigeon to pigeon by the hippoboscid (louse fly) *Lynchia maura* (and others), and it was concluded that all haemoproteids were transmitted by hippoboscid flies. However, Fallis and his colleagues demonstrated that biting flies of the genus *Culicoides* (Diptera:Ceratopogonidae) were vectors of a number of species of haemoproteids, including *H. nettionis* of ducks (Fig. 20.1), *H. canachites* (= *H. mansoni*) of grouse, *H. velans* of woodpeckers, and *H. fringillae* of the fringillid sparrows. Recent studies have

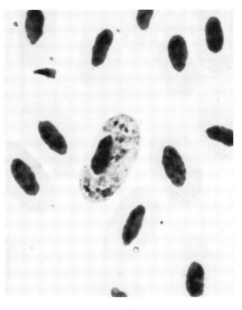

Fig. 20.1. Mature macrogametocyte of *Haemoproteus nettionis* of ducks and geese (infected cell approximately 14 μm long).

shown that *H. meleagridis* of turkeys and *H. desseri* of parrots are also transmitted by ceratopogonids. More haemoproteids are known to be transmitted by ceratopogonids (7 species) than by hippoboscids (3 species, 1 questionable). Detailed investigations of the life cycles of these parasites, together with the study of their development in the vector, led Bennett et al. (1965) to propose the genus *Parahaemoproteus* for the ceratopogonid-vectored haemoproteids. This genus was subsequently reduced to subgeneric rank by Levine and Campbell (1971). Morphologically, the gametocytes in thin-film preparations from both groups are indistinguishable and can be referred to broadly as the genus *Haemoproteus sensu latu*.

Life Cycle

Invertebrate Host. Sporogony occurs in either louse flies of the family Hippoboscidae for *Haemoproteus* (*Haemoproteus*) or ornithophilic species of *Culicoides* of the family Ceratopogonidae for *Haemoproteus* (*Parahaemoproteus*). Sporogony occurs in 3–5 days; large oocysts (hippoboscids) producing numerous sporozoites or small oocysts (ceratopogonids) producing 16 to 32 sporozoites are formed. Transmission is via the bite of the vector.

Vertebrate Host. The prepatent period takes 14–21 days; only gametocytes are found in peripheral blood. The intensity of parasitemia can be acute, with 60–90% erythrocyte involvement. Exoerythrocytic schizogony occurs in the lungs; schizonts are elongated and branched, producing numerous merozoites. High-intensity infections can persist for 6–9 months or longer; recrudescence of infections in natural populations is seen during the breeding season with up to 65% erythrocyte involvement during recrudescence in wild songbirds. Transmission occurs on the breeding grounds, with the young of the year showing highest parasite prevalence. Under natural conditions, 60% of infected birds retain infection for 1 or more years (Bennett et al. 1977). Prevalence of infection varies markedly from continent to continent and region to region (Greiner et al. 1975; White et al. 1978).

Clinical Signs. Species of *Haemoproteus* have rarely been incriminated as the causal agents of mortality in avian populations (Bennett et al. 1976). Despite high erythrocyte involvement (96% of erythrocytes averaging 3.5 parasites per infected cell in a young sapsucker), few deaths or symptoms have been ascribed to members of this genus. Julian and Galt (1980) reported that in Ontario *H. nettionis* caused high mortality in a flock of Muscovy Ducks (*Cairina moschata*) but did not produce a patent parasitemia. Kucera et al. (1982) also reported that an unknown haemoproteid caused mortality among Muscovies in Czechoslovakia. Considering that haemoproteids represent the majority of the reported blood parasite infections in birds, these few cases indicate that this genus of parasites does not pose a serious veterinary problem. The ducks that did succumb were described as listless and anorexic.

Differential Diagnosis. The few life history studies to date indicate that species of *Haemoproteus* tend to be family specific. However, specific diagnosis of the numerous species described requires careful examination of the gametocytes in the peripheral blood. Separation of haemoproteids from the avian species of *Plasmodium* is frequently difficult and often rests on the tenuous evidence of the absence of erythrocytic schizonts. Diagnosis is best confirmed by a specialist in the field. A pictorial guide to some species of haemoproteids is provided by Greiner and Bennett (1975).

Treatment. Little is known about the treatment of avian haemoproteid infections. Coatney (1935) demonstrated that Atebrin and Plasmochin reduced the number of gametocytes of *H. columbae* circulating in the blood of pigeons but did not attack the tissue schizonts and effect a cure. Large doses of Atebrin were toxic to the pigeons. In view of the fact that haemoproteids are not extremely pathogenic, treatment is probably not necessary. Control of the parasites is probably best achieved by the exclusion of the *Culicoides* and hippoboscid vectors.

Genus *Leucocytozoon* (Apicomplexa:Leucocytozoidae)

Synopsis. The considerable confusion surrounding the early taxonomy of this group was clarified by Bennett et al. (1975). The genus with its approximately 96 species and varieties was recently reviewed in depth by Fallis et al. (1974). Members of this genus (Fig. 20.2) have a cosmopolitan distribution and have been recorded in over 1000 species of birds of 98 families. Prevalence of infection is highest in birds from northern regions or from areas where numerous rivers and streams provide breeding sites for the simuliid vectors. The group, strangely, is lacking in South and Central America and islands of the West Indies. Positive records from these areas primarily represent North American birds taken on winter migration (White et al. 1978).

Life Cycle

Invertebrate Host. Sporogony occurs only in blackflies (Diptera:Simuliidae) and is complete in 3–5 days. The oocytes produce numerous sporozoites, which migrate to the salivary glands and infect a host when the fly feeds.

Vertebrate Host. The prepatent period takes 5–9 days, and gametocytes occur only in the circulating blood. Infection can be intense but normally ranges from 1 to 10 parasites per 10,000 erythrocytes. The first schizogonic cycle is hepatic; subsequent cycles are hepatic and other organs. Studies by Greiner et al. (1977) have shown that the hepatic cycle of *Leucocytozoon simondi* of ducks produces a round gametocyte and that renal schizogony produces fusiform gametocytes. Hepatic schizonts can be large and visible as small white dots to the naked eye; in intense infections large creamy white patches can be found in the liver (Fig. 20.3). Intense infections persist for 2–6 weeks, then reduce to as few as 1 to 2 parasites per blood film. Recrudescence of infection may occur in the spring, experimentally initiated by long days and/or the onset of egg laying. Parasite transmission occurs on the hosts' breeding grounds, with the young of the year showing the highest prevalences. Under natural conditions, 60% of the birds retain their infection from year to year.

Two species of *Leucocytozoon*, *L. simondi* of

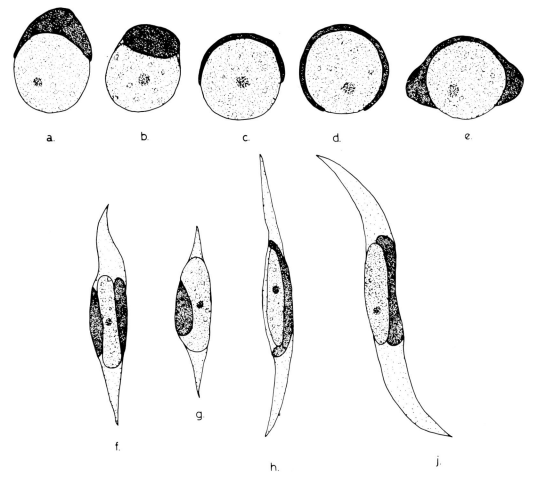

Fig. 20.2. Typical forms of *Leucocytozoon:* a. *fringillinarum* of passerines; b. *vandenbrandeni* of anhingid screamers; c. *majoris* of parids; d. *sakharoffi* of corvids; e. *dubreuili* of thrushes; f. *smithi* of turkeys; g. *toddi* of hawks; h. *ziemanni* of owls; i. *simondi* of ducks and geese.

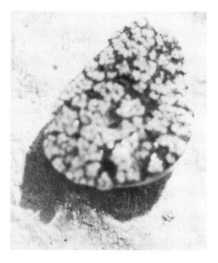

ducks and geese and *L. smithi* of turkeys, cause heavy mortality in domestic flocks (as high as 100%) and probably contribute to mortality in wild anatid populations. Frank (1965) reported an unspecified *Leucocytozoon* causing mortality in parrots in West Germany. The impact of other species of the genus is not well known but is considered minimal. *Leucocytozoon simondi,* a holarctic parasite, is transmitted in North America by the ornithophilic blackflies *Simulium rugglesi* and *Eusimulium anatinum,* usually north of the 43rd parallel. *Leucocytozoon smithi,* originally described from turkeys in France, has

Fig. 20.3. *Leucocytozoon simondi* of ducks. Megaloschizonts cause the large white patches in the liver. (×2.5)

been introduced to various parts of the world, where a wide range of simuliid vectors transmit the parasite. *Leucocytozoon smithi* in North America is transmitted by *Simulium slossonae, Eusimulium johannsoni,* and *E. congareanarum* among others.

Clinical Signs. Symptoms of both *L. simondi* and *L. smithi* include listlessness, anorexia, somnolence, watery eye discharge, and severe convulsions before death. Characteristically, the onset of leucocytozoonosis is sudden, with birds appearing normal one day and dead within 24–48 hours. Anemia and a greatly reduced packed cell volume and hemoglobin content are characteristic; numerous parasites are seen on blood films. At necropsy, the liver and spleen are found to be grossly enlarged, up to 10 times the normal volume; tissue sections contain megaloschizonts up to 160 μm in diameter. Birds surviving the initial crisis usually recover, showing a slower growth rate but eventually attaining a normal size. Reports that the "sporocyst" stage of leucocytozoids cause cysts in the cardiac and skeletal muscles are completely unfounded. These reports arise out of infections in caged psittacines in the United Kingdom that have yet to be identified as to the causal agent but are not members of the genus *Leucocytozoon*.

Differential Diagnosis. The limited experimental studies show that most *Leucocytozoon* spp. are host family specific and only a few avian families harbor more than a single species. Specific diagnosis is based on gametocyte morphology in a stained peripheral blood film. A pictorial atlas of *Leucocytozoon simondi* was published by Herman et al. (1977) and a pictorial guide of other species of this genus is provided by Greiner and Bennett (1975), but specific diagnosis should be confirmed by an expert.

Treatment. No effective treatment is known. Fallis (1948) showed that Atebrin, Paludrin, and sulfamerazine had no prophylactic or therapeutic effects on birds infected with *L. simondi* and *L. sakharoffi.* Control is best achieved by elimination of the simuliid vectors.

Genus *Akiba*
(Apicomplexa:Leucocytozoidae)

Synopsis. The monotypic genus *Akiba* was erected to contain *Akiba caulleryi,* a leucocytozoidlike parasite of domestic fowl in southeast Asia and Japan. This genus differs from the related genus *Leucocytozoon* in two essential features. First, the gametocytes frequently exit the host erythrocyte on maturity and circulate in the peripheral blood as intercellular parasites. Second, the vector is the ceratopogonid midge *Culicoides arakawae* (and its close relatives). Other than in Asia, the genus has rarely been recorded, only Bennett and Borrero (1976) citing a record of an *Akiba*-like parasite in a Colombian bird. This parasite has not been a problem in aviary or cage birds. Recent reports that a species of *Akiba* caused heavy mortality in caged psittacines in England during the late summer should be treated with utmost caution until the identity of the pathogen has been clearly established. This pathogen has been widely confused with *Leucocytozoon* and the condition referred to as "leucocytozoonosis." This conclusion is unwarranted at this time as neither group of organisms has been demonstrated in the afflicted psittacines. Furthermore, the epidemiology associated with the infections is totally inconsistent with either group of parasites. Such reports emphasize the importance of having expert advice before making specific diagnoses.

Life Cycle

Invertebrate Host. Sporogony occurs in the biting midge *Culicoides arakawae* (Diptera:Ceratopogonidae) and related species of *Culicoides.* Sporogony is complete in 3–5 days at optimal temperatures, with transmission via the bite of an infected vector.

Vertebrate Host. The prepatent period takes 14 days, and gametocytes only appear in erythrocytes of the peripheral circulation. On maturity, gametocytes frequently break out of their host cell and circulate as intercellular parasites (Fig. 20.4). Schizogony occurs in nearly all the internal organs, with megaloschizonts ranging in size from 26 to 300 μm in diameter. The megaloschizonts rupture and release merozoites, which invade erythrocytes or reinvade the tissues to produce new megaloschizonts.

Clinical Signs. Affected birds are listless, anemic, and diarrheic, and the combs and wattles appear pallid. On autopsy, gross hemorrhage from the lungs, liver, and kidneys has been noted in the peritoneal cavity, possibly due to the rupture of the megaloschizonts. Death can occur before a patent parasitemia has been established.

Treatment. Little can be done to cure birds infected with these parasites. There has been some success in using a variety of sulfa derivatives (sulfaquinoxaline, sulfadimethoxine) as preventative medicine. These drugs did not affect either the schizonts or the gametocytes and did not cure infected birds. Control, therefore, is

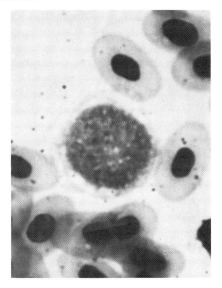

Fig. 20.4. Free mature macrogametocyte of *Akiba caulleryi* in peripheral circulation (approximately 15 μm in diameter).

best accomplished by elimination of *Culicoides* vectors.

Genus *Plasmodium*
(Apicomplexa:Plasmodidae)

Synopsis. Since Ross's historic work in 1898, some 35 species of avian malaria have been described and placed in the subgenera *Novyella, Haemamoeba, Giovannolaia,* and *Huffia.* The genus *Plasmodium* is cosmopolitan in distribution, with the highest prevalence in areas where populations of suitable vectors are large. Some avian malarias are host specific, such as *P. durae* and *P. hermani* of turkeys and *P. kempi* of quail, while others such as *P. circumflexum, P. relictum,* and *P. vaughani* occur in a wide range of avian species and families (Bennett et al. 1982). Effects of avian malaria on their hosts are variable. Under appropriate conditions probably all species will cause the death of the host. The canary (*Serinus canaria*), for example, appears to be highly vulnerable to most malarias under experimental conditions. Malarial species such as *P. gallinaceum, P. lophurae,* and *P. relictum* are more virulent than the relatively benign *P. vaughani.* Birds coming from areas where *Plasmodium* is natively absent and placed in a zoo/aviary situation are extremely susceptible to malarial attack. The devastating effect of *P. relictum* on captive penguins is well recorded (Stoskopf and Beier 1979).

Life Cycle

Invertebrate Host. All species of avian *Plasmodium* are transmitted by mosquitoes, usually by those in the genera *Aedes, Culex,* and *Culiseta,* although vectors from nearly every genus except *Anopheles* are known. Gametocytes are ingested by the insect and on reaching the stomach exit the host erythrocyte and the microgametocytes fertilize the females. Following fertilization, ookinetes are formed, move through the stomach wall, and form oocysts, which produce sporozoites. The sporozoites, released into the hemocoel, flood through the body and some reach and penetrate the salivary glands from which they are injected into a host during feeding.

Vertebrate Host. Following infection, the sporozoites move to the liver where they form exoerythrocytic schizonts, which on maturity rupture to release numerous merozoites into the circulatory system. A portion of these reenter hepatic, splenic, renal, or pulmonary cells to form new megaloschizonts while others penetrate the erythrocytes to initiate the erythrocytic cycle. In the peripheral blood, the merozoites within the red cells form trophozoites, which mature to form the erythrocytic schizonts that contain a number of merozoites (the number characteristic of the species, ranging from 3 to 5 for *P. juxtanucleare* to 30 to 40 for *P. gallinaceum*). This formation of the erythrocytic schizont separates *Plasmodium* from the other hemosporidian genera and also permits the passage of *Plasmodium* from host to host via blood inoculation. Some merozoites, on entering an erythrocyte, form either male or female gametocytes, which continue the life cycle when ingested by a suitable vector mosquito. The prepatent period is highly variable for the genus but fairly specific for the individual species, ranging from 8 to 18 days. *Plasmodium* infections tend to be most severe at the onset of the disease, rapidly declining in intensity (if the host survives the initial crisis) until a chronic low-level parasitemia is established. Stress conditions can lead to recrudescence of the infection.

Clinical Signs. The birds become listless and anorexic and stop preening and other normal behavioral activities. Anemia, edema of the eyelids, emaciation, and sudden death are frequently seen. Necropsies frequently reveal serous hemorrhage and hepato- and splenomegaly.

Differential Diagnosis. Specific diagnosis is carried out by examination of a thin, stained blood film. The species of *Plasmodium* most likely to be encountered in cage or aviary birds

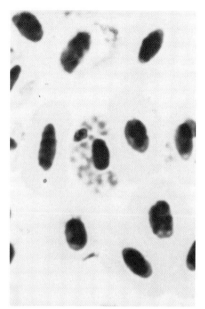

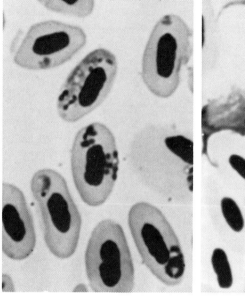

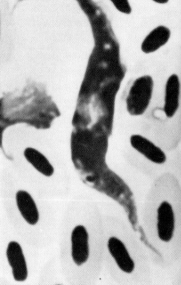

Fig. 20.5. Erythrocytic schizont of *Plasmodium circumflexum* (infected cell approximately 13 μm long).

Fig. 20.6. Erythrocytic schizont and macrogametocyte of *Plasmodium vaughani* (infected cell approximately 13 μm long).

Fig. 20.7. Trypanosome of the *T. avium* complex (uninfected erythrocytes 12–13 μm long).

are *P. circumflexum* (Fig. 20.5), *P. relictum,* and *P. vaughani* (Fig. 20.6); but due to the broad host range of avian malarias and the species and geographic location of host birds, almost any species of malaria can be involved. While a number of guides to the species of avian *Plasmodium* exist (Garnham 1966; Greiner et al. 1975), specific identification is probably best left to the specialist.

Treatment. Avian malarias such as *P. gallinaceum* tend to respond to treatments with antimalarial drugs (chloroquine at 5 mg/kg body weight and proguanil at 7.5 mg/kg body weight). However, the same drugs with other avian malaria species have little or no effect (Peters 1980). Treatment, therefore, is a somewhat ad hoc affair. Control is best achieved by the elimination of mosquito vectors.

Genus *Trypanosoma*
(Trypanosomatidae)

Synopsis. Since Danilewsky first described *Trypanosoma avium* (Fig. 20.7) in 1885, some 90 species of avian trypanosomes have been described. Studies by Bennett (1961) showed that trypanosomes from a single infected bird were transmissible to several bird species of a number of families and orders. Trypanosomes of identical morphology had different abilities to

develop in a range of vectors and subsequently infect new avian hosts. The avian trypanosomes exhibit extreme pleiomorphism, and specific identification is difficult on the basis of specimens seen in blood smears.

Life Cycle

Invertebrate Host. Transmission is by a blood-feeding arthropod, probably via the posterior station. Studies on certain strains of *T. avium* (Bennett 1961, 1970a,b) have shown that they multiply and produce infective stages in blackflies, mosquitoes, and ceratopogonid midges; reproduction (but not infective forms) also occurred in both tabanid flies and reduviid bugs. Other studies (Baker 1956) have shown that another strain of *T. avium* is transmitted by the hippoboscid fly *Ornithomyia avicularia,* although Bennett's strains would not multiply in this genus. Trypanosomes assume the promastigote and epimastigote stages on ingestion by a suitable arthropod and rapidly multiply by binary fission in the insect's stomach. When the digested blood meal is eliminated, a proportion of the trypanosomes remain in the hindgut and presumably infect a new host when the arthropod feeds again.

Vertebrate Host. Trypanosomes are intercellular parasites in the circulatory system and presumably have a tissue-oriented stage in their avian host. Neither the nature and location of this stage nor division of trypanosomes in the peripheral blood have yet been seen.

Clinical Signs. Avian trypanosomes are not incriminated as causing harm to their avian hosts. No symptoms are reported.

Specific Diagnosis. Trypanosomes usually occur in low numbers in blood films, and frequently there are only a few specimens per slide, making specific diagnosis tenuous. More accurate results are obtained using the hematocrit centrifuge techniques of Bennett (1962) and Woo (1969). Another excellent diagnostic approach is mixing fresh blood with physiological saline and examining the preparation under a coverslip for movement of trypanosomes. Specific diagnosis is currently based on morphological attributes of stained specimens and culture and serological techniques.

Treatment. Treatment is not warranted.

Microfilariae (Nematoda:Filarioidea)

Synopsis. The microfilariae found in the peripheral circulation of birds present a serious problem in species identification. During the first half or so of this century it was assumed that filariids were highly host specific and many species of filariids were described (under the genus designation *Microfilaria* or *Microfilarium*). Recent research by Anderson and his colleagues suggests that avian filariids have a broad host range with only a relatively few species with a wide geographical distribution.

Life Cycle

Invertebrate Host. Filarial worms are transmitted by a variety of biting flies, including blackflies (Simuliidae), mosquitoes (Culicidae), and biting midges (Ceratopogonidae). The biting flies ingest microfilariae in a blood meal; the microfilariae pass through the digestive tract into the body cavity and frequently lodge in the thorax. The parasites grow and pass through three larval molts in 9–15 days; the infective third stage migrates to the head, where it enters the vertebrate host when the insect feeds.

Vertebrate Host. On entry into the vertebrate host the filariid establishes in the appropriate tissue or organ (arterial wall, eyelid) and matures into the adult. The females, when fertilized, produce microfilariae, which are released into the circulating blood. The prepatent period is usually long; 75–90 days have been reported.

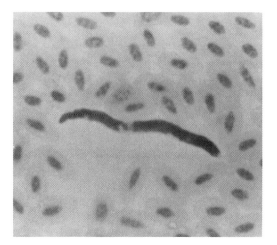

Fig. 20.8. Microfilaria found in the peripheral circulation of a psittacine. (*Courtesy of Walter J. Rosskopf, Jr., Hawthorne, Calif.*)

Clinical Signs. No signs have been reported.

Differential Diagnosis. Diagnosis is based on detection of microfilariae in the blood (Fig. 20.8); parasitemia is frequently low and detection enhanced by use of a hematocrit centrifuge or a similar technique (Bennett 1962; Woo 1969). Specific identification is best carried out by a specialist and requires the adult worms.

Treatment. Treatment is not warranted.

Avian Hematozoa of Uncertain Status

A variety of avian blood parasites are ascribed to the genera *Atoxoplasma, Babesia, Haemogregarina, Hepatozoon, Lankesterella,* and *Toxoplasma.* The taxonomy, life cycles, and relationships of these groups are poorly known in the avian context, and little consensus among various authorities can be found. Parasites of these groups are rarely encountered, and their effect on their avian hosts is seldom documented. Baker et al. (1972) have summarized knowledge on the avian blood coccidians (*Atoxoplasma, Haemogregarina*) and Box (1971) the *Lankesterella-Atoxoplasma* group; Peirce (1975) has reappraised the avian piroplasms. *Toxoplasma gondii* occurs in a wide variety of mammals and birds; in the latter hosts they apparently cause little problem (Levine 1985) and parasitemias rarely persist longer than 2 weeks. No satisfactory treatment is known for these parasites although some promising results using pyrimethamine and sulfonamides in combination have been obtained in mammals (Levine 1985). Diagnosis is by identification of the organism in tissue or blood preparations.

References

Adie, H. A. 1915. The sporogony of *Haemoproteus columbae. Indian J. Med. Res.* 2:671–80.

Aragao, H. B. 1907. Sobre o cyclo evolutio do halteridia do pombe. Nota preliminar. *Bras.-Med.* 21:141–42.

Baker, J. R. 1956. Studies on *Trypanosoma avium* Danilewsky 1885. II. Transmission by *Ornithomyia avicularia* L. *Parasitology* 46:335–52.

Baker, J. G., G. F. Bennett, G. W. Clark, and M. Laird. 1972. Avian blood coccidians. *Adv. Parasitol.* 10:1–30.

Bennett, G. F. 1961. On the specificity and transmission of some avian trypanosomes. *Can. J. Zool.* 39:17–33.

———. 1962. The haematocrit centrifuge for the laboratory diagnosis of haematozoa. *Can. J. Zool.* 40:123–25.

———. 1970a. *Trypanosoma avium* Danilewsky in the avian host. *Can. J. Zool.* 48:803–7.

———. 1970b. Development of trypanosomes of the *T. avium* complex in the invertebrate host. *Can. J. Zool.* 48:954–57.

Bennett, G. F., and J. I. Borrero. 1976. Blood parasites of some birds from Colombia. *J. Wildl. Dis.* 12:454–58.

Bennett, G. F., P. C. C. Garnham, and A. M. Fallis. 1965. On the status of the genera *Leucocytozoon* Ziemann, 1898, and *Haemoproteus* Kruse, 1890 (Haemosporidia: Leucocytozoidae and Haemoproteidae). *Can. J. Zool.* 43:927–32.

Bennett, G. F., M. Laird, R. A. Khan, and C. M. Herman. 1975. Remarks on the status of the genus *Leucocytozoon* Sambon, 1908. *J. Protozool.* 22:24–30.

Bennett, G. F., E. C. Greiner, and W. Threlfall. 1976. Impact of parasitic diseases on wildlife populations: Protozoans. In *Wildlife Diseases*, ed. L. A. Page, pp. 25–33. New York: Plenum.

Bennett, G. F., E. C. Greiner, M. F. Cameron, and C. M. Herman. 1977. Hematozoos de aves passeriformes silvestres muestreadas en anos sucesivos. *Bol. Dir. Malariol Saneamiento Ambiental* 16:313–19.

Bennett, G. F., M. Whiteway, and C. Woodworth-Lynas. 1982. *Host-Parasite Catalogue of the Avian Haematozoa.* Mem. Univ. Occas. Pap. Biol. 5:1–243.

Box, E. D. 1971. *Lankesterella (Atoxoplasma).* In *Infectious and Parasitic Diseases of Wild Birds,* ed. J. W. Davis, R. C. Anderson, L. H. Karstad, and D. O. Trainer, pp. 309–12. Ames: Iowa State University Press.

Coatney, G. R. 1935. The effect of Atebrin and Plasmochin on the *Haemoproteus* infection of the pigeon. *Am. J. Hyg.* 21:249–59.

Danilewsky, B. 1885. Zur Parasitologie des Blutes. *Biol. Zentralbl.* 5:529–37.

Fallis, A. M. 1948. Observations on *Leucocytozoon* infections in birds receiving Paludrine, Atebrin and sulphamerazine. *Can. J. Res. Sect. D Zool. Sci.* 26:73–76.

Fallis, A. M., S. S. Desser, and R. A. Khan. 1974. On species of *Leucocytozoon.* In *Advances in Parasitology,* vol. 12, ed. B. Dawes, pp. 1–67. New York: Academic.

Frank, W. 1965. Eine *Leucocytozoon:* Infektion bei Pennantsittichen (*Platycercus elegans*). *Gefiederte Welt* 89:93–94.

Garnham, P. C. C. 1966. Malaria parasites and other Haemosporidia. Oxford, Engl.: Blackwell Scientific Publications.

Greiner, E. C., and G. F. Bennett. 1975. Avian haematozoa. I. A color pictorial guide to some species of *Haemoproteus, Leucocytozoon* and *Trypanosoma. Wildl. Dis.* No. 66 (52 color figures on microfiche).

Greiner, E. C., G. F. Bennett, M. Laird, and C. M. Herman. 1975. Avian haematozoa. 2. Taxonomic keys and colour pictorial guide to species of *Plasmodium. Wildl. Dis.* No. 68 (44 color figures on microfiche).

Herman, C. M., S. S. Desser, G. F. Bennett, and I. B. Tarshis. 1977. Avian haematozoa. 3. Color atlas of *Leucocytozoon simondi* Mathis and Leger, 1910. *Wildl. Dis.* No. 70 (48 color figures on microfiche).

Julian, R. J., and D. E. Galt. 1980. Mortality in Muscovy Ducks (*Cairina moschata*) caused by *Haemoproteus* infection. *J. Wildl. Dis.* 16:39–44.

Kucera, J., K. Marjankova, V. Rachac, and J. Vitovec. 1982. Haemosporidiosis as a fatal disease in Muscovy Ducks (*Cairina moschata*) in South Bohemia. *Wildl. Dis.* No. 70 (48 color figures on microfiche).

Levine, N. D. 1985. *Veterinary Protozoology.* Ames: Iowa State University Press.

Levine, N. D., and G. R. Campbell. 1971. A check-list of the species of the genus *Haemoproteus* (Apicomplexa:Plasmodidae). *J. Protozool.* 18:475–84.

Manwell, R. D., and G. S. Rossi. 1975. Blood protozoa of imported birds. *J. Protozool.* 22:124–27.

Peirce, M. A. 1969. Blood parasites found in imported birds at post-mortem examination. *Vet. Rec.* 84:113–16.

———. 1975. *Nuttallia* Franca, 1909 (Babesidae), preoccupied by *Nuttallia* Dall, 1898 (Psammobiidae): A reappraisal of the taxonomic position of the avian piroplasms. *Int. J. Parasitol.* 5:285–87.

Peirce, M. A., and B. J. Bevan. 1977. Blood parasites of imported psittacine birds. *Vet. Rec.* 100:282–85.

Peters, W. 1980. Chemotherapy of malaria. Part B. Avian malaria. In *Malaria,* vol. 1, ed. J. P. Kreier, pp. 176–82. New York: Academic.

Poelma, F. G., and P. Zwart. 1972. Toxoplasmose bis kroonduiven en andere vogels in de Koninklijke Rotterdamse diergaarde "Blijdorp." *Acta Zool. Pathol. Antverp.* 55:29–40.

Ross, R. 1898. Preliminary report on the infection of birds with *Proteosoma* by the bites of mosquitoes. Calcutta: Government Press, Oct. 11.

———. 1899. Mosquitoes and malaria: The infection of birds by mosquitoes. *Br. Med. J.* 1:432–33.

Stoskopf, M. K., and J. Beier. 1979. Avian malaria in African Black-footed Penguins. *J. Am. Vet. Med. Assoc.* 175:944–47.

White, E. M., E. C. Greiner, G. F. Bennett, and C. M. Herman. 1978. Distribution of the haematozoa of neotropical birds. *Rev. Biol. Trop.* 26:43–102.

Woo, P. K. T. 1969. The haematocrit centrifuge for the detection of trypanosomes in the blood. *Can. J. Zool.* 47:921–23.

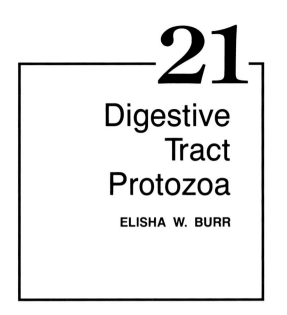

21

Digestive Tract Protozoa

ELISHA W. BURR

PROTOZOA of the digestive tract are an important cause of disease in birds kept by humans. For many centuries falconers have known the disease "frounce," caused by *Trichomonas. Histomonas,* likewise, has been known for decades as a cause of disease in galliforms. Also of economic importance are diseases caused by *Coccidia,* which are found in a wide range of avian hosts and probably more important in exotic birds than previously realized. Individual hosts may harbor several species of coccidiae and all parasitize the digestive tract except renal coccidiae of geese. The pathogenicity of digestive protozoans in the host depends on the parasite species, immunity, and genetic susceptibility of the host. Acquired immunity in highly susceptible flocks may limit the disease naturally. Birds are susceptible to protozoal diseases at any age but are usually more resistant to infection if they are previously exposed adult birds. The subject area is broad; only the more important diseases are discussed in this chapter.

Trichomoniasis

Etiology. Trichomoniasis is a common disease affecting pigeons and occasionally raptors (e.g., falcons), canaries, finches, and other small passerines. Large psittaciforms appear resistant to the infection: Budgerigars, however, may contract the disease in epidemic proportions. *Trichomonas gallinae* is the most common organism causing the disease although other trichomonads may occasionally be isolated. Some strains of the disease are highly virulent while others remain latent. Adult birds previously infected may be carriers of the disease. Direct contact via crop milk is a common mode of transmission among pigeons. Stress conditions may predispose to disease (overcrowding, poor hygiene, cold). The protozoa do not survive long outside of the host and therefore strict sanitation reduces disease incidence. Infection in raptors is caused by eating infected pigeons. Total eradication is not possible, as some trichomonads are always present in the mouth and crop (Perry 1983). Cecal trichomonads are usually nonpathogenic although they may destroy the integrity of the cecal mucosa, causing secondary bacterial invasion (Harrigan 1981).

Clinical Signs. The disease usually affects young birds, causing high mortality. Two types of lesions may be found, diphtheritic (wet canker) and necrotic (dry caseous necrosis). In adult birds, the disease is usually chronic, causing few mortalities. Weight loss and weakness may be seen in these birds, with wet canker ulcerations in the mouth, esophagus, larynx, and pharynx (Fig. 21.1). Bacterial invasion of the lesions ex-

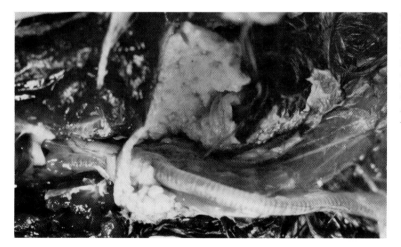

Fig. 21.1. Trichomonad esophagitis in a Budgerigar (*Melopsittacus undulatus*). The diphtheritic membranes became so extensive that complete obstruction occurred. (*Courtesy of David J. Schultz, Hawthorn, South Australia, Aust.*)

acerbates the disease and may produce lesions in the skin muscles or central nervous system. *Trichomonas* spp. are also the cause of a number of cases of moist and dry skin necrosis in the beak area, esophagus, and crop in pigeons and Budgerigars. Young birds are most often affected. Clinical symptoms of disease usually do not appear until after 4 weeks of age. Certain species of birds (pheasants, peafowl) appear to be extremely resistant to disease and may act only as carriers. Less often, similar lesions are seen around the vent and ventral aspects of squabs, with gross fecal contamination of the plumage. When esophageal lesions are severe, labored breathing and respiratory rales may be present. In the necrotic form of the disease, yellow caseous nodules are seen in the respiratory and digestive tracts. The conjunctiva is also occasionally affected. Virulent forms are sometimes evidenced by necrotic lesions in the liver and abdominal viscera. Vomiting and severe diarrhea may also be seen with the virulent form of the disease.

Diagnosis. Wet smear preparations of fresh specimens are the easiest method of diagnosing the disease. Oocysts are susceptible to heat drying and chemicals, so care must be taken when preparing slides (Jackson and Cooper 1981). Wet mounts of scrapings in warmed dextrose saline show organisms smaller than heterophils and of varying motility (Schultz 1978). Irregular twisting movements noticed on the smear are characteristic of the protozoa. If the "tails" are not flicking, they can sometimes be seen if the microscope condenser is racked down. The organism dies rapidly outside of the host, so immediate collection from a recently dead bird may be necessary for positive identification. In cases where liver involvement is suspected (especially in Budgerigars), isolation of trichomonads from the esophagus by crop tube and suction is usually successful.

Treatment. Dimetridazole is the most effective treatment for the disease (Fowler 1978; Schultz 1978; Steiner and Davis 1981; Woerpel and Rosskopf 1981; Burr 1982; Scholtens 1982) at 2 g/l in the drinking water for 7 days. Enheptin can also be used at 2 g/l in the drinking water. Medicated drinking water should not be made available to breeding birds with young for longer than 2 hours per day because of their increased water intake. Signs of overdose are ataxia, staggering, apparent blindness, and death. When the digestive tract is blocked by cankerous lesions, the birds must be treated by using 5 mg metronidazole/100 g body weight suspended in a glucose solution and tube fed for 7 days. Supplementary therapy may be necessary in extremely debilitated birds or in birds suffering from chronic weight loss (Fudge 1981). If a flock is severely infected, prophylactic use of dimetridazole may be indicated, along with culling of birds not likely to recover. Birds that recover may develop an immunity and perpetuate the disease. Protection can be transferred from immune to nonimmune birds via plasma or serum (Perry 1983). To prevent contamination of food and water, strict sanitation measures must be followed.

Giardiasis. *Giardia* is a protozoan closely related to *Hexamita*. Birds become infected via contaminated feces; therefore poor sanitation and hygiene predispose a bird to infection. Budgerigars are very susceptible to infection, and the disease is frequently seen in this species (Panigrahy et al. 1978). The disease is almost exclusively seen in small passerines and psittacines housed under intensive conditions. Natural infections are not known to occur.

Clinical Signs. Chronic diarrhea, weight loss, and occasionally death are seen in affected birds. The small intestine may be filled with a semisolid material and contain a large number of organisms. Necropsy reveals enteritis and mucosal ulceration (Perry 1983). In acute cases, a foamy, foul-smelling, yellow-brown diarrhea is seen. Mortality can be 20–50% in untreated cases. *Giardia* spp. infection can also contribute to a feather problem by blocking absorption of fat-soluble vitamins (Perry 1983). Elevated lactate dehydrogenase (LDH) and serum glutamic oxaloacetic transaminase (SGOT) levels associated with a leucopenia may be seen on the blood profile.

Diagnosis. Intestinal scrapings of duodenal loop is the best method of demonstrating the organism in freshly killed birds. The motile, pear-shaped trophozoite or thick-walled cysts can be seen in the scraping (Fig. 21.2). Demonstrating the organism in the feces is erratic and often frustrating since only the cyst form is shed in the droppings.

Treatment. Dimetridazole is placed in the drinking water at the rate of 2 g/l for 7 days. Adequate hygiene and sanitation help to prevent reinfection. Sulfonamides may be effective in mild infections but are not recommended for treating an outbreak. Treatment may have to be repeated in chronic cases to avoid a relapse. A good diet and a nonstressful environment should also be provided (Steiner and Davis 1981).

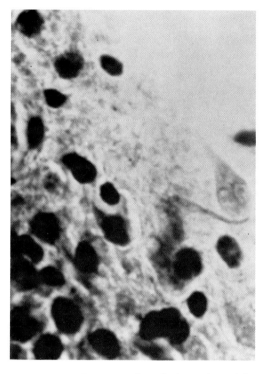

Fig. 21.2. Intestinal scrapings of the duodenal loop stained with Lugol's iodine, revealing motile, pear-shaped trophozoites of *Giardia* spp. from a psittacine. (*Courtesy of Walter J. Rosskopf, Jr., Hawthorne, Calif.*)

Histomoniasis

Etiology. This protozoan parasite frequently occurs in captive galliforms. Young birds are most susceptible to the disease. Pigeons, turkeys, quail, pheasants, partridge, and peafowl may be infected. The disease is caused by *Histomonas meleagridis* and spread by eating an infected cecal helminth egg (*Heterakis* spp.) or eating an invertebrate host. Invasion of the cecal mucosa by the heterakis larvae is thought to aid infection by *Histomonas meleagridis.*

Clinical Signs. Young birds are most often affected. Clinical symptoms of disease usually do not appear until after 4 weeks of age. Certain species of birds (pheasants, peafowl), appear to be extremely resistant to disease and may act only as carriers. Loose, blood-tinged feces are commonly seen. The liver may exhibit necrotic circular areas up to 1 cm in diameter (Fig. 21.3). The abdomen may be hard, swollen, and painful due to an enlarged cecum (Schultz 1981). The droppings are frequently yellow-green, indicating liver involvement. If enteritis is severe, emaciation and dehydration are evidenced. The disease is often rapid, producing high mortality. At necropsy, caseous casts may be found in the cecum and local peritonitis around the affected area.

Diagnosis. Definite diagnosis is only made on histopathological examination of the liver and cecum. Diagnosis of the heterakis egg in the

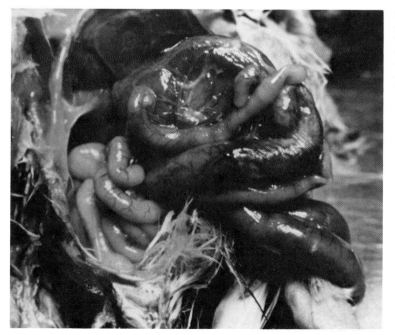

Fig. 21.3. Typhlitis and circular necrotic areas in the liver of a peachick (*Pavo cristatus*), caused by *Histomonas* spp. (*Courtesy of David J. Schultz, Hawthorn, South Australia, Aust.*)

feces may suggest *Histomonas* infection in galliforms.

Treatment. The protozoa can be treated using dimetridazole in the drinking water at 2 g/l for 5–7 days. To treat acute infection, Enheptin may be administered at 2 g/l water for 7 days. For chronic infection, longer treatments with this drug are necessary, which may result in drug toxicity. In commercial turkey operations, nitrophenylarsonic acid is placed in the feed at 375–500 g/t feed (Amand 1978). This is fed at 6 weeks of age and continued as a preventive medication until 1 week before slaughter. Nithiazide can also be used to treat chronic infections. *Heterakis* spp. can be treated using levamisole at 25 mg/kg subcutaneously (Arnall and Keymer 1975). Control is often difficult because it involves detecting the organism in the feces of carrier birds. Domestic poultry carry the organism and should not be run with game birds.

Complete control is best achieved by providing adequate sanitation, especially disinfecting cages and rotating birds periodically to clean premises. Young birds should not be reared near older birds. Adult birds do not generally require treatment if provided with adequate sanitation. Burning floors or raising birds on wire also help to control the disease (Schultz 1981).

Toxoplasmosis. The disease toxoplasmosis, caused by *Toxoplasma gondii,* occurs naturally in numerous avian species. Prior to the identification of *Lankesterella* (*Atoxoplasma*), certain infections caused by these species were described as toxoplasmosis (Harrigan 1981). In captive bird collections small passerines and penguins are most commonly affected (Obendorf and McColl 1980). Parrots, ducks, and crows can also be occasionally infected. Munday (1970) found the infection in 37% of 184 ravens in Tasmania. The disease appears to be of little importance to most cage bird species (Hasholt 1969). Outbreaks may occur, but usually individual specimens are involved.

Clinical Signs. Birds usually die rapidly before clinical symptoms appear. Occasionally neurological symptoms such as tremors and torticollis are seen a few days to hours before death. Digestive disturbances (rarely seen with the disease) consist of greenish, watery feces, probably due to liver involvement. At necropsy lesions may be found in the spleen, liver, kidney, brain, and intestine. Chronic cases of the disease are rare. Encephalitis and eye disorders may be seen in chronic cases.

Diagnosis. Histopathological examination reveals comma-shaped protozoan organisms associated with necrotic foci. Because the disease is seldom encountered, clinical symptoms alone may not suggest the disease. Definite diagnosis must be made by biological transmission.

Treatment. Treatment is unknown. Since the mode of transmission is also unknown, proper hygiene and sanitation are the only methods to control the disease. Cat feces often contain *T. gondii* oocysts and may aid in transmission through contamination of food. Cats, however, appear to be an insignificant cause of the disease in birds (Huchzermeyer 1983).

Hexamitiasis. This disease, caused by *Hexamita meleagridis,* affects galliforms and closely associated orders, most commonly turkeys, quail, pigeons, and pheasants. Occasionally other orders of birds are also affected. Adults tend to remain carriers and act as a reservoir to infect young birds. Emaciation and a fluid diarrhea may be the only clinical symptoms seen. Diagnosis is made by the demonstration of large numbers of rapidly motile organisms in wet smears of affected intestines from recently dead birds (Harrigan 1981). Control of the disease is based on isolation of carrier birds and maintaining proper sanitation. Treatment consists of dimetridazole placed in the water at recommended dosages.

Coccidiosis

Etiology. Numerous species of coccidiae occur in birds (Munday 1977; Marcus and Munday 1978; Thompson and Wright 1978; Ward 1978; Williams 1978; Harrigan 1981). These protozoans infect the small intestine of birds and produce oocysts that are passed in the feces. Differences in morphology of the sporulated oocyst result in classification of the organism into the following different genera (Harrigan 1981):

1. *Eimeria* spp. have sporulated oocysts containing four sporocysts, each with two sporozoites.
2. *Isospora* spp. have sporulated oocysts containing two sporocysts, each with four sporozoites.
3. *Dorisiella* spp. have sporulated oocysts containing two sporocysts, each with eight sporozoites.
4. *Wenyonella* spp. have sporulated oocysts containing four sporocysts, each with four sporozoites.
5. *Tyzzeria* spp. have sporulated oocysts con-

taining eight sporozoites free within the oocyst and not confined in any sporocyst.

6. *Sarcocystis* spp. have sporulated oocysts containing four sporozoites.

The life cycle for all the above species is similar. After ingestion of a sporulated oocyst, they hatch in the intestine and undergo several asexual generations. This schizogonous cycle is followed by a sexual (gametocytic) generation that passes nonsporulated oocysts in the feces (Harrigan 1981). Exposure to a warm environment allows them to hatch and become infective. Most coccidians live within the host without producing any pathological condition. The disease is most important in pigeons, quail, peafowl, ducks, and occasionally psittacines. It is seldom encountered in zoological collections because birds are not housed under intensive conditions, as are domestic poultry.

Clinical Signs. Enteritis may be the only clinical sign seen. The feces are frequently blood tinged and watery. Weight loss associated with chronic diarrhea may suggest the disease if many birds are housed together. Death may occur after heavy infestation for several months. Sudden deaths seldom occur. Lesions (sarcocysts) of *Sarcocystis* spp. are sometimes seen in the skeletal muscle and are visible with the naked eye (Fig. 21.4).

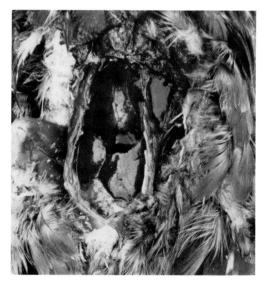

Fig. 21.4. Necropsy of a Princess Parakeet (*Polytelis alexandriae*) revealing small skeletal and visceral cysts that proved to be caused by *Sarcocystis* spp. (*Courtesy of George A. Smith, Peterborough, Engl.*)

Diagnosis. Diagnosis is made by clinical symptoms suggestive of the disease and demonstration of large numbers of organisms in the feces. Demonstration of a few oocysts in routine fecal examination is insignificant. Specific diagnosis of the feces must be made by laboratory methods.

Treatment. Numerous drugs that are available to treat domestic poultry have been used in captive birds. Treatment should include the use of sulfa drugs or amprolium, combined with improved sanitation (Dolensek and Bruning 1978). Amprolium at 3 ml/l water for 2 weeks is very safe and efficient to use in all species of birds. Sulfaquinoxaline 0.05% can also be used at 6 g/l water for 7 days (Williams 1978). This dosage must be increased by 50% in small birds, and a second treatment may have to be given. Resistance and toxicity to sulfonamides are known to occur in birds that have been treated continuously or overdosed (Burr 1983).

References

Amand, W. B. 1978. Fowl, quail, pheasant (Galliformes). In *Zoo and Wild Animal Medicine,* ed. M. E. Fowler, pp. 309–18. Philadelphia: W. B. Saunders.

Arnall, L., and I. F. Keymer. 1975. *Bird Diseases.* Neptune City, N.J.: T.F.H. Publications.

Burr, E. W. 1982. *Diseases of Parrots.* Neptune City, N.J.: T.F.H. Publications.

_____. 1983. Parasites of psittacine blood. *Mod. Vet. Pract.* 64(4):333–36.

Dolensek, E., and D. Bruning. 1978. Ratites. In *Zoo and Wild Animal Medicine,* ed. M. E. Fowler, pp. 167–80. Philadelphia: W. B. Saunders.

Fowler, M. E. 1978. Psittacines. In *Zoo and Wild Animal Medicine,* ed. M. E. Fowler. Philadelphia: W. B. Saunders.

Fudge, A. 1981. *Assoc. Avian Vet. Newsl.* 2(4):15.

Harrigan, K. E. 1981. Parasitic diseases of birds. In *Refresher Course for Veterinarians on Aviary and Caged Birds,* pp. 337–96. University of Sydney, Post-Graduate Committee in Veterinary Science, Proceedings no. 55. Sydney, Aust.

Hasholt, J. 1969. Toxoplasmosis. In *Diseases of Cage and Aviary Birds,* ed. M. L. Petrak, pp. 331–38. Philadelphia: Lea and Febiger.

Huchzermeyer, F. W. 1983. Personal communication (Veterinary Research Institute, Onderstepoort, South Africa).

Jackson, C. A. W., and K. Cooper. 1981. Trichomoniasis. In *Refresher Course for Veterinarians on Aviary and Caged Birds,* pp. 623–38. University of Sydney, Post-Graduate Committee in Veterinary Science, Proceedings no. 55. Sydney, Aust.

Marcus, M. B., and P. J. Munday. 1978. Intestinal sarcocystis in vultures and its significance. *Parasitology* 79:39.

Munday, B. L. 1970. The epidemiology of toxoplasmosis with particular reference to the Tasmanian environment. M.V.Sc. thesis, Faculty of Veterinary

Science, University of Melbourne.

———. 1977. A species of sarcocystis using owls as definite hosts. *J. Wildl. Dis.* 13:205–17.

Obendorf, D. L., and K. McColl. 1980. Mortality in Little Penguins (*Eudyptula minor*) along the coast of Victoria, Australia. *J. Wildl. Dis.* 16:251–59.

Panigrahy, B., G. Elissalde, L. C. Grumbles, and C. F. Hall. 1978. Giardia infection in parakeets. *Avian Dis.* 22:815–18.

Perry, R. A. 1983. *Vade Mecum. Diseases of Birds.* University of Sydney, Post-Graduate Foundation in Veterinary Science. Sydney, Aust.

Poelma, F. G., P. Zwart, G. M. Dorrestein, and C. M. Iordens. 1978. Cochlosomosis: A problem in raising waxbills kept in aviaries. *Tijdschr. Diergeneeskd.* 103:586–90.

Scholtens, R. G. 1982. *Assoc. Avian Vet. Newsl.* 3(3):53–54.

Schultz, D. J. 1981. Alimentary tract disease. In *Refresher Course for Veterinarians on Aviary and Caged Birds,* pp. 535–62. University of Sydney, Post-Graduate Committee in Veterinary Science, Proceedings no. 55. Sydney, Aust.

———. 1978. Diseases of parrots. In *Refresher Course for Veterinarians on Fauna,* pp. 223–44. University of Sydney, Post-Graduate Committee in Veterinary Science, Proceedings no. 36. Sydney, Aust.

Steiner, C. V., and R. B. Davis. 1981. *Caged Bird Medicine.* Ames: Iowa State University Press.

Thompson, E. J., and I. G. A. Wright. 1978. Coccidiosis in Kiwis. *N.Z. Vet. J.* 26:166–69.

Ward, F. P. 1978. Parasites and their treatment in birds of prey. In *Zoo and Wild Animal Medicine,* ed. M. E. Fowler, pp. 276–83. Philadelphia: W. B. Saunders.

Williams, R. B. 1978. Notes on some coccidia of peafowl, pheasants and chickens. *Vet. Parasitol.* 4:193–94.

Woerpel, R. W., and W. J. Rosskopf, Jr. 1981. Avian therapeutics. *Mod. Vet. Pract.* 62(12):947–49.

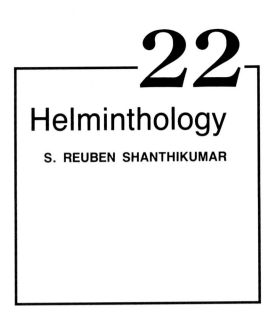

22

Helminthology

S. REUBEN SHANTHIKUMAR

HELMINTH PARASITE INFECTIONS are one of the most common conditions a veterinary practitioner encounters in cage and aviary bird practice. Helminth parasites of importance in captive birds are the nematodes or roundworms (class Nematoda, phylum Nemathelminthes), the cestodes or tapeworms (subclass Cestoda, phylum Platyhelminthes), and trematodes or flukes (class Trematoda, phylum Platyhelminthes). Acanthocephalids or thorny-headed worms (phylum Acanthocephala) are also of clinical significance in some species.

General Considerations. Parrots, finches, canaries, pigeons, and other birds are increasing in popularity as pet birds in North America, Europe, Australia, and other countries. Export and import control regulations have given rise to captive breeding, intensive rearing, and sale of many exotic birds.

Helminth infections in captive-bred birds are usually less prevalent than in wild-caught or newly imported birds. Infections are also more common in birds kept in outdoor aviaries, especially in zoos, where contact with wild birds and intermediate hosts is difficult to control.

Nematodes of the Digestive Tract

Capillaria contorta

General Biology. *Capillaria contorta*, the crop worm, occurs in the mouth, esophagus, and crop of a wide variety of birds. Major hosts are psittacines, passerines, galliforms, and anseriforms.

The male is 6–45 mm long, the size depending on the host species. The female is 15–46 mm long.

Life Cycle. *C. contorta* has a direct life cycle although sometimes earthworms may act as mechanical hosts. The eggs are passed in the feces of the bird and reach the infective stage after 4–6 weeks incubation. Birds are infected by the ingestion of the eggs, mostly by contaminated water and feed, and occasionally by mechanical hosts. The life cycle is completed in a minimum of 60 days.

Clinical Signs. Clinically the bird may show listlessness, weight loss, reduced water intake, feather loss, anorexia, anemia, or inflammation of the buccal mucosa. Drooping of the head, a penguinlike stance, and frequent swallowing attempts may also be seen.

Heavy infestations produce marked thickening, severe inflammation, a mucopurulent exudate, and sloughing of the mucosa. Chronic emaciation is frequently followed by death. Contents of the esophagus and crop may be hemorrhagic, and a large number of parasites may be found in the mucosa and necrotic membranes.

Diagnosis, Treatment, and Control. Diagnosis is based on the clinical signs and the demonstration of capillaria eggs in the feces of the bird. The eggs are lemon-shaped; have protruding transparent polar plugs and slightly barrel-shaped asymmetrical side walls; are thick, brown, and smooth-shelled; and have granular unsegmented contents. They measure 50–65 μm by 22 to 28 μm (Fig. 22.1).

At necropsy, lesions are readily seen in the esophagus and crop. The nematodes are difficult to see with the naked eye but readily detected when lesions are examined microscopically under low power.

Treatment has been successful in raptors, galliforms, columbiforms, and psittacines given

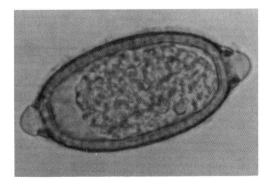

Fig. 22.1. *Capillaria* spp. eggs from a White-backed Magpie (*Gymnorhina hypoleuca*). (*Courtesy of K. E. Harrigan, University of Melbourne Veterinary School, Melbourne, Aust.*)

levamisole at 20 mg/kg body weight orally or 10 mg/kg body weight subcutaneously.

Control consists of preventing contamination of feed and water containers and eliminating mechanical hosts. New arrivals should be isolated and dewormed before introduction into an aviary. Routine treatment with anthelmintics reduces infection.

Dispharynx nasuta

General Biology. The nematode *Dispharynx nasuta* (syn.: *D. spiralis, Acuaria spiralis*), the gizzard worm, is found in the gizzard and proventriculus of Budgerigars and other psittacines, passerines, and game birds. The male is 7–8 mm long, the female 9–10 mm long with the body usually rolled into a spiral. The eggs are ellipsoidal, 36–40 μm long and 21 μm wide, and are embryonated when passed in the feces of the bird (Fig. 22.2).

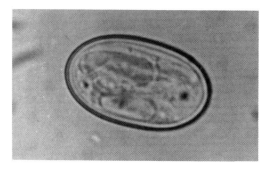

Fig. 22.2. *Dispharynx nasuta* eggs from a White-backed Magpie (*Gymnorhina hypoleuca*). (*Courtesy of K. E. Harrigan, University of Melbourne Veterinary School, Melbourne, Aust.*)

Life Cycle. Arthropods, pillbugs, sowbugs, beetles, and ants act as intermediate hosts. These invertebrates ingest embryonated eggs passed in the feces, and larvae are found in avian tissues. The third stage infective larvae develop within the invertebrate in about 26 days. Birds are infected by eating the infected intermediate host. The life cycle is completed in a minimum of 57 days.

Clinical Signs. Infected birds show droopiness, dullness, and ruffled feathers. There is inhibition of growth, anorexia, and inability to thrive, sometimes leading to emaciation and death in 2–3 weeks.

At necropsy, lesions are found that consist of ulceration and inflammation of the proventriculus. In heavy infestation, there is marked hypertrophy of the wall of the proventriculus, which may be as large as the gizzard (Fig. 22.3). The mucous membrane shows catarrhal inflammation and is often completely destroyed. The parasites may be buried in a mass of degenerated and necrotic tissue. In such cases the lumen of the proventriculus can be occluded.

Diagnosis, Treatment, and Control. Diagnosis is based on clinical signs, demonstration of eggs in the feces, and the presence of parasites in the proventriculus and gizzard.

Injectable levamisole can be used to treat gizzard worms at 20 mg/kg body weight orally or 10 mg/kg subcutaneously. Levamisole soluble powder has also been used in small passerines at 2.0 g/gal (4.5 l) drinking water for 5 days.

Control is based on preventing the ingestion of intermediate hosts, which is difficult in outdoor aviaries. The use of mild insecticides like pyrethrin preparations helps to reduce the arthropod intermediate hosts.

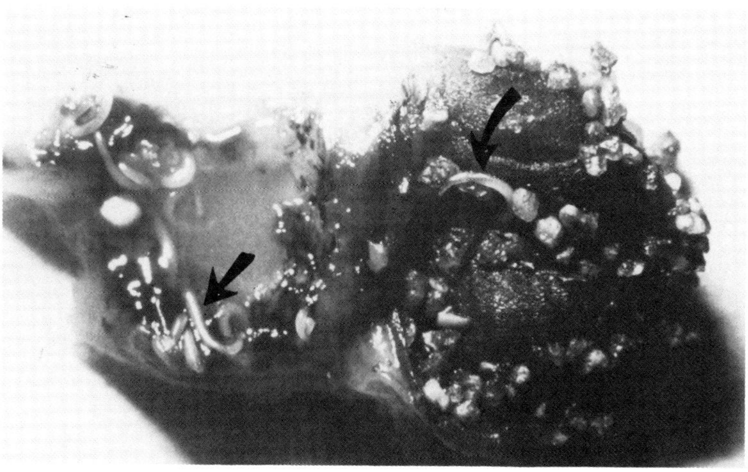

Fig. 22.3. *Dispharynx nasuta* (gizzard worms) (*arrows*) in the proventriculus and gizzard of an amazon parrot. (*Courtesy of F. W. Huchzermeyer, Onderstepoort, Republic of South Africa*)

Spiroptera incerta

General Biology. *Spiroptera incerta* (syn.: *Cyrnea incerta, Habronema incerta*) is one of the most important nematodes pathogenic to cage and aviary birds. It has been reported in numerous psittacine and other bird species.

Life Cycle. The life cycle of *S. incerta* is not well understood. It is possible that it is indirect, involving an arthropod intermediate host.

Clinical Signs. *S. incerta* infection may produce clinical symptoms similar to other nematode infections. Inability to thrive, emaciation, diarrhea, mucus in the droppings, and death after an acute attack may be seen.

At necropsy, *S. incerta* worms may be seen in the proventriculus. They cause swelling of the mucus membrane and interference with food passage. Adenomatous mucus membrane hyperplasia associated with peritonitis may be seen if the worms penetrate through the proventriculus into the air sacs. Immature worms are also sometimes found under the horny lining of the gizzard. Degeneration of the gizzard lining may be evidenced if the infection is severe (Fig. 22.4).

Diagnosis, Treatment, and Control. Clinical signs, detection of eggs in the feces, and necropsy findings help to diagnose the condition. Thiabendazole or levamisole may prove useful in treatment.

Tetrameres Fissispina

General Biology. *Tetrameres fissispina* is a nematode parasite principally found in the proventriculus of pigeons and aquatic birds, but it may also occur in galliforms. It is white and slender. The male is 3–6 mm long, the female 2.5–3 mm long and 1–2 mm wide. The males are filiform, the females globular. The eggs are thick shelled, 48–56 μm by 26–30 μm, and contain an embryo when passed in the feces.

Life Cycle. Amphipods, fleas, grasshoppers, cockroaches, and earthworms act as intermediate hosts. The larva is fully developed when the egg is laid; on ingestion of the eggs by the intermediate host, it hatches out and develops into the infective stage. Birds are infected by eating this stage. The complete cycle takes a minimum of 22 days.

Clinical Signs. Infection causes diarrhea, weight loss, emaciation, and anemia and may lead to death.

At necropsy, the proventriculus shows desquamation of epithelium and excessive mucus production. A marked catarrhal inflammation is evident. The mucosa is thickened and covered with tenacious mucus under which the female worms appear as discrete hematomas (30 to 50 worms may be present in the wall of the proventriculus). There are also soft nodules in the musculature, proventriculus, and intestine.

Diagnosis, Treatment, and Control. Diagnosis is based on clinical signs, detection of worm eggs in the feces, and the presence of worms in the proventriculus.

T. fissispina infection in pigeons has been successfully treated with levamisole at 15–30 mg/kg body weight orally. For effective control, eradication of intermediate hosts and regular deworming are necessary.

Capillaria obsignata

General Biology. *Capillaria obsignata* (syn.: *C. columbae*), the intestinal hair worm, is mostly found in wild and domestic pigeons. It is

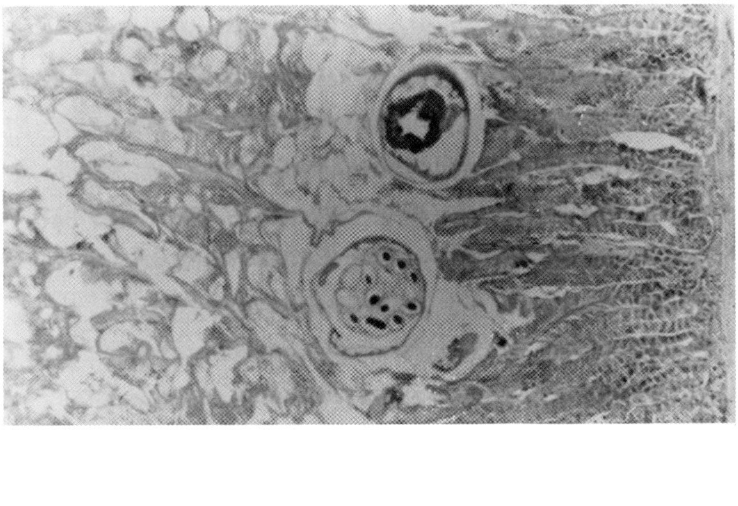

Fig. 22.4. Degeneration of the gizzard lining of a Blue-faced (Parrot) Finch (*Erythrura trichroa*) caused by *Cheilospirura* sp. (*Courtesy of K. E. Harrigan, University of Melbourne Veterinary School, Melbourne, Aust.*)

a parasite of the intestine. The male is 8.6–10 mm long, the female 10–12 mm.

Life Cycle. The life cycle is direct; infection occurs by ingestion of eggs in contaminated feed and water. The infective stage develops within the eggshell in about 8 days. The life cycle is completed in a minimum of 19–26 days.

Clinical Signs. Clinical signs consist of droopiness, weakness, emaciation, incoordination, and diarrhea. Younger birds are more susceptible and may die within 8–10 days of the onset of clinical signs. In chronic cases, there is diarrhea with mucus and blood; in severe cases this also contains numerous epithelial cells. The diarrhea may improve, birds may regain normal appearance, and feces may become firm, but unless treated, birds will continue to lose weight and become markedly emaciated and debilitated.

At necropsy extensive destruction of the intestinal mucosa can be seen and the intestine contains large quantities of dark brown hemorrhagic fluid. In chronic cases, there is marked thickening of the intestinal wall and edema.

Diagnosis, Treatment, and Control. The infection can be diagnosed by the clinical signs and the detection of eggs in the feces. The eggs are similar to *C. contorta*. They are lemon-shaped with protruding transparent polar plugs (both ends) and have a thick, brown, smooth shell and granular, unsegmented contents. They are 50–62 μm long and 20–25 μm wide.

Treatment can be attempted with levamisole at 15–30 mg/kg body weight orally.

Control is best achieved by maintenance of good hygiene and covering aviaries to prevent contamination by wild birds. Routine deworming is also important.

Ascaridia galli

General Biology. *Ascaridia galli* occurs in the small intestine of Budgerigars, other psittacines, galliforms, anseriforms, and various wild birds. They are whitish yellow worms. The male is 5–7.5 cm long, the female 7–11.5 cm. There are three large lips around the mouth, and the esophagus has no posterior bulb. The eggs are ellipsoidal with slightly barrel-shaped side walls and have a thick, smooth, three-layer shell with the middle layer most developed. The eggs measure 75–80 μm long and 45–50 μm wide, and the contents are unsegmented when passed in the feces.

Life Cycle. This parasite may have a direct life cycle or an indirect one through earthworms or grasshoppers. The eggs are passed in the feces of the bird, and the infective second stage larvae develop within the egg in 8–10 days under optimal conditions (30–33°C, 80% relative humidity). The eggs are then ingested by birds with contaminated feed or water, and larvae are liberated inside the intestine. Earthworms or grasshoppers may ingest the eggs and act as mechanical vectors and also spread the infection. The cycle is complete in a minimum of 35 days.

Clinical Signs. Clinical symptoms in infected birds include diarrhea, constipation, lethargy, exhaustion, and anemia. Young birds are affected more than adults. In heavy infections, intestinal lesions include acute congestion and hemorrhagic enteritis. In less severe infections, there are catarrhal inflammation and chronic enteritis. Secondary effects are obstruction or perforation of the intestines, and mature worms are occasionally found inside the oviduct, causing blockage and egg peritonitis. Liver scarring is sometimes seen.

Diagnosis, Treatment, and Control. Ascaridia infection can be diagnosed by the clinical symptoms and by the demonstration of eggs in the feces.

Treatment is successful with piperazine at 175–400 mg/kg body weight in feed or water, to be repeated after 21 days. Levamisole can also be used at 20 mg/kg body weight orally or 10 mg/kg subcutaneously.

Control is by maintenance of good hygiene, minimized contact with wild birds, and elimination of earthworms. Routine deworming is also advised.

Ascaridia columbae

General Biology. The nematode *Ascaridia columbae* is found in the small intestine of wild and domestic pigeons and has also been reported in a Barraband Parakeet (*Polytelis swainsonii*). It is similar to *A. galli* but smaller, the male 1.6–3.1 cm long and the female 2.0–3.7 cm. The eggs also appear similar to *A. galli* and are 68–90 μm by 40–50 μm.

The life cycle, clinical features, diagnosis, treatment, and control are similar to *A. galli* infection.

Ascaridia hermaphrodita

General Biology. *Ascaridia hermaphrodita* is the most commonly found ascarid worm in cage and aviary birds. It occurs in the small intestine of numerous psittacines and other avian species.

The worms and eggs are similar in appearance to *A. galli.*

The life cycle, clinical features, diagnosis, treatment, and control are similar to *A. galli* infection.

Heterakis gallinarum

General Biology. *Heterakis gallinarum* is a nematode found commonly in the ceca of a wide variety of birds including Budgerigars, passerines, game birds, peafowl and other galliforms, and anseriforms. It is a small white worm. The male is 7–13 mm long, the female 10–17 mm. The mouth is surrounded by three small lips, and the esophagus ends in a well-developed bulb. The eggs are thick shelled and ellipsoidal, have unsegmented contents, and are 63–75 μm long and 36–48 μm wide.

Life Cycle. The life cycle is usually direct, but earthworms may act as intermediate transport hosts. The eggs are passed in the feces, and birds are infected by ingestion of contaminated feed and water. Earthworms may ingest the eggs and act as "concentrating" transport hosts. Eggs reach the infective stage in 12–15 days under optimal conditions. A minimum of 36 days are required for the parasite to complete its life cycle.

Clinical Signs. Clinical signs of infection are anorexia, diarrhea, emaciation, stunting, and cessation of egg laying.

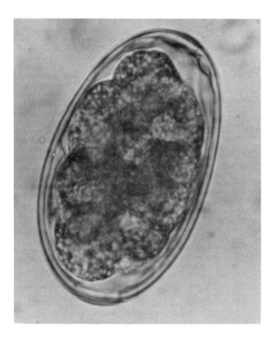

At necropsy prominent lesions are seen only in heavy infection; they consist of slight thickening of the cecal mucosa, with petechial hemorrhage. The principal importance of *H. gallinarum* is its role as a carrier of *Histomonas meleagridis,* the protozoan parasite that causes enterohepatitis (blackhead). The protozoan parasite remains viable in the eggs of *H. gallinarum,* and birds that ingest them develop blackhead.

Diagnosis, Treatment, and Control. A diagnosis of *H. gallinarum* infection is made by the detection of eggs in the feces and worms in the cecum.

Levamisole at 20 mg/kg body weight orally has been found effective. Thiabendazole can also be used at 25–50 mg/kg body weight.

The parasite is normally nonpathogenic but can be controlled by reducing food and water contamination.

Nematodes of the Respiratory System

Syngamus trachea

General Biology. *Syngamus trachea,* called gapeworms due to the gaping they produce in infected birds, are parasitic nematodes found in the trachea or bronchi of a wide variety of birds, especially passerines and game birds.

S. trachea is a bright red worm, the male 2–6 mm long, the female 5–20 mm. They form a Y shape because they are found constantly in copula. The eggs are ellipsoidal, operculated at either pole, and 78–100 μm long and 43–60 μm wide. The egg, when passed in the feces, usually contains a morula with 8 to 16 blastomeres (Fig. 22.5).

Life Cycle. The life cycle may be direct or indirect. The eggs are liberated in the trachea or bronchi and are coughed up by the bird, where they may drop to the ground or be swallowed and passed out in the feces. Under optimal conditions (25°C, 85–90% relative humidity), the third stage infective larvae develop within the eggshell in 1–2 weeks. Then the cycle may take one of three courses: (1) the egg is ingested directly, (2) the larvae hatch and are ingested, or (3) the larvae are ingested by an intermediate host (earthworm, slug, snail, myriapod, housefly, other invertebrate) and passed

Fig. 22.5. *Syngamus trachea* eggs from a White-backed Magpie (*Gymnorhina hypoleuca*). (*Courtesy of K. E. Harrigan, University of Melbourne Veterinary School, Melbourne, Aust.*)

on to the bird when eaten. Once in the bird's intestine, larvae reach the trachea and bronchi via the bloodstream. The life cycle is completed in a minimum of 21 days.

Clinical Signs. The disease is most severe in young birds. The worms may cause partial blockage of the trachea, which causes marked dyspnea, the bird fighting for breath with the mouth gaping open. The birds may show cough, head shaking, inappetence, emaciation, and anemia. The respirations can become laborious, leading to death by suffocation. Although a major pathogenicity is due to adult worms causing obstruction, the larvae migrating in the lung may cause a lobular bronchopneumonia. In less acute forms of the disease, local nodular inflammatory reactions may be seen at the site of attachment of the worm.

Diagnosis, Treatment, and Control. The typical gaping position of the bird is diagnostic of *S. trachea* infection, although diagnosis is more difficult in less acute cases and in the pulmonary form. Presence of characteristic eggs in the feces is confirmative of the infection.

Treatment has been attempted with several drugs. Disophenol was found to be effective in pheasants at 10 mg/kg body weight subcutaneously but was toxic and caused 11% mortality in the birds. Better results could be expected with Ivermectin, although there are no reports of usage in cage and aviary birds. Thiabendazole has been found to be effective at 25–50 mg/kg body weight orally. Thibenzole, a premix containing 25% W/V thiabendazole and normal feed ingredients to 100% can be used for treatment in pheasants and other ground birds at 4 kg/t feed. Medicated feed should be given for 2–3 weeks. Mebendazole at 125 mg/kg feed for 3 days controlled the infection in young pheasants. Levamisole injectable solution 13.65% given in drinking water at 1.25 ml/l water was effective in geese (medicated water was the only water provided for 24 hours, and treatment was repeated after 3 weeks). Good hygiene can control *S. trachea* infection in pet birds kept indoors. A covered roof in outdoor aviaries can help to prevent infection from wild birds. Soil floors in aviaries provide a source of infection through intermediate hosts.

Nematodes of the Circulatory System

Filarial Roundworms

General Biology. Filarial roundworms are long, thin, threadlike nematodes that live in the lymph, blood, connective tissue, air sacs, and thoracic and abdominal cavities. They produce larvae (microfilariae) that are found in the blood and tissues of birds. Numerous species of filarial worms have been found in passerines, psittacines, falconiforms, and anseriforms. The Corvidae and Coracidae families in particular harbor several species. *Splendidofilaria passerina* is a pathogenic species found in House Sparrows and *Diplotriaena* spp. have been reported in thrushes, grackles, and crows. Microfilariae have been detected in the blood of many captive birds; of 183 birds of 21 species that died in one zoo, 12% had microfilariae.

Life Cycle. The life cycle of many species is unknown, but generally speaking, the parasites live in the lymph, blood, and tissues of the bird and the females produce ova, which give rise to microfilariae (larvae). These microfilariae enter the bloodstream and are transmitted by bloodsucking insects such as simulids, culicoids, midges, and lice. The microfilariae, on entering the insect intermediate host, encyst in the thoracic muscles. After further development, the infective larvae emerge and enter the proboscis of the insect and are transmitted to birds when they bite the host. The larvae enter the bloodstream, reach the appropriate site, and mature to adults.

Clinical Signs. Very little information is available. One report regarded *D. tricuspis* as pathogenic to jays, causing pneumonia and consolidation of the lungs. Fits and sudden death have been reported due to microfilariae plugging cerebral capillaries or due to rupture of blood vessels.

At necropsy, subserosal cysts in intestines, enlargement and thickening of arterial walls, and fibrosis, necrosis, and stenosis of blood vessels may be seen. Filarial worms may also be seen inside air sacs and the thoracic and abdominal cavities.

Diagnosis, Treatment, and Control. Filarial infections can be diagnosed in the live bird by the detection of microfilariae in the blood. Examination of a drop of blood as a wet preparation or of a thick, Giemsa-stained blood smear usually reveals microfilariae. When a wet preparation is examined with a low-power microscope, microfilariae are seen wriggling actively. A thick, stained blood smear allows detailed examination of the microfilariae. Since microfilariae often exhibit periodicity, blood should be examined at 8-hour intervals.

No satisfactory treatment is available. Some control is possible by the elimination of biting flies (simulids, culicoids).

Filarial Nematodes of the Subcutaneous Tissues

Avioserpens taiwana

The nematode *Avioserpens taiwana* (syn.: *Oshimaia taiwana*) is found in ducks. It causes subcutaneous nodules under the mandible and other parts of the body. The female worm is 25 cm long.

Life Cycle. The developmental cycle is indirect via various species of cyclops. The filarial larvae pass through an opening in the skin made by the female worm when the bird enters water. The infective larvae occur in the body cavity of the cyclops, and birds become infected by ingesting infected cyclops.

Clinical Signs. Clinically, there are swellings under the skin on all parts of the body, but particularly under the mandible. The nodules become hard and painful, may reach the size of a hazel nut, and interfere with respiration and swallowing. Severe cases lead to emaciation and asphyxia. Swellings may occur on the leg, interfering with movement, and when parasites die in the nodules, abscesses may form.

Diagnosis, Treatment, and Control. Diagnosis is based on clinical symptoms and seasonal incidence. It is most common in the dry season. Successful treatment has been achieved by the surgical removal of the worms from the nodules and local antibiotic therapy. Control measures consist of providing ducklings with water free of cyclops.

Pelecitus clavus

General Biology. *Pelecitus clavus* (syn.: *Eulimdana clava*), a filarial nematode parasite of pigeons, is found in the subcutaneous connective tissue of the neck. It is a small nematode, the male 6–7 mm long and the female 17–20 mm. The microfilariae are 80 μm long and 6 μm in diameter. The microfilariae of *P. mazzanti,* another filaria of pigeons, is 140–180 μm long.

Life Cycle. The microfilariae are found in the blood. The life cycle probably involves an intermediate host, but nothing is known.

Clinical Signs. This nematode generally is not very pathogenic, but there are reports of anorexia, wasting, and anemia. Local lesions consist of congestion and subcutaneous hemorrhage in the peritracheal region. General lesions of congestion, necrosis of the liver and pancreas, and punctiform intestinal hemorrhages, all due to microfilariae, have also been seen.

Diagnosis, Treatment, and Control. No treatment is available, and control is not known because of lack of knowledge of the life cycle.

Ornithofilaria fallisensis

This is a filarial nematode found in the subcutaneous tissues of birds, especially ducks and geese. It is transmitted by simulids (blackflies), and the infection is seasonal in occurrence.

Nematodes of the Eye

Oxyspirura mansoni

General Biology. This parasitic nematode is found under the nictitating membrane and sometimes in the nasal sinus of numerous bird species.

The male nematode is 10–16 mm long, the female 12–19 mm. The eggs are embryonated when deposited and are 50–60 μm by 45 μm.

Life Cycle. The life cycle is indirect and involves the cockroach (*Pycnoscelus surinamensis*) as the intermediate host. Eggs are deposited underneath the nictitating membrane and washed down the lachrymal ducts into the nasal cavity, swallowed, and passed out in the feces of the bird. The eggs are ingested by the cockroach along with fecal material and hatch in the digestive tract of the insect. After migration and growth, they become third stage infective larvae in approximately 50 days and encyst in various parts of the insect. Birds are infected when they ingest the infected cockroaches. The larvae are liberated in the crop, migrate anteriorly, and reach the nictitating membrane via the esophagus, pharynx, and lachrymal duct.

Clinical Signs. The birds are uneasy and frequently scratch their eyes. There is marked lachrymation with conjunctivitis and later ophthalmia and blindness. Lesions depend on the number of worms present, varying from a mild conjunctivitis to total destruction of the eye in severe cases. The nictitating membrane becomes swollen and protrudes from the corner of the eyelids. The eyelids may be stuck together with exudate, and caseous material may collect underneath them due to bacterial infection. Parasites are usually not present in the later stages of infection due to the marked reaction.

Diagnosis, Treatment, and Control. Diagnosis is based on clinical symptoms and detection of eggs in the feces. Parasites may be also detected in the eye. Treatment consists of the removal of the worms with fine forceps, under general anesthetic. After removal, antibiotic eyedrops are helpful in controlling secondary bacterial infections. Control is by the destruction of cockroaches with a suitable insecticide (e.g., pyrethrin derivatives) and preventing ingestion of the insects.

Acanthocephalids. Acanthocephalids
(thorny-headed worms) are cylindrical helminth parasites that are covered with a thick cuticle, do not possess an alimentary canal, and absorb nutrients through the body wall. Anteriorly they have a retractable proboscis that is usually inserted into the intestinal mucosa of the host to provide a firm anchor. The eggs are thick shelled and have a hooked embryo (acanthor). Various intermediate hosts, usually arthropods, are required for the developmental cycle to be completed.

Polymorphus boschadis

Polymorphus boschadis (syn.: *P. minutus*) occurs in the small intestines of various anseriforms and passerines. The male is 3 mm long, the female up to 10 mm. It has a most distinctive bright orange color when fresh, and the cuticle is covered with anterior spines. The proboscis is spindle-shaped and carries sixteen rows of seven to ten hooks each. The eggs are fusiform, measure 110 μm by 20 μm, and have a yellowish red embryo.

Life Cycle. In anseriforms, the developmental cycle is indirect through the freshwater shrimp *Gammarus pulex* or *G. lacustris.* The infective juvenile form may also reencyst in fish that serve as transport hosts. The birds become infected by the ingestion of these crustaceans. In passerines, annelids and terrestrial insects act as intermediate hosts.

Clinical Signs. Infection with this parasite produces a general debility associated with diarrhea. The bird becomes emaciated and gradually dies. At necropsy, parasites may be found in the terminal part of the intestine. White or yellowish pea-sized nodules may be visible on the surface of the intestinal wall. There is inflammation of the mucosa with catarrhal enteritis and hemorrhagic spots.

Diagnosis, Treatment, and Control. Infection is difficult to diagnose clinically due to the indistinct clinical signs presented. Fecal examination may show the characteristic eggs, or at necropsy parasites and nodules may be found. Treatment with thiabendazole has been found to be useful. Control is by the elimination of freshwater crustaceans and other intermediate hosts, such as annelids.

Fillicollis anatis

General Biology. *Fillicollis anatis* is a thorny-headed worm found in the small intestine of various anseriforms. The male is white, 6–8 mm long and 1–2 mm in diameter. The female is yellow, 10–25 mm long and up to 4 mm in diameter. The proboscis of the male is ovoid, carrying eighteen longitudinal rows of ten or eleven hooks each. The female has a long slender neck; the proboscis is spherical, 2–3 mm in diameter, and there are eighteen rows of ten or eleven hooks each, arranged in a star-shaped pattern. The eggs are ovoid, 60–70 μm by 20–25 μm.

Life Cycle. The life cycle of *F. anatis* involves the crustacean *Asellus aquaticus.* Infection of birds occurs when they ingest these crustaceans carrying the infective stage.

Clinical Signs. Clinical signs are general debility, associated with diarrhea, emaciation, and death. At necropsy, parasites are found in the middle part of the intestine. Well-developed white or yellowish nodules, catarrhal enteritis, and hemorrhagic spots may be found.

Diagnosis, Treatment, and Control. Diagnosis is by the demonstration of eggs in the feces and of parasites and nodules at necropsy. Thiabendazole has been useful in treating the infection. Control is by the elimination of the crustacean intermediate host.

Other Important Acanthocephalids

Other acanthocephalids of significance are *Plagiorhynchus formosus, Prosthorhynchus* spp. and *Centrorhynchus* spp. found in passerines, and *Mediorhynchus grande,* which has been reported in a Varied Lorikeet (*Psitteuteles versicolor*).

Cestodes

General Biology. Cestodes (tapeworms) are flattened (tapelike), segmented helminth parasites found in psittacines, passerines, raptors, pigeons, and a variety of other birds (Fig. 22.6). They have a scolex (anterior end) and a neck that produces segments (proglottids) collectively called "strobila." Most taenioid tapeworms have a retractile organ with hooks

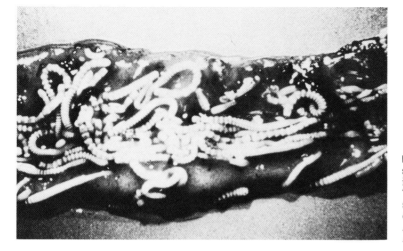

Fig. 22.6. Tapeworm segments in the small intestine of a psittacine. The tape- or ribbonlike segments (strobila) are evident. (*Courtesy of F. W. Huchzermeyer, Onderstepoort, Republic of South Africa*)

(the rostellum). Tapeworms vary in length according to species. They do not have an alimentary system and absorb nutrients through the body wall. Most tapeworms are found in the small intestine, attached to the mucosa by the scolex. In a heavy infestation, however, the entire intestine can be full of them. Newly captured birds have been found to have large masses of tapeworms in their intestines, without apparently any ill effects.

Tapeworms of importance in cage and aviary birds belong to the families Davaineidae, Hymenolepididae, Dilepididae, and Anoplocephalidae. Davaineidae are found in various birds, including passerines and psittacines. Hymenolepididae are found in anatids, passerines, and other birds. Dilepididae are common in passerines. Anoplocephalidae are mainly mammalian parasites but sometimes are found in psittacines.

Since tapeworms require an intermediate host for transmission, they are more common in insect-eating birds than in birds feeding predominantly on seeds and fruits. Infection also occurs in nestlings fed insects as a protein and supplement.

Life Cycle. The life cycle is indirect and involves an intermediate host such as annelids (earthworms), mollusks, and aquatic and terrestrial arthropods (ants, beetles). When the eggs are ingested by the invertebrate, the hexacanth embryo penetrates the intestinal wall and eventually develops into the cysticercus (bladder worm), the part of the invertebrate depending on the species of cestode. Birds become infected by ingestion of the invertebrate.

Clinical Signs. Clinical manifestations of cestode infections are not always clear, varying from diarrhea to general debility and even death. Only a few tapeworms may be pathogenic while at other times large numbers may be present without causing any ill effects. At necropsy, lesions can be seen consisting of catarrhal or hemorrhagic enteritis, especially where the scolex is attached to the mucosa. Large numbers of tapeworms occasionally cause intestinal obstruction.

Diagnosis, Treatment, and Control. The presence of tapeworm eggs or proglottids in the feces is diagnostic of the infection. At necropsy, large masses of tapeworms are sometimes found.

Niclosamide is used for oral treatment of small passerines and psittacines at 500 mg/kg body weight. Praziquantel administered orally is quite effective in parrots and raptors. Dichlorophen has also been used at 600 mg/kg body weight. Control consists mainly of elimination of potential intermediate hosts, whenever possible.

Trematodes. Trematodes (flukes) are dorsoventrally flattened helminth parasites (flatworms) with leaflike bodies. Exceptions are amphistomes, which are thick, fleshy flukes, and schistosomes, which are elongate forms. They have a cuticle, which may be smooth or spinous. In most trematodes, there is an oral sucker at the anterior end and a ventral sucker placed ventrally. The orifice at the anterior end also serves as the mouth and leads into the pharynx, which in turn leads into the alimentary canal. The worms are hermaphrodites except in schistosomes (where the sexes are separate). The eggs are yellowish or brown

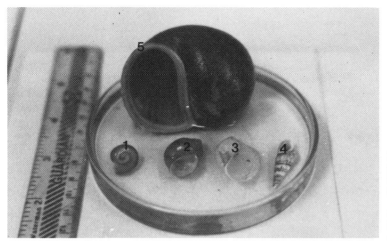

Fig. 22.7. Shells of snails that are intermediate hosts in the life cycle of trematodes: *Planorbis* sp. (*1*), *Viopara* sp. (*2*), *Lymnaea* sp. (*3*), *Melania* sp. (*4*), *Pila* sp. (*5*). (*Courtesy of Elisha W. Burr*)

to dark brown and possess a thin shell with an operculum.

The eggs are passed out in the feces of the host, and the larvae enter an appropriate molluscan intermediate host, usually snails (Fig. 22.7). After development and multiplication within the snail, the final larval stage (cercaria) leaves the snail and reaches the final host by being ingested or by penetration of the host skin. A second intermediate host, such as dragonflies or other invertebrates or fish, may be necessary for completion of the life cycle in some species of flukes.

Flukes in birds may parasitize the digestive tract, respiratory system, eye, reproductive system, skin, kidney, or blood vessels. All trematodes found in birds belong to the suborder Prosostomata, order Digenea, class Trematoda.

Trematodes of the Reproductive System

Prosthogonimus ovatus

General Biology. This fluke is found in the bursa of Fabricius and oviduct of passerines, anseriforms, and other wild birds. It is 3–6 mm long and 1–2 mm wide. The ventral sucker is almost double the size of the oral sucker. The eggs are small, thin shelled, and measure 22–24 μm by 13 μm.

Life Cycle. The life cycle requires two intermediate hosts for completion. The first is a water snail, the second the nymphal stage of dragonflies. Three species of water snails may act as intermediate hosts for *P. ovatus*: *Bithynia leachi*, *Gyraulus albus* or *G. gredleri*. After liberation from the snail, the cercariae swim about in the water and are drawn into the anal openings of dragonfly naiads by the breathing movement of these insects. The cercaria sheds the tail and the metacercaria migrates from the rectal respiratory chamber into the muscles and finally becomes encysted in the hemocoel. The metacer-

cariae reach the infective stage about 2 months after infection. In North America species of dragonflies of the genera *Tetragoneuria*, *Leucorhynia*, *Epicordulia*, and *Mesothermis* act as second intermediate hosts. In other countries, the genera *Libellula*, *Platycnemis*, *Epicordulia*, *Anax*, and *Sympetrum* may serve as second intermediate hosts.

The cercaria persists in the hemocoel until the dragonfly becomes an adult. Birds become infected by ingesting the infected naiad or adult dragonfly. The metacercariae are liberated in the small intestine and migrate to the cloaca (in young birds, the bursa of Fabricius), where they become adults. When the bursa of Fabricius begins to atrophy, the parasite enters the oviduct. In the case of passerines, the intermediate hosts are land snails and insects. Captive birds become infected by eating a dragonfly, the dragonfly being part of the wild bird cycle.

Clinical Signs. Clinically, birds may show malformed eggs, anorexia, dullness, and emaciation. Birds show a tendency to sit on the nest and may adopt a penguin stance due to increased distension of the abdomen. In acute infections, marked inflammation of the oviduct causes the eggs to be ejected rapidly without shells. A milky fluid, consisting of secretions from the calcium glands in the uterus, may also be discharged and adhere to the feathers around the anus. Where retroperistalsis has resulted in peritonitis, a marked distension of the abdomen is evident and the birds appear obviously ill, become prostrate, and die. There is acute inflammation of the oviduct, and eggs have either no or very thin shells. As a result of retroperistalsis, the broken yolk, albumin, bacteria, and parasites enter the peritoneal cavity, producing an often-fatal acute peritonitis.

At necropsy, flukes may be seen embedded in the mucosa or free in the lumen. In chronic cases, distension of the oviduct and thickened walls are seen and the mucosa is covered with a sticky exudate containing albumin, blood, and fibrin. Rupture of the oviduct may take place. The abdomen is often markedly swollen and discolored. The infection is often seasonal, occurring in spring and early summer because of the life cycle of dragonflies.

Diagnosis, Treatment, and Control. Diagnosis is based on evidence of malformed eggs, abdominal distension, or the discharge of eggs without shells from the cloaca. Diagnostic lesions seen at necropsy are an excessively distended oviduct and "egg peritonitis." In acute infections, the trematodes are seen as small, reddish flukes embedded in the inspissated material in the oviduct. Trematode eggs can also be seen on a fecal examination.

There is no satisfactory treatment. Control is by preventing birds from ingesting intermediate hosts.

Trematodes of the Skin

Collyriclum faba

General Biology. *Collyriclum faba* is a trematode parasite causing skin lesions in passerines, galliforms, and other birds. It is a plump, spiny form 3–5 mm long by 4.5–5.5 mm wide. The oral sucker is subterminal, the ventral sucker absent. The eggs are 19–21 μm by 10–11 μm. The parasite occurs in cysts in the subcutaneous tissue. The cysts are about 4–6 mm in diameter; each contains two worms of unequal size with their ventral surfaces applied to each other, and there is a central opening through which the eggs escape.

Life Cycle. The life cycle is not well understood, but it is possible that the dragonfly naiads are infected by the cercariae, similar to *Prosthogonimus* spp.

Clinical Signs. The subcutaneous cysts are found mainly around the cloaca but may occur elsewhere in the body. In heavy infestations, birds show wasting and anemia, and die. The cysts may discharge a darkish fluid. Obstruction of the cloaca by *C. faba* cysts leading to death has been reported in wood thrushes (*Hylocichla mustelina*).

Diagnosis, Treatment, and Control. The presence of cysts in the skin of birds, especially around the cloaca, and the detection of flukes on necropsy are diagnostic of *C. faba* infection. There is no drug available for treatment. However, the condition can be treated by the surgical removal of the flukes from the subcutaneous

cysts. Control is not possible without understanding the life cycle.

Trematodes of the Circulatory System

Gigantobilharzia spp.

General Biology. *Gigantobilharzia* spp. (schistosomes) are flukes that live in the blood vessels of psittacines, passerines, anseriforms, and other birds. *G. hurensis* has been recorded in the North American Goldfinch (*Spinus tristis tristis*) and in cardinals. A *Gigantobilharzia* species of trematode has also been recovered from a Nanday Conure (*Nandayus nenday*).

Life Cycle. The life cycle is indirect and involves snails as intermediate hosts.

Clinical Signs. An infection of *Gigantobilharzia* spp. in a Nanday Conure was characterized by weight loss, blood-flecked diarrhea, and death. At necropsy lesions have been seen consisting of hemorrhagic ulcerative colitis and cloacitis. The mucosal surface of the cloaca was roughened and appeared to be covered with a diphtheritic membrane. Schistosome eggs may be seen in the feces, cloaca, lungs, liver, and kidneys (Fig. 22.8).

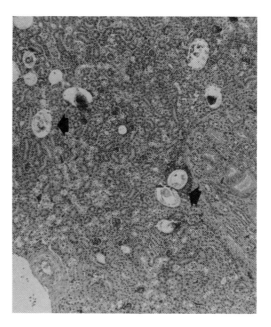

Fig. 22.8. Schistosome (*Gigantobilharzia* sp.) eggs embedded in the renal parenchyma of a Nanday Conure (*Nandayus nenday*). (×64) (*From Greve et al. 1978, by permission*)

Diagnosis, Treatment, and Control. Diagnosis is made by examination of feces for oval eggs with a single spine (Fig. 22.9). Parasites may also be seen at necropsy, and lesions are of diagnostic value. There is no known treatment. Control is by preventing ingestion of snails by birds or by using molluscicides in aviaries.

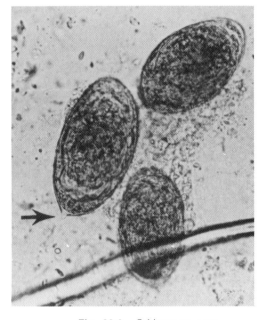

Fig. 22.9. Schistosome eggs recovered from the feces of a Nanday Conure (*Nandayus nenday*). (×370) (*From Greve et al. 1978, by permission*)

Trematodes of the Alimentary Tract

Echinostoma revolutum

This trematode occurs in the cecum, rectum, and small intestine of pigeons and waterfowl. It is 10–20 mm long and up to 2.0–2.5 mm wide. The eggs are 97–126 μm by 59–70 μm. The life cycle involves intermediate hosts such as snails and tadpoles. Pigeons with heavy infections may show hemorrhagic diarrhea leading to emaciation and death.

Trematodes of the Kidney

Tamerlania bragai

This fluke occurs in the kidneys and ureters of pigeons.

Other Trematodes

Platynosomum proxillicens

This fluke has been reported to occur in the liver of Sulphur-crested Cockatoos. As many as 100 parasites may be seen in the liver of birds, causing bile duct hyperplasia, inflammation, and necrosis.

Diagnosis is by the detection in the feces of broadly oval, darkly pigmented eggs with a flat operculum at one end. The egg is embryonated when laid.

Reference

Greve, J., et al. 1978. Bilharziasis in a Nanday Conure. *J. Am. Vet. Med. Assoc.* 172(10):1212–14.

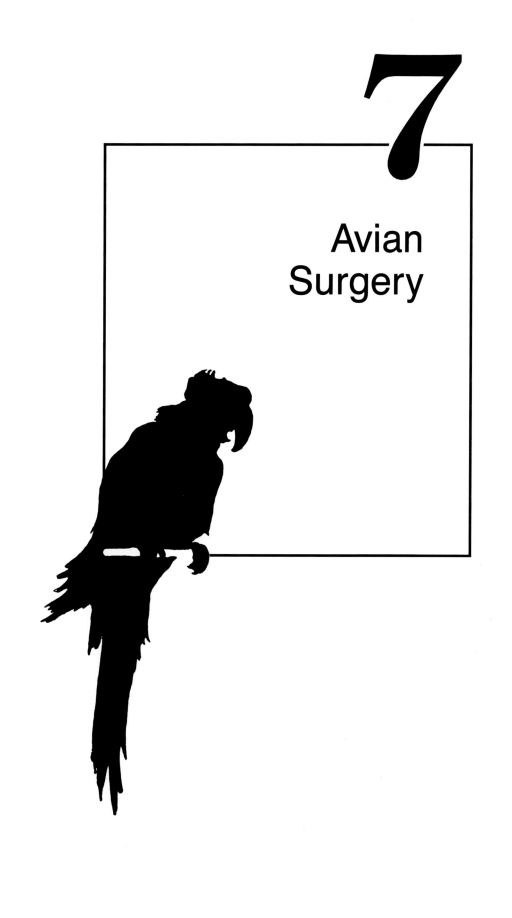

7

Avian
Surgery

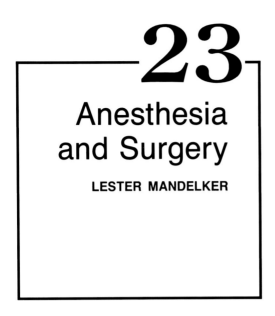

23

Anesthesia and Surgery

LESTER MANDELKER

AVIAN ANESTHETIC and surgical techniques have progressed greatly in the last decade. Many avian practitioners today routinely perform a variety of surgical procedures, including exploratory surgery, fracture repair, and surgical sexing. Microsurgery has just surfaced as a new and exciting procedure ideally suited to avian patients.

The choice of anesthesia and administration is often as important for success as the surgical procedure itself. Good surgical technique, proper hemostasis, and adequate postsurgical care are also essential for a favorable outcome.

Presurgical Evaluation. A thorough examination of the patient prior to surgery is vital to determine health status and surgical risk (see Chapter 4 for methods of physical restraint). During the preanesthetic evaluation, diagnostic tests can be performed (blood exams, radiographs) to determine illness or injury. A minimum data base prior to surgery should include measures of packed cell volume (PCV), total protein, clotting time (for liver suspects), and blood glucose levels. A PCV above 55 indicates dehydration, and those surgical candidates should be rehydrated prior to surgery. A PCV below 20 indicates anemia, and those patients should be withheld from surgery until the condition is resolved or a blood transfusion given. Blood glucose levels below 200 mg/100 ml indicate low serum levels and require treatment with dextrose prior to surgery. Fluid therapy can be given safely in the pectoral muscles before and during surgery. It is recommended that the avian patient be brought in the night before or at least 12 hours prior to surgery to acclimatize to the new environment. Whenever pos-

sible, the bird should stay in its own cage. It is helpful to provide warm, quiet quarters (85–90°F or 29–32°C) and to offer food and water. Fasting a granivorous bird is not necessary and often increases the surgical and anesthetic risks. Due to birds' high metabolic rate, fasting depletes the glycogen reserves in their livers that are needed to help detoxify and eliminate the toxic levels of drugs. In frugivorous birds (e.g., lorikeets), however, fasting for 4–10 hours prior to surgery is a must to prevent fluid aspiration into the respiratory system. Aspirated fluid can cause rapid death (1–2 hours postsurgery) or lead to aspiration pneumonia 3–4 days later.

Anesthesia

Restraint. Physical restraint (see Chapter 4) is necessary before an examination or administration of an anesthetic. Unmanageable patients may be restrained without handling by covering a small cage or enclosure (e.g., a fish tank) and introducing volatile anesthetics with oxygen.

Preanesthesia. For the most part, preanesthetics are not administered before surgery. Atropine, however, is recommended by some authors to decrease the flow of respiratory secretions, at 0.04 to 0.1 mg/kg body weight, injected in the pectoral muscles 5–10 minutes before induction. For short-term procedures, using injectable anesthetics (ketamine, atropine) is not necessary. A short, small-gauge needle (25–27 gauge) and a tuberculin or insulin syringe is recommended.

Local Anesthesia. Local anesthesia is not often used because birds are noted for poor cutaneous sensation. Local anesthesia is useful, however, for certain areas, such as the head, joints, parts of the legs, and vent. Most local agents have had limited use because of the need for manual restraint for both application of the agent and the surgical procedure. Local anesthetic agents, such as cetacaine or ethyl chloride, have been used effectively for superficial procedures (wart removal, feather cyst removal, incision and drainage of abscesses). Proparacaine is useful as an anesthetic for detailed eye examinations. Procaine has had limited usage because many avian patients are very sensitive to its application (this may be more an overdosage problem than actual sensitivity to the drug).

A new, popular local anesthetic and skin refrigerant, Medi-Frig, freezes the skin by application of its chilled (14°F, or −10°C) agent, dichlorodifluoromethane. It is useful for minor surgery and cryosurgery and prior to electrocautery. The quick freezing before electro-surgery reduces heat necrosis. It has proved beneficial in many minor surgical procedures; birds tolerate it well, and it is nontoxic. In summary, unless one is familiar with safe, local anesthetic dilutions, it is best to avoid their use in cage birds.

Oral Anesthesia. Anesthetics have received little use due to their unpredictability and length of application. Agents such as chloral hydrate and barbiturates applied in water or food have occasionally been used in capturing wild birds.

General Anesthesia. General anesthesia is desirable for most surgical procedures. General anesthetics reduce the need for physical restraint, danger of trauma, and shock. An understanding of induction stages and general anesthesia is essential for safe usage. The general anesthetics are divided into two categories, injectable agents and inhalation agents. Lightly anesthetized birds may be classified as being in a state of narcosis. Narcosis differs from anesthesia in that birds can be aroused from this drug-induced sleep. In early narcosis, the eyelids droop and the bird appears lethargic. Although deep narcosis characteristically resembles general anesthesia, fluttering and activity can be easily invoked by painful stimuli. Therefore, it is important to achieve a surgical level of anesthesia when administering general anesthetics.

There are two methods for estimating the level of anesthesia, the rate of respiration and the reflex response to stimuli. The best gauge to monitor anesthesia is the rate, pattern, and depth of respiration. Reflexes are helpful but not always reliable; the toe pinch reflex is the most accurate. Light anesthesia is characterized by a mild depression of all reflexes (palpebral, corneal, toe pinch). Respiration is deep and rapid, and there is no voluntary movement. Medium anesthesia is evidenced by absence of some reflexes (palpebral) and general depression of other reflexes (corneal, toe pinch). Respiration that is slow, deep, and regular is the ideal surgical level. Deep anesthesia exists when all voluntary movements and reflexes are abolished. Respiration is slow and regular but shallow. This level of anesthesia is unsafe for surgery because stress may result in respiratory and cardiac arrest.

Injectable Anesthetics. For the most part, injectable agents are less desirable than are inhalation agents. There is an inherent danger of overdosing, since once given, they cannot be reversed. A surgical level of anesthesia is difficult to maintain for extended periods without causing cardiac and respiratory depression, and injectable agents depend on a bird's metabolism, uptake, and elimination to insure safe recovery. Therefore, accurate dosages and bird weights must be assessed before injectable drugs are administered. A gram scale should be used to weigh birds. Injectable agents can be given intraperitoneally (IP), subcutaneously (SC), intravenously (IV), or intramuscularly (IM). Most are given IM. Often the required dose of anesthetic agent is so small that a microliter syringe must be used. A tuberculin syringe can also be used to dilute (e.g., tenfold in saline) or to administer a small quantity (<0.2 cc) anesthetic. The recommended injectable agents include Equithesin, pentobarbital, and various combinations of ketamine, acepromazine, Valium, and Rompun.

Anesthetics

Sodium Pentobarbital. Sodium pentobarbital can be given orally to birds at 1.5 mg/30 g body weight or 4 mg/100 g body weight IP or IM. As with most barbiturates, there is significant cardiac and respiratory depression and recovery is often prolonged. For these reasons, barbiturates are not routinely used in cage bird medicine.

Equithesin. Equithesin, a mixture of chloral hydrate, magnesium sulfate, and pentobarbital, was formerly the injectable anesthetic of choice. It can be given IM or IV. The IM dosage is 2.5 cc/kg (0.2–0.25 ml/100 g), while the IV dose is reduced by one-third. Duration lasts 30–60 minutes, and a surgical level of anesthesia persists for 7–10 minutes.

Ketamine. Ketamine and ketamine combinations with acepromazine, Valium, or Rompun are the most effective injectable agents available today. Ketamine treatment in birds was first used in Budgerigars in 1972 as a sole agent and proved effective for minor surgical procedures. A dosage of 2 mg ketamine (0.066 mg/g body weight) is satisfactory for minor surgical procedures; a surgical level of anesthesia is obtained for 5–12 minutes. A dosage of 3 mg (0.1 mg/g body weight) is capable of maintaining a surgical level of anesthesia for 20 minutes or more in most small birds. Dosages higher than 3 mg in small birds (<100 g) cause cardiac and respiratory depression, extended recoveries, and even death. Other published reports detail dosage rates ranging from 0.1–0.2 mg/g body weight. Using the higher range (0.2 mg/g), an injection of 6 mg in a 30-g Budgerigar produces profound depression and increased recovery time, often lasting greater than 2 hours. In a toxicity study of ketamine in parakeets, the lethal dose was 0.5 mg/ g (15 mg/30-g bird). In large birds (>100 g), the mg/g dosage of ketamine must be reduced. Doses of 0.025–0.1 mg/g are effective for parrots and larger birds.

Ketamine used alone often produces an excitatory phase during recovery, manifested by flapping and thrashing. The phase lasts several minutes and does not appear to be detrimental unless injury occurs. To minimize the possibility of injury, the bird can be placed in a small cannister, such as a mailing tube, or wrapped with a small towel or stockinette and placed in a dark recovery area.

Ketamine Combinations. Ketamine combinations with acepromazine, Valium, or Rompun improve muscle relaxation and reduce the excitatory phase of recovery. Ketamine combined with acepromazine (1 part acepromazine to 10 parts ketamine) is the most ideal injectable anesthetic agent. Using this mixture, dose according to the ketamine component at 0.066–0.1 mg/g body weight for small birds. For larger birds, dose at 0.025–1 mg/g body weight, adding 1 part Valium per 10 parts ketamine. Both these drugs appear safe in birds, with no more risk than with ketamine used alone. Rompun, for the most part, is unreliable when used alone and capable of causing bradycardia and heart block (A-V block).

Ketamine-Rompun mixtures are an effective and dependable anesthetic mixture but more potent than ketamine alone, and dosages of either agent have to be reduced. The recommended dose of ketamine (100 mg/ml) is 0.05 mg/g mixed with Rompun (20 mg/ml) at a dose of 0.01 mg/g (Table 23.1). This would equilibrate to a mixture of 0.015 cc of each drug.

Ketamine Toxicity. In debilitated patients, ketamine dosage must be reduced. Since ketamine is eliminated via the kidneys, fluid therapy is also indicated for dehydration. In a study of ketamine toxicity in parakeets, the debilitated patients and those that lost blood (2 to 3 drops) during surgery displayed a prolonged recovery time at least double that of healthy birds. If blood is lost during surgery, fluid therapy should be given IM or IP (IV in large birds). However, IP injections are difficult to administer and are not recommended for most procedures. The right side near the anterior cloaca is the area used for IP injections. The paralumbar fossa is not used for fear of liver puncture. Another complication is injection into the bowel. When blood loss occurs, IV transfusions should be given.

Pigeon blood can be used if a homologous blood donor is not available. Using heparin as an anticoagulant (rinse syringe only), 0.2–0.3 cc/30 g body weight is given for smaller birds and 2–3 cc for average-sized parrots. To obtain blood from a donor parakeet, the jugular vein is used. Daily repeated transfusions from different species are a dangerous practice, since antibodies can form and hemolyze the blood.

Other Injectable Agents. Other injectable agents include phencyclidine hydrochloride, Telazol (CI-744), and Saffan (CT-1341). Phencyclidine at 1–2 mg/kg body weight has been an effective immobilizing drug in several avian species. Telazol is still an experimental drug that appears in research animals to be equal or superior to ketamine. Saffan is a steroid anesthetic available in England but not yet in the United States. It has a wide safety margin but is very short acting. These anesthetics are not routinely used in the United States but if they become available, should provide an additional regimen of short-term injectable anesthetic agents.

Volatile Anesthetics. For most surgical procedures, volatile anesthetics are preferable to injectable agents in birds because they are easily controlled and reversed as necessary. The most frequently used agents are methoxyflurane and halothane (Table 23.2). Nitrous oxide is often helpful to augment anesthetic agents but is not useful as a sole agent. Inhalation agents can be

Table 23.1. Recommendations for the use of ketamine and Rompun in psittacines

Species	Amount of Ketamine (ml)[a]
Budgerigar	0.01
Conure	0.05
Cockatiel	0.02
African Gray Parrot	0.08–0.1
Macaw	0.15–0.20
Amazon	0.05–0.1
Lory, rosella	0.07
Cockatoo	0.12–0.15

[a]Solution containing 100 mg/ml mixed with an equal volume of Rompun containing 20 mg/ml.

Table 23.2. Volatile agents

Halothane
  Mask induction 2% (with oxygen)
  Maintenance 1–1.5%
  Oxygen flow 1–2 l/min
  Precise monitoring of anesthesia necessary

Methoxyflurane
  Mask induction 3–4% (with oxygen)
  Maintenance 1.5–2%
  Oxygen flow 1–2 l/min
  Wide margin of safety

given directly via a nose cone or following pre-anesthesia with an injectable agent. Following induction of anesthesia, all birds over 100 g should be intubated. In large birds, the endotracheal tube can be easily passed once it is moistened. Cole endotracheal tubes (size 10 French or larger) are most often used. While intubation is difficult in small passerines and Budgerigars, a bent paper clip can be used as a mouth speculum to prevent the tongue from occluding the glottis (see Fig. 4.5). This procedure is especially helpful in calming excitable birds.

Halothane. Halothane has the quickest induction and shortest recovery time of the volatile agents but requires precise monitoring. Induction is usually introduced at 2% with a high oxygen flow of 1–3 l/minute with or without nitrous oxide. A nonrebreathing system should be used in smaller birds (<100 g), due to the increased dead space. A safe induction method has been reported using methoxyflurane in large birds (>250 g) via a face cone and then switching to halothane anesthetic via a nonrebreathing system. This technique employs the use of methoxyflurane-impregnated cotton. The use of a face cone for induction using halothane presents more risk due to the high volatility of the gas. The face mask can induce respiratory or cardiac arrest in excitable birds, and therefore it is not recommended. Another method of halothane induction is the use of an enclosure (e.g., a plastic bag covering the cage) with a high oxygen flow. The depth of anesthesia must be monitored visually to avoid anesthetic overdosage. Following induction, halothane is maintained at a level of 1–1.5%.

Methoxyflurane. Methoxyflurane is the safest volatile agent for induction of anesthesia. It is popular because it is less toxic but requires a longer induction and recovery time than halothane. Many practitioners routinely use methoxyflurane-soaked cotton and a small cup or face mask as the sole anesthesia. This procedure is not without risk, especially in excitable birds, but is still safer than a similar application with halothane. Liquid methoxyflurane has been applied, one drop at a time, directly in the nares or mouth using a tuberculin syringe. With this method it is difficult to maintain an accurate dosage and it also irritates the mucous membranes; therefore it is generally not recommended. Methoxyflurane induction concentration is 3.5–4% (full open) using a face mask with oxygen or a plastic covering. Methoxyflurane can be used to induce anesthesia by using a plastic bag over the cage; following its removal, the bird is put on maintenance anesthesia (using a converted face mask or cone or a baby nipple with the end cut and glued to a plastic bag, which is then placed over the bird's head). Maintenance levels of methoxyflurane are 1.5–2%, which would equilibrate to a reading of 6–8 on an anesthetic machine. Budgerigars and parrots have been kept on safe levels of methoxyflurane anesthesia for well over 1 hour.

Anesthesia Problems. Problems with anesthesia rarely occur in healthy birds, but it is always best to prepare for them so immediate action can be taken if they occur. Overdosage of injectable agents can only be treated symptomatically since they must be excreted and metabolized. Fluid therapy given either IM or IV may be helpful in maintaining blood pressure and kidney perfusion. If Rompun has been used with ketamine, Dopram at 0.007 mg/g or 0.2 mg/30 g body weight IM may be a helpful stimulant and partially reverse the effects of Rompun.

Volatile agents often cause apnea during induction. This is best prevented and/or treated by administration of high oxygen flow. Artificial respiration may be attempted for respiratory arrest using digital pressure on the sternum. Again, Dopram given IM may be helpful to stimulate respiration. In emergencies, a tracheostomy may be necessary, using an IV catheter and removal of the needle following penetration. Cardiac arrest usually follows respiratory arrest. Intracardiac or IV injections of heart stimulants may be tried. Recent field reports indicate norepinephrine is superior to adrenalin for cardiac arrest in avian species. Anesthesia should be monitored throughout the surgical procedure. The rate and depth of respiration must be visualized at all times, so draping smaller patients is generally avoided unless transparent drapes are utilized. The bird's respiration and cardiac rate are monitored with a stethoscope. The use of an oscilloscope or electrocardiogram is reported to be of great value in complicated surgical procedures in the larger birds (e.g., macaws).

During anesthesia and subsequent surgery, there is considerable heat loss from the avian body. It is therefore imperative to conserve as much body heat as possible to prevent hypothermia. Birds should never be placed on cold surgical tables. Heating pads or towels are very helpful during surgery, and heated recovery units are often necessary postoperatively. Baby incubators are also useful for this purpose. The application of a hot water bottle or a circulating-water heating pad is recommended. The application of hot compresses several minutes postoperatively has proven satisfactory when incubators were not available. A rapid return to normal body temperature upon cessation of anesthesia indicates that prolonged application of heat is not warranted. A quiet, warm, darkened environment with supplemental oxygen is helpful in providing a smooth and safe recovery. Inserting the bird in stockinette will help prevent trauma and struggling during recovery.

At the other extreme, some birds may get hyperthermia following use of injectable agents such as ketamine. This is due to postanesthetic hyperactivity. Cloaca temperature is an excellent indicator of high body temperature. An electronic thermometer is the most accurate, provided there is good contact with cloacal tissue rather than stool or air. Hyperthermia is treated symptomatically by providing oxygen and IM dextrose and reducing body temperature as necessary (e.g., with alcohol spray).

Surgery

Surgical Preparation. Once the bird is anesthetized, the feathers should be plucked from the surgical site. Breaking off feathers may lead to self-mutilation. Individual feathers should be plucked out in the direction in which they lie rather than cut close to skin level, so that new feathers will be stimulated to grow immediately. Plucking clusters of feathers incurs the risk of tearing the skin. Any excessive plucking subjects the bird to a prolonged risk of hypothermia both during and subsequent to surgery. A light mist of water applied before plucking will reduce feather contamination when preparing the surgical site. Although birds are quite resistant to infection, sterile surgical technique should be performed to avoid introducing resistant bacteria or gross contamination. Because the skin of small avian patients is thin and fragile, excessive trauma during scrubbing should be avoided. Soft cotton swabs or cotton tip applicators are useful for this purpose, and circular scrubbing patterns are recommended. Several types of surgical scrubs have been employed, including povidone-iodine preparations, zephiran and alcohol, and tincture of merthiolate. The application of sterile K-Y jelly to surrounding feathers often is beneficial to keep feathers out of the surgical area following scrubbing.

Surgical Equipment. Eye instruments are preferred for avian surgery. They should include small dissecting (strabismus) scissors (4 in. curved), iris scissors (4 in. straight), plain and rat tooth forceps, several mosquito forceps and small hemostats, and a needle holder/scissors combination. A pointed blade (number 15 or 11) is most often used to make the initial incision.

Recently, electrosurgery has become very popular and ideally suited for avian surgery. Usually, ophthalmic suture material is satisfactory for abdominal closure, including 3-0 to 6-0 Dexon, 3-0 to 6-0 catgut (atraumatic needle), and even multifilament wire for hernia repair. For skin closure, 3-0 to 4-0 silk is commonly used, but 4-0 to 5-0 Prolene has also been found very effective. Recently, Tissue-Glue has been found very useful in skin closure and even for deep internal usage in birds. Tissue-Glue, which is used in human medicine, is nontoxic and consists of methylcyane acrylate. It is similar to the "super-glue" products but not toxic like these commercial glues.

An adequate number of sterile cotton swabs should be available for use as sponges and for blunt dissection. The wooden side of a cotton swab can also be used to break down air sacs when necessary for surgical exposure. Warm, sterile saline or lactated Ringer's solution should be available to rinse suture material and moisten tissue during surgery.

Hemostasis is essential in surgery, especially in small birds. Whenever possible, visible blood vessels should be clamped and ligated. Cut large vessels must be ligated immediately. Silver nitrate, dilute adrenalin (1:10,000), Clotisol, or Kwik-Stop can be used on bleeding surfaces but are not safe in deep wounds or body cavities. Gelfoam or dilute adrenalin are more suited for internal usage. The use of Gelfoam has been reported to be dangerous in small birds due to significant amounts of blood absorbed before coagulation. An ophthalmic cautery unit (Concept Inc., Clearwater, Fla.) has also been found to be ideally suited for hemostasis in the avian species.

Electrosurgery is probably the preferred method of performing surgery in birds. The advantages are (1) reducing surgical time by enhancing speed, (2) reducing the need for blunt dissection and ligation, (3) maintaining better hemostasis, and (4) having the ability to reach areas that are unreachable by other techniques. If alcohol is used, it must have completely dried before activation of the electrodes. The main disadvantage of the technique is the offensive burnt odor of tissue.

Several electrosurgical units are available but the Ellman Surgitron is preferred because it is useful both for electrosurgery and for electrocoagulation. Another good electrosurgical unit is the Cameron-Miller machine. Both machines have different currents available for skin surgery, coagulation, biopsy, and destruction of tissue (e.g., feather cysts). An electrosurgical unit is highly recommended for the practitioner contemplating extensive avian surgery. It is advisable, however, to avoid the use of electrosurgery in the cervical area due to close proximity of vital blood vessels, the trachea, and the esophagus. Cryosurgery has also been found to be useful in avian surgery, especially for removal of granulation tissue.

Surgical Procedures. Numerous surgical procedures are performed on caged birds. Some of the more common procedures and newer surgical techniques will be briefly described. Fracture repair (orthopedics) and endoscopic examination are discussed in Chapters 24 and 25.

Dental acrylics commonly used by dentists for tooth repair have been adapted to the repair of damaged or cracked beaks in the larger birds. They also have been used in stabilizing fractures since they are inert and nontoxic. They are available at a variety of dental supply houses.

Crop disease is a common problem in Budgerigars, while impaction is more of a problem in parrots and macaws. Sour crop in Budgerigars responds well to nonsurgical cleaning and massage. Impaction often requires surgical intervention and can be accomplished with little or no anesthesia. Cryosurgery (e.g., with Medi-Frig) provides excellent local anesthesia. An incision is made following feather removal and site preparation. Upon removal of foreign material, the crop wall is sutured using inverted sutures of 3-0 to 5-0 Dexon or gut. Similarly, the skin is closed using nylon, Prolene, silk, or Tissue-Glue. Occasionally crop fistula, a postoperative complication, may occur, necessitating surgical intervention. After surgery, water and food are withheld for several hours and dextrose and lactated Ringer's solution ($2\frac{1}{2}$ + $\frac{1}{2}$R) are given IM.

Exploratory surgery is often necessary to obtain biopsies, remove neoplasias, extract egg contents from the abdomen, repair hernias or ruptured oviducts, and retrieve intestinal foreign objects. A liver biopsy technique has recently been described for birds with liver disease or when further diagnostic information is needed. The bird is best positioned in the left lateral recumbency using a small biopsy needle just anterior to the right femur and between the articulation of the ribs with the sternum. Extreme care must be used around bowel tissue because it may not respond well to anastomosis. In small birds abdominal surgery has been disappointing. Proventriculotomy can be performed for removal of foreign bodies from the proventriculus and gizzard. Incision is made in the proventriculus and a small metal spoon passed to scoop out the debris (metal coke spoons, sold legally in novelty shops, are ideal).

The use of fiber-optic endoscopes and of otoscopes has made abdominal exploration and visualization easier and less traumatic (see Chapter 25). They can preclude the need for exploratory surgery, be used to obtain biopsies, and also are very useful for anatomical translumination.

Following intense straining, prolapse of the cloaca or oviduct may occur. If simple replacement is not successful, the bird may be anesthetized or sprayed with a local anesthetic. A purse-string suture is placed around the vent and left until straining has ceased. In a cockatoo, surgical repair of a chronic prolapse or an everted cloaca in a cockatoo using a cloacapexy technique is possible. The cloaca is secured to the abdominal wall using wire sutures to withstand the stress of straining. Hysterectomy can also be performed to prevent egg laying or correct ovarian disease causing prolapse. Abdominal hernias are more common in female birds and may be related to egg-laying stress. Once a true hernia is determined using radiographs or endoscopic examination, repair may be attempted. Using a midline incision, abdominal muscles are sutured together with small multifilament wire or Dexon.

Microsurgery has recently gained significant attention in avian and small animal surgery. Several factors, however, still restrict the use of microsurgery, including cost, lack of specialized training in techniques, and a need for understanding the application of microsurgery and microdiagnostics. Several microscopes are soon to come on the market, some of which may be applicable to avian surgery.

Skin surgery is often necessary to remove tumors and other growths. Occasionally, trauma and bite wounds (e.g., from cats) also require surgical repair. When removing growths, the blood supply must be considered, as well as the availability of adequate skin for closure. The initial incision is made with a scapel or electrosurgical wire. Bleeding vessels should be cauterized or compressed with Gelfoam. With small sutures, an atraumatic needle and a continuous suture pattern is used. Tissue-Glue lends itself well to closing skin in areas where there is little stress on the incision site. Bite wounds are often serious; damage, infection, and hemorrhage may occur in the deep tissues; they must be treated carefully with fluids, antibiotics, and steroids. The patient should be hospitalized and kept warm, with stress avoided. Such injuries always warrant a guarded prognosis. Feather cysts are easily recognized and may be removed surgically by curettage and chemical cauterization. Gelfoam is helpful in controlling hemorrhage. Electrocauterization may also be employed to destroy feather cysts. The application of intense heat is necessary, using a fulgurating current.

Prophylactic Therapy. Following routine surgery, prophylactic chemotherapy is not routinely practiced. If an infection develops, broad spectrum antibiotics should be administered orally or IM. For complicated or stressful surgery, IM antibiotic prophylaxis is advisable. Postsurgically, sutures may be picked at, and wound infection and self-mutilation may occur. Sutures and collars are necessary only for those that attempt self-mutilation. X-ray film or plastic sheets of vinyl can be cut to fit around the head. The application of Vetrap around the neck is also recommended to prevent picking at sutures.

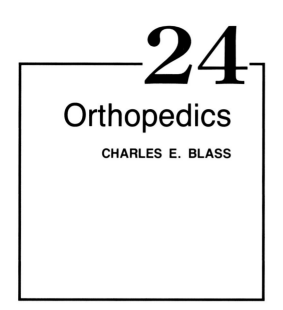

24
Orthopedics

CHARLES E. BLASS

THE TYPES of orthopedic diseases encountered in birds include those caused by trauma, nutritional deficiencies or imbalances, infection, and metabolic disturbances. The difficulties encountered in avian orthopedics include problems with stress, restraint, anesthesia, and a lack of suitable orthopedic equipment and qualified avian veterinarians.

The goal of fracture treatment in avian orthopedics is to restore full function rapidly. Healing may take place, but function does not always follow. The postrepair function of small companion birds is usually not critical, due to limited opportunity or demand for flight. In birds of prey, however, a significant malunion or joint stiffness can produce a disadvantage in its function.

A bird that has sustained a fracture is usually in a physiologic state of maximum stress. Many surgical repairs are successful, but the bird may die as a result of stress associated with injury and therapy. See Bush and James (1975), Montali and Bush (1975), Bush et al. (1976), Redig and Roush (1978), Roush (1980), Altman (1982), and Bush (1983).

Avian Fracture Healing. It has been reported that medullary bones heal more rapidly than pneumatized bones. However, others report that air sacs do not retard fracture healing.

The basic mechanism for repair in a well-aligned, stable fracture is the formation of an intramedullary callus. While periosteal callus does form, it is less entensive than in mammals and mainly provides secondary support.

The time required for clinical union to occur varies depending on the location, fracture type, bird size, infection, and treatment method. The bones of small birds tend to heal more quickly than those of larger species. Union occurs in the presence of infection; however, healing may be delayed. Delayed union may also result from a nonstable fracture and/or a repair technique that disrupts the endosteal callus. Bridging callus formation may be seen 2 weeks postoperatively in well-aligned fractures. See Arnall and Keymer (1975), Bush et al. (1976), Bush (1977), James et al. (1978), and Gandal and Amand (1982).

General Considerations. Diagnosis of a fracture or of a luxation is based on physical examination and confirmed by radiographs. Radiographic examination should always be performed to determine the extent of fracture and the technique necessary for repair. Fractures and luxations are characterized by abnormal angulation, exceptional and uncontrolled mobility, and a grinding sound on manipulation. A fractured wing is usually held low, most noticeably at the tip. The patient should be stabilized prior to fracture repair. Supportive therapy includes antibiotics, fluid replacement, corticosteroids, and temporary stabilization by splinting and/or bandaging the fracture. The bird should be placed in a small, warm, dark cage with low perches. Wild birds with fractures that are several days old are hypoglycemic and should receive intravenous and/or oral glucose solutions to meet their immediate metabolic needs. Glycogen storage capacity in birds is considerably less than in other species, and this increases the possibility of hypoglycemia. See Arnall and Keymer (1975), Bush and James (1975), Altman (1981, 1982), and Bush (1983).

If surgical therapy is indicated, standard aseptic technique should be adhered to. The lack of subcutaneous connective tissue makes accessibility to muscle, bone, and underlying structures in birds simple and relatively avascular (Figs. 24.1, 24.2, 24.3, and 24.4).

External Coaptation. Treatment of fractures in small birds usually consists of some form of coaptation splinting in which the wing is bound to the body (wing fractures) or simple tape splints are applied (leg fractures). External coaptation is also used in combination with internal fixation to provide additional support. See Bush et al. (1976), Bush (1977), and Gandal and Amand (1982).

Many techniques using adhesive tape as "flap splints" have been described (Fig. 24.5). These flap splints can be contoured to fit any leg shape at any location (Figs. 24.6 and 24.7). When applying splints the fracture should be re-

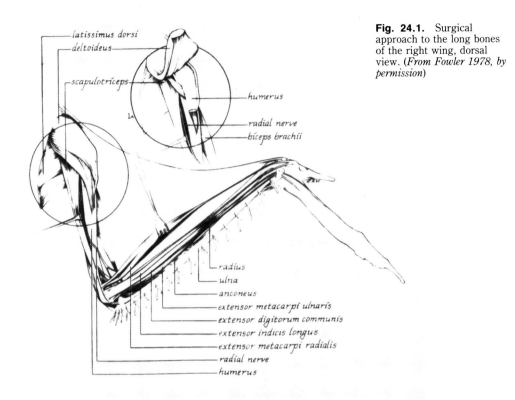

Fig. 24.1. Surgical approach to the long bones of the right wing, dorsal view. (*From Fowler 1978, by permission*)

latissimus dorsi
deltoideus
scapulotriceps
humerus
radial nerve
biceps brachii
radius
ulna
anconeus
extensor metacarpi ulnaris
extensor digitorum communis
extensor indicis longus
extensor metacarpi radialis
radial nerve
humerus

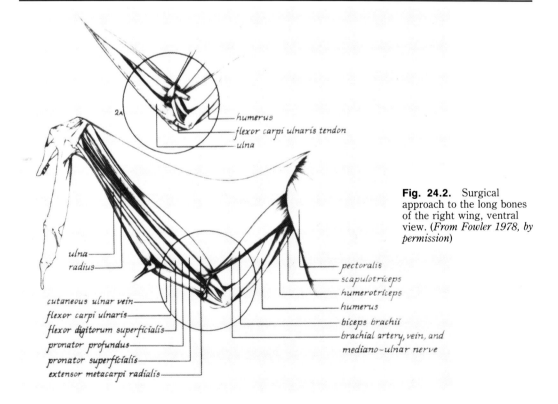

Fig. 24.2. Surgical approach to the long bones of the right wing, ventral view. (*From Fowler 1978, by permission*)

humerus
flexor carpi ulnaris tendon
ulna

ulna
radius

pectoralis
scapulotriceps
humerotriceps
humerus
biceps brachii
brachial artery, vein, and
mediano-ulnar nerve

cutaneous ulnar vein
flexor carpi ulnaris
flexor digitorum superficialis
pronator profundus
pronator superficialis
extensor metacarpi radialis

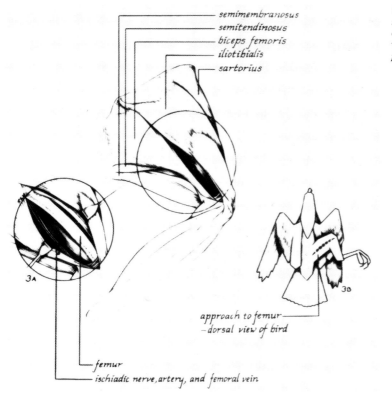

semimembranosus
semitendinosus
biceps femoris
iliotibialis
sartorius

3A

approach to femur
—dorsal view of bird

femur
ischiadic nerve, artery, and femoral vein

Fig. 24.3. Surgical approach to the long bones of the right leg, lateral view. (*From Fowler 1978, by permission*)

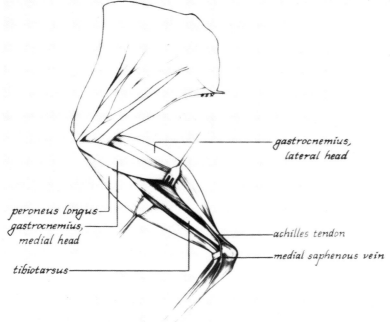

gastrocnemius,
lateral head

peroneus longus
gastrocnemius,
medial head

tibiotarsus

achilles tendon
medial saphenous vein

Fig. 24.4. Surgical approach to the long bones of the right leg, medial view. (*From Fowler 1978, by permission*)

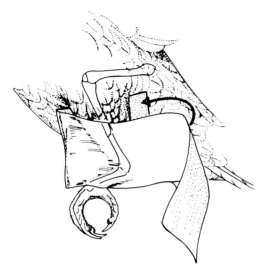

Fig. 24.5. Applying a flap splint. It is begun medially and then folded around the leg in several more layers. (*From Kirk 1977, by permission*)

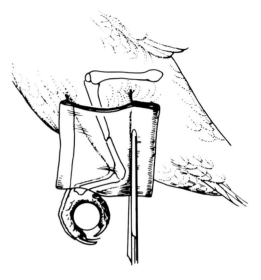

Fig. 24.6. Applying a flap splint. The tape is compressed with a hemostat to secure it. (*From Kirk 1977, by permission*)

duced manually and feathers plucked from the area. Small wooden sticks or metal pins may be incorporated into the splint for added strength. Anesthesia is rarely necessary for splint application. See Bush (1974), Roush (1980), and Gandal and Amand (1982).

Wing fractures may also be supported by adhesive tape splinting (Fig. 24.8). The wings are taped against the body in their normal flexed position (Fig. 24.9). This type of fixation is not rigid and allows small amounts of movement. All but large birds (>5 kg) can be splinted in this method. Body splints may also be used to stabilize wing fractures, but care must be taken to avoid compromising respiration by putting excessive pressure on the abdomen and chest. Initially, this type of splint may render the bird unstable; however, after 4–12 hours they usually learn to balance well. In adequately reduced and supported fractures where external coaptation is used for repair, the minimum time for splint removal is 3 weeks. See Altman (1981, 1982), Gandal and Amand (1982), and Putney et al. (1983).

In larger species of birds, adhesive tape splints are not suitable because of their lack of strength, their inability to support the limb, and the tendency of some birds to chew them. For larger birds, therefore, fiberglass and plastic resins (e.g., Hexcelite orthopedic tape) can be used. These materials have replaced plaster since they are lighter and more easily applied

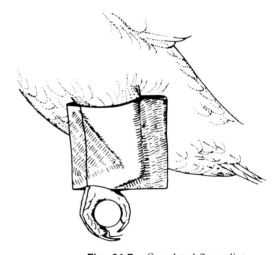

Fig. 24.7. Completed flap splint. This splint is applied with the leg held in extension. (*From Kirk 1977, by permission*)

and dry faster. Only one or two layers are required. The application of fiberglass, plastic resins, or plaster splints usually requires anesthesia. See Altman (1977, 1981).

All splints should be examined at least once a week for adjustments (Altman 1977, 1982). Gravel should be removed from the cage bottom, and perches left to encourage the bird to perch.

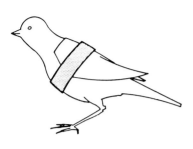

Fig. 24.8. Applying a body splint. The first strip of adhesive tape is placed under the fractured wing at the anterior margin, then carried dorsally over the wing and wound around the body, also confining the normal wing. (*From Kirk 1977, by permission*)

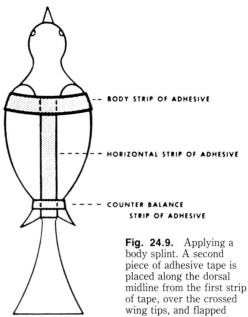

-- BODY STRIP OF ADHESIVE

--- HORIZONTAL STRIP OF ADHESIVE

--- COUNTER BALANCE STRIP OF ADHESIVE

Fig. 24.9. Applying a body splint. A second piece of adhesive tape is placed along the dorsal midline from the first strip of tape, over the crossed wing tips, and flapped under the wing tips. More adhesive tape is added over the first strip to secure the dorsal strip of tape to it. A third strip of adhesive tape is placed around the wing tip. (*From Kirk 1977, by permission*)

Most problems associated with splinting fractures are created by disuse of the limb. In medium-sized and large birds, excessive periosteal callous formation may result in decreased or lost function and joint stiffness. When used as the sole means of fixation for serious fractures, external coaptation is unsatisfactory because the ability to fly may be lost. These types of splints are also not very effective in larger birds such as parrots, macaws, and cockatoos. See Spink (1978) and Gandal and Amand (1982).

Internal Fixation. Surgical treatment of avian fractures is undertaken only to accomplish a better end result than would be expected with conservative treatment. Avian fractures present unique problems: avian bone is very brittle, most fractures tend to be comminuted, and birds have pneumatized bones with larger intramedullary spaces, which complicates stabilization. The objective of fracture repair includes rigid fixation, good anatomical alignment and apposition, absence of infection, and an early return to function. Blood loss and tissue handling should be kept to a minimum. In smaller birds, the total blood volume may be only 2–4 ml. Electrosurgery minimizes capillary bleeding. It is important to avoid stripping any muscle or fascial attachments from bone fragments. Even if devitalized these fragments act as cortical bone grafts and offer structural support. Although some of these fragments may sequestrate, they will support the fracture site while being replaced by new bone. The sequestra can be removed after cancellous union. See Bush et al. (1976), Bush (1977, 1983), Newton and Zeitlin (1977), Spink (1978), Galvin (1980), Alt- man (1981, 1982), and Gandal and Amand (1982).

Open, comminuted, and intraarticular fractures are difficult to immobilize properly and are less likely to result in a good functional result. These fractures generally require surgical correction. Open fractures should be debrided and closed as soon as possible. See Roush (1980) and Altman (1982).

Intramedullary Pinning. The advantages of intramedullary pinning include simplicity, economy, accurate alignment of fractures, and ease of implant removal. The disadvantages include poor rotational stability in some situations, invasion of the fracture site, weight of the apparatus, disruption of medullary callus, potential for joint invasion and damage, and necessity of a second surgery to remove the intramedullary pin. A pathologic sequela associated with intramedullary fixation is ischemia leading to necrosis of bone. This condition may occur when the intramedullary pin is too large. Placement of intramedullary pins is critical so that damage to muscles, tendons, and the joint is avoided (Figs. 24.10 and 24.11). The Jonas splint should be avoided. External coaptation may be used in conjunction with intramedullary pinning to minimize rotation. When external coaptation is used, pin removal as early as 1 week may be indicated to prevent disruption of the endosteal callus. See Bush (1974, 1977, 1983), Newton and Zeitlin (1977), Roush (1980), Gandal and Amand (1982), and MacCoy (1983).

External Skeletal Fixation. Fracture immobilization by external skeletal fixation offers a viable alternative to internal fixation. Half-pin and full-pin techniques have been used (Figs. 24.12 and 24.13). The advantages of external skeletal fixation include rigid fixation, short surgery and anesthesia time, minimal special equipment necessary, ease of application, early return to function, minimal postoperative care, and ease of adjustment. The disadvantages include the greater weight of the device and the possibilities of ascending infection, damage to the external device, and stress fractures at the pin-bone interface. See Bush (1983), Kock (1983), MacCoy (1983), and Putney et al. (1983).

Bone Plating. Plating is most applicable to leg fractures in large birds. When bone plates are used, additional support is not required and function returns almost immediately. This type of fixation is rigid, and joints are avoided. Problems associated with plate fixation include the potential for splintering small cortices, the large surgical exposure required, and a prolonged anesthetic time. The cortices of the bones of the leg are thicker than those in the wings. Plate removal after bone healing is preferable.

Other Means for Internal Fixation. Roush (1980) described use of monofilament stainless steel wire (interfragmentary, cerclage, and hemicerclage). The wires may be used to prevent rotation, provide interfragmentary compression, or incorporate small fragments into the fracture area. Suture material has been used to hold small fragments at the fracture site.

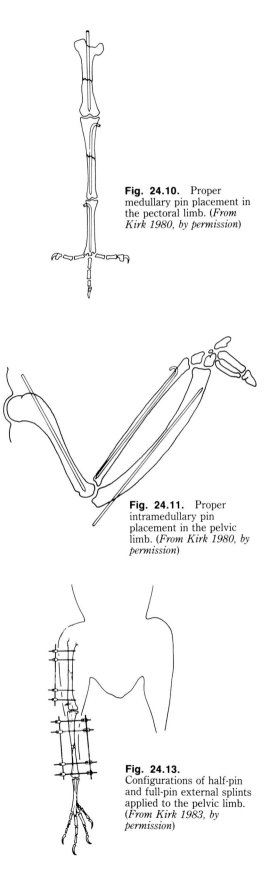

Fig. 24.10. Proper medullary pin placement in the pectoral limb. (*From Kirk 1980, by permission*)

Fig. 24.11. Proper intramedullary pin placement in the pelvic limb. (*From Kirk 1980, by permission*)

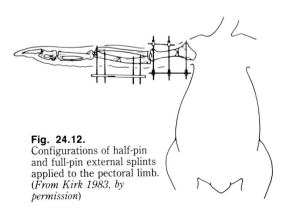

Fig. 24.12. Configurations of half-pin and full-pin external splints applied to the pectoral limb. (*From Kirk 1983, by permission*)

Fig. 24.13. Configurations of half-pin and full-pin external splints applied to the pelvic limb. (*From Kirk 1983, by permission*)

MacCoy (1983) described using polymer rods for intramedullary placement. The rods are lightweight and compatible with tissue and therefore do not require removal. These rods are placed using a "shuttle pin" technique, which requires some practice. Stress concentration and diaphyseal fulcrums produced can result in further fragmentation at the fracture ends. Diaphyseal fractures with minimal comminution are best suited for this technique.

Methyl methacrylate has been used to stabilize avian fractures (Borman and Putney 1978; Putney et al. 1983). Bone cement is placed in the medullary cavity, the fractures reduced and held together until the cement hardens.

Fracture prognosis depends on the age of the patient and accompanying damage to soft tissue, vessels, and nerves. Damage severe enough to cause necrosis is usually evident within the first week. See Altman (1977, 1982).

Most badly distracted extremity fractures are open and comminuted; as a result, contamination is a problem. Infection at the fracture site may cause a delayed union as well as affect the bird systemically. Osteomyelitis is not a common sequela, and when it does occur, it is usually a local phenomenon. See Altman (1977, 1982), Newton and Zeitlin (1977), and Gandal and Amand (1982).

Treatment of nonunions consists of reestablishing the medullary canal at the fracture site, freshening up the fracture ends, and achieving rigid fixation (Roush 1980).

Fractures of the Pectoral Limb. Wing fractures occur with less frequency than leg fractures. When a wing is injured it must undergo precise repair to maintain function. Fractures of the wing most frequently involve the radius, ulna, and humerus. See Arnall and Keymer (1975) and Altman (1977).

For fractures of the pectoral extremities, adhesive tape splints may be used to support and confine the wing in its natural resting position. This method is most applicable in small and medium-sized birds. These splints are usually removed after 3–5 weeks. Birds should not be allowed to fly for at least 2 weeks after splint removal. On occasion, external coaptation of wing fractures has been found to be superior to intramedullary pinning. See Richards et al. (1972), Bush (1974), Altman (1977, 1982), Spink (1978), and Gandal and Amand (1982).

Humeral fractures in larger birds require surgical repair since immobilization by external coaptation allows too much motion at the fracture site (Fig. 24.14). Internal fixation of humeral fractures is most frequently accomplished by intramedullary pinning. The pins are usually normograded from the anterior cortex with proximal humeral fractures. Midshaft and distal fractures can be pinned in a retrograde manner (Redig and Roush 1978). The pin is driven from the fracture site so that it emerges from the anterior cortex of the proximal segment. After the fracture is reduced, the pin is anchored into the distal segment. External coaptation may be combined with intramedullary pinning for added stability.

Humeral fractures may also be stabilized by external skeletal fixation (Fig. 24.15). This can be accomplished using standard equipment or by connecting fixation pins with acrylic connecting bars. The half-pin splint should be placed on the dorsolateral aspect of the humerus (Bush 1983).

The radius and ulna usually fracture together (Fig. 24.16). In the absence of severe soft

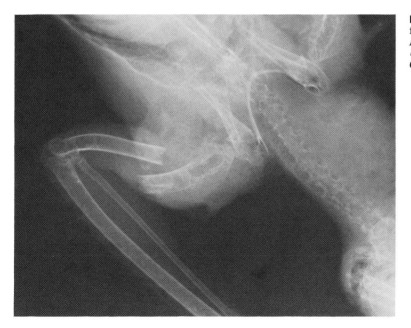

Fig. 24.14. Humeral fractures. (*Courtesy of E. L. Egger, Colorado State University, Fort Collins, Colo.*)

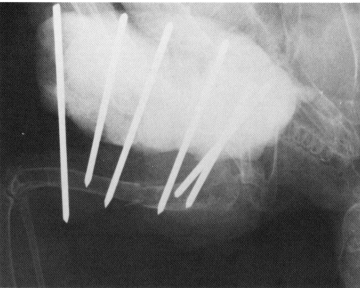

Fig. 24.15. Humeral fracture in a kestrel, stabilized with an external fixation device using stainless steel pins and methyl methacrylate. (*Courtesy of E. L. Egger, Colorado State University, Fort Collins, Colo.*)

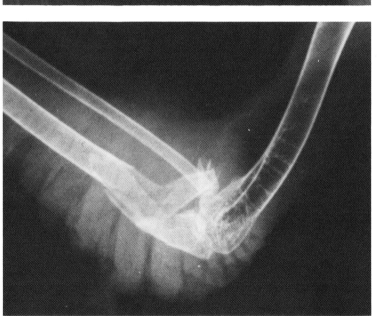

Fig. 24.16. Fracture of the radius and ulna.

tissue damage or infection, external coaptation is recommended. The ulna is larger than the radius and is more acceptable for internal fixation. Intramedullary pinning is the most common method of internally stabilizing fractures of the radius and ulna. Generally, only the ulna is stabilized (Fig. 24.17). Careful pin placement is necessary to avoid entry to the elbow joint. Intramedullary pinning is frequently combined with external coaptation for fractures of the radius and ulna. See Newton and Zeitlin (1977) and Redig and Roush (1978).

Radius and ulnar fractures in larger birds may also be stabilized by external skeletal fixation. Either half-pin or full-pin splints may be used (Bush 1983).

Fractures of the carpus, metacarpal bones, and phalanges are most often treated by external coaptation. The wing is usually splinted for 10–14 days. Although this portion of the wing bears the bulk of the flight feathers, limited flying is possible even if these bones are badly damaged. See Arnall and Keymer (1975) and Redig and Roush (1978).

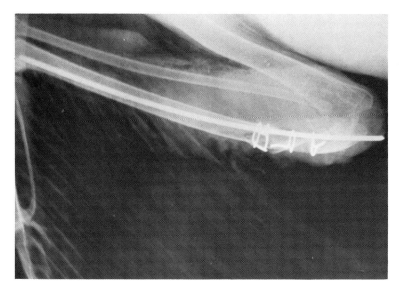

Fig. 24.17. Stabilization of a severely comminuted ulnar fracture in a Red-tailed Hawk (*Buteo jamaicencis*), using an intramedullary pin and interfragmentary wire. Note the persistent malalignment of the proximal radial fracture.

Bone plate fixation of wing fractures is usually not practical because of the thinness of the cortices, size of the implant, and difficulty of implant removal.

Fractures of the Pelvic Limb. Fractures of the femur are uncommon because it is incorporated within the contour of the body and is better protected. Unless surgical treatment is contemplated, immobilization by means of a body splint is frequently necessary (Altman 1982). The leg is held flexed completely against the body. In this position, the fracture fragments will generally align sufficiently to permit union. Alternately, confinement in a small dark cage may allow healing.

Internal fixation of femoral fractures can be provided for by intramedullary pinning, bone plating, or external skeletal fixation. While an intramedullary pin maintains excellent alignment, some form of external coaptation such as a body splint may be necessary to prevent rotation. Simple coaptation splinting (a flap splint) of the femur is impossible because the femur lies within the body confines. The femurs of larger birds are large enough to allow the use of very small bone plates. Femoral fractures can also be stabilized by external skeletal fixation, utilizing half-pin splintage placed on the lateral side of the leg. See Redig and Roush (1978), Altman (1982), and Bush (1983).

Fractures of the proximal aspect of the tibiotarsus, like femoral fractures, are too high for external coaptation and should be surgically stabilized like femoral fractures (Altman 1982). These fractures are more difficult to reduce

with flexion of the leg. For this reason, many of these fractures are treated by intramedullary pinning. Fortunately, fractures of the proximal tibiotarsus are uncommon.

Fractures of the middle and distal aspect of the tibiotarsus are amenable to external coaptation, such as with the flap splint. This type of splint can be used in birds up to the size of an average parrot. Larger birds require surgical stabilization by intramedullary pinning, external skeletal fixation, or external coaptation with fiberglass, plastic resin, or plaster. When external coaptation is used, it should be applied so that the tarsometatarsal-phalangeal joint is movable. With fractures near the tibiotarsal-tarsometatarsal joint, care should be taken to ensure that angulation of the limb occurs at the joint rather than at the fracture site. Surgical management of tibiotarsal fractures usually involves intramedullary pinning or external skeletal fixation (Fig. 24.18). Small Steinmann pins, Kirschner wires, and occasionally hypodermic needles may be used as intramedullary pins. Stabilization by external skeletal fixation usually involves full-pin splintage (through-and-through) on the lateral and medial aspects of the leg (Fig. 24.19). See Altman (1977, 1982) and Bush (1983).

Fractures of the tarsometatarsus are most often stabilized by flap-type external coaptation. This is the method of choice because of the proximity of the bones to the skin and the ease of immobilizing the joint above and below the fracture. Immobilization of the metatarsal-phalangeal joint is accomplished by placing a strip of tape under the claws and carrying it up the

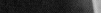

Fig. 24.18. Tibiotarsal fracture.

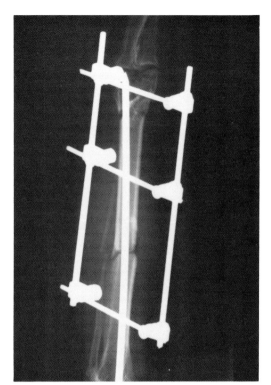

Fig. 24.19. Comminuted, segmental fracture of the tibiotarsus in an eagle, repaired with an intramedullary pin and a through-and-through external skeletal fixation device.

lateral and medial side of the metatarsal bone prior to application of the flap splint. The splint must be tight enough to support the bone without inhibiting circulation. See Altman (1977, 1982) and Roush (1980).

Fractures of the toe or phalanx are frequently not noticed until the bone heals, usually malaligned. If the fracture is detected early, the toe should be immobilized in an extended position by taping a large ball of soft gauze within the grasp of the foot or by fixing it to an adjacent digit with flexible colloidin or colloidin and cotton. Flap splints placed in the horizontal plane may also be used. See Arnall and Keymer (1975), Altman (1977, 1982), and Galvin (1980).

Dislocations. Dislocations or luxations produce obvious deformities. They are less common than fractures because of the pneumatized structure of the bones and the well-developed ligaments. Dislocations are usually of traumatic origin; however, congenital dislocations are not uncommon in Budgerigars. See Arnall and Keymer (1975) and Altman (1982).

Luxations should be treated as soon as pos-

sible. If a joint has been luxated for several days it can be fibrosed into the luxated position and closed reduction may be difficult or impossible. Closed reduction is accomplished by manipulation of the limb, coupled with gentle squeezing of the joint between the finger and thumb. This is usually sufficient to replace the articular surfaces (producing an audible click), after which normal joint movement is present. See Redig and Roush (1978), Roush (1980), and Kock (1983).

The shoulder joint is rarely dislocated. Repair, which is difficult, consists of closed reduction and fixation of the wing to the body. Transarticular pinning has been performed when closed reduction failed. The elbow joint can luxate with or without ligamentous rupture. If these ligaments are intact, closed reduction with bandaging in flexion is usually successful. If the ligaments have ruptured, open reduction with ligamentous repair is recommended. Luxation of the carpus and more distal joints usually responds well to closed reduction. See Roush (1980).

Coxofemoral luxations are uncommon and

can be managed by closed reduction and slinging, or by open reduction and slinging. Transarticular pinning may also be performed. Forces applied in the area of the stifle almost always produce fractures rather than luxations. Luxations of the lower leg are treated by closed reduction and splinting. See Roush (1980) and Altman (1982).

It is important that the joint be held in anatomic reduction for enough time to allow repair of the joint by fibrosis. Joint motion usually returns 1–2 weeks after reduction; physical therapy may be necessary to regain full motion. It is important to allow return of joint motion before stiffness becomes overwhelming. This is usually done every other day, using chemical immobilization. See Roush (1980).

During anesthetic recovery, the bird should be kept in a warm, dark, quiet environment with a minimum of human contact. All splints should be checked and adjusted at least once a week. See Galvin (1980) and Gandal and Amand (1982).

References

Altman, R. B. 1977. Fractures of the extremities of birds. In *Current Veterinary Therapy VI,* ed. R. W. Kirk, pp. 717–20. Philadelphia: W. B. Saunders.

_____. 1981. General principles of avian surgery. *Compend. Cont. Educ. Pract. Vet.* 3:177–83.

_____. 1982. Disorders of the skeletal system. In *Diseases of Cage and Aviary Birds,* ed. M. L. Petrak, pp. 382–94. Philadelphia: Lea and Febiger.

Arnall, L., and I. F. Keymer. 1975. *Bird Diseases.* Neptune City, N.J.: T.E.H. Publications.

Borman, E. R., and D. L. Putney. 1978. Repair of a wing fracture with methyl methacrylate bone cement. *Vet. Med. Small Anim. Clin.* 73:794.

Bush, M. 1974. Avian orthopedics. In *Annu. Proc. Am. Assoc. Zoo Vet.,* pp. 111–13.

_____. 1977. External fixation of avian fractures. *J. Am. Vet. Med. Assoc.* 171:943–46.

_____. 1983. External fixation to repair long bone fractures in larger birds. In *Current Veterinary Therapy VIII,* ed. R. W. Kirk, pp. 630–33. Philadelphia: W. B. Saunders.

Bush, M., and A. E. James. 1975. Some considerations of practice of orthopedics in exotic animals. *J. Am. Anim. Hosp. Assoc.* 11:587–94.

Bush, M., R. J. Montali, G. R. Novak, and A. E. James. 1976. The healing of avian fractures: A histologic xeroradiographic study. *J. Am. Anim. Hosp. Assoc.* 12:768–73.

Fowler, M. E., ed. 1978. *Zoo and Wild Animal Medicine.* Philadelphia: W. B. Saunders.

Galvin, C. 1980. Care and treatment of captive wild birds. In *Current Veterinary Therapy VII,* ed. R. W. Kirk, pp. 692–96. Philadelphia: W. B. Saunders.

Gandal, C. P., and W. B. Amand. 1982. Anesthetic and surgical techniques. In *Diseases of Cage and Aviary Birds,* ed. M. L. Petrak, pp. 320–23. Philadelphia: Lea and Febiger.

James, A. E., R. J. Montali, G. R. Novak, and M. Bush. 1978. The use of xeroradiographic imaging to evaluate fracture repair in avian species. *Skeletal Radiogr.* 2:161–68.

Kirk, R. W., ed. 1977. *Current Veterinary Therapy VI.* Philadelphia: W. B. Saunders.

_____. 1980. *Current Veterinary Therapy VII.* Philadelphia: W. B. Saunders.

_____. 1983. *Current Veterinary Therapy VIII.* Philadelphia: W. B. Saunders.

Kock, M. D. 1983. The use of a modified Kirschner-Ehmer apparatus in avian fracture repair. *J. Small Anim. Pract.* 221:383–90.

MacCoy, D. M. 1983. High density polymer rods as an intramedullary fixation device in birds. *J. Am. Anim. Hosp. Assoc.* 19:767–72.

Montali, R. J., and M. Bush. 1975. Avian fracture repair, radiographic and histologic correlation. In *Annu. Proc. Am. Assoc. Zoo Vet.,* pp. 150–54.

Newton, C. D., and S. Zeitlin. 1977. Avian fracture healing. *J. Am. Vet. Med. Assoc.* 170:620–25.

Putney, D. L., E. R. Borman, and C. L. Lohse. 1983. Methyl methacrylate fixation of avian humeral fractures: A radiographic histologic study. *J. Am. Anim. Hosp. Assoc.* 19:773–82.

Redig, P., and J. C. Roush. 1978. Orthopedic and soft tissue surgery in raptorial birds. In *Zoo and Wild Animal Medicine,* ed. M. E. Fowler, pp. 246–53. Philadelphia: W. B. Saunders.

Richards, D. A., P. J. Hinko, and E. M. Morse. 1972. Orthopedic procedures for laboratory animals and exotic pets. *J. Am. Vet. Assoc.* 161:728–32.

Roush, J. C. 1980. Avian orthopedics. In *Current Veterinary Therapy VII,* ed. R. W. Kirk, pp. 662–73. Philadelphia: W. B. Saunders.

Spink, R. R. 1978. Fracture repair in rehabilitation of raptors. *Vet. Med. Small Anim. Clin.* 73:1451–55.

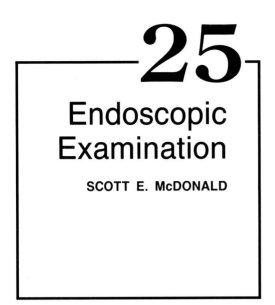

25

Endoscopic Examination

SCOTT E. McDONALD

ENDOSCOPY, one of the major recent advances in avian medicine and husbandry, is the inspection of any body cavity by means of an endoscope. Its primary functions are to be a management tool for sex determination and a diagnostic aid to evaluate medical problems. While the surgical skills required are not difficult, it is imperative that the veterinarian gain proficiency by practicing the procedure on inexpensive birds before performing it on valuable exotics. Endoscopy performed in the presence of the owner allows a better appreciation of the technique and the veterinary skills required, as well as giving the owner an opportunity to view the internal structures of the bird.

Endoscopic Equipment. The basic equipment required for avian laparoscopy includes a small-diameter rigid endoscope with corresponding-sized cannula and trocar, light source, and fiber-optic cable. The endoscopes of choice are the Needlescope and the LUMINA-SL telescope.

The Needlescope used routinely in avian laparoscopy is either 1.7 mm in diameter (16 gauge) or 2.2 mm in diameter (14 gauge) and is available in lengths of 100 mm or 150 mm. The lens system, a 20-power magnification microscope, utilizes optical fibers developed for high light-carrying capacity to provide sharp imagery with either a straight (0°) or angled (27°) field of view. The small, 1.7-mm-diameter, 100-mm-long, angled view, Needlescope is preferred in birds because there is less risk of puncturing the abdominal viscera; birds weighing as little as 30 g can be safely examined with this method. The shorter lens is also preferred because it is less fragile and is not normally inserted more than

50 mm (except in larger birds, such as cranes).

As the endoscope is withdrawn, the magnification decreases while the field of view increases. A 6-ft flexible fiber-optic cable brings light to the instrument from a tungsten-halogen light source. The trocar is pyramid-shaped and, because of its sharpness and small size, is inserted easily and virtually trauma-free in any size bird.

The LUMINA-SL telescope is available in diameters of 2.2 mm and 2.7 mm. These instruments use a rod-lens optical system, which provides sharp imagery, magnification, and a wide (10°) field of view. In large birds, a 5-mm telescope may be used. This diameter instrument permits photography when connected to a photo light source. Photography through the smaller-diameter telescopes is difficult because little light is transferred to the target organ.

The 2.7-mm LUMINA-SL telescope is the instrument most widely purchased by avian veterinarians. This instrument is more durable than the Needlescope and its larger diameter allows more light to illuminate the field of view. It can be used to sex most avian species; however, caution is warranted in birds weighing less than 200 g. In small birds it is recommended to dissect through the abdominal musculature with hemostats before insertion of the telescope. This size instrument is also more versatile and can be used for examination of cats and dogs.

Sexing of Birds. No sexual dimorphism is evident in many species, especially psittacines, which has led to frequent pairing in birds of the same gender. Two male or two female birds housed together may be highly compatible, groom and feed each other, attempt copulation, and in the case of females, even lay infertile eggs. With no clue as to the bird's sex other than behavior in monomorphic species, the aviculturist can become frustrated waiting for them to reproduce. Sex determination can enhance propagation, prevent lost time by properly pairing birds, and increase their value. This chapter discusses sexing by endoscopic methods. Other methods are discussed in Chapter 28.

Surgical Sexing by Laparoscopy. Laparoscopy, an endoscopic examination of the abdominal cavity without gross surgical invasion, is a safe and accurate method to determine sex, the stage of maturity, and disease in large and small species (Satterfield 1980) (Table 25.1.).

Presurgical Considerations. Careful evaluation of the patient prior to laparoscopy can minimize inherent risks that accompany anesthesia. Each

Table 25.1. Avian laparoscopy at the San Diego Zoo

Sexing Results	Clear Diagnoses	Questionable
Males	53.8% (n = 176)	6.1% (n = 20)
Females	34.3% (n = 112)	1.2% (n = 4)

Unidentifiable birds = 4.6% (n = 15)
Complications relating to morbidity = 21.4% (n = 70)
　Immaturity　(n = 21)　　Respiration (n = 5)
　Hemorrhage (n = 14)　　Anatomical (n = 3)
　Anesthesia　(n = 13)　　Equipment　(n = 3)
　Obesity　　(n = 9)　　Pathology　(n = 2)
Profile of postoperative mortality
　1.5% (n = 5) within 24 hours
　0.6% (n = 2) within　7 days
　0.9% (n = 3) within 15 days
Confirmed errors (only from questionable sexings)
　0.3% (n = 1) verified by necropsy
　0.6% (n = 2) verified by fecal steroid analysis

Source: Drs. Arden Bryan Bercovitz and Phillip Ensley and the San Diego Zoo veterinary staff.

Note: The number of birds in each category is indicated (n). Results were accumulated over a 5-year period, 1978–1983. All omnivores, carnivores, and herbivores were generally fasted prior to surgery and parenteral administration of ketamine hydrochloride (variable dosage, 15–90 mg/kg body weight).

bird should be visually or manually inspected for evidence of lethargy, depression, labored breathing, emaciation, or palpable abnormalities. The abdomen should always be palpated before examination to ensure the bird is not in egg. Birds in egg are difficult to sex by laparoscopy due to lack of space to position the scope and anatomical changes present. If a bird with obvious or potential problems is identified, laparoscopy may be postponed until the patient is considered a better surgical risk.

Initial physical restraint of the patient should be accomplished with as little stress on the bird as possible. If a bird escapes capture and flies about the room, it should be returned to its cage to calm down. Fatal cardiac arrest can occur due to stress or hyperventilation if immediate induction with inhalation anesthesia is attempted.

Preoperative fasting varies with the size and species of bird. Small specimens (<300 g) usually are not fasted because hypoglycemia may occur. Exceptions include fruit and nectar eaters (e.g., lories), in which passive regurgitation commonly occurs if food is not withheld. All fruit and nectar eaters and birds weighing more than 300 g should be fasted for several hours before surgery to allow emptying of the crop and upper digestive tract. This prevents regurgitation and inadvertent trocar puncture of an enlarged stomach. Raptors, in particular, should not be examined for 24–36 hours after consuming a large meal.

Restraint. The decision of whether to use anesthesia during avian laparoscopy is left to the discretion of the veterinarian. Anesthesia should always be used when the technique is being learned or if diagnostic laparoscopy is being performed.

A method using manual restraint for laparoscopic sexing of birds has been reported in which the patient is positioned in right lateral recumbency (Fig. 25.1) and secured to a restraint board (Harrison 1978). It is essential to maintain a true lateral position to assure a consistent anatomical relationship.

The legs and head are held in place with masking tape, wire, or strips of Velcro. The wings are brought behind the bird in full extension and twisted one over the other so that they interlock. (Care must be taken not to tape the

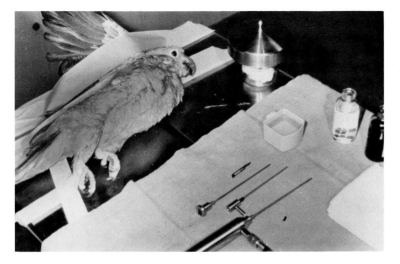

Fig. 25.1. Bird properly positioned and restrained for laparoscopy. The instruments are placed on a sterile drape adjacent to the patient.

wings flush against the table as this causes the body to rotate dorsally.) The left leg is extended caudally as far as possible and held in place with tape while the right leg is pushed beneath the abdomen and left unsecured. The objective of leg displacement is to expose the site for insertion of the endoscope. If a bird is fractious, a towel can be used to decrease visual stimulation. Another technique requires an assistant to manually restrain the bird in lateral recumbency by holding the wings together at the humerus and pulling them over the back while extending the legs posteriorly (Satterfield 1980). The disadvantage of this technique is that the humerus of a struggling bird can fracture if the wings are held at the carpus.

Physical restraint may be adequate for rapid sexing if the bird is calm and the species anatomy is known. In fractious birds under physical restraint, there may be difficulty in maintaining proper positioning and trauma may occur. In these cases, anesthesia is used. The various methods of chemical restraint are discussed in Chapter 23.

Surgical Procedure and Technique. Avian laparoscopy should be performed using sterile instruments and technique. The laparoscopic instruments are initially sterilized by cold sterilization for 15 minutes in a disinfecting solution. Before entering the abdominal cavity, the instruments are rinsed of the disinfectant using sterile water or saline and then dried with sterile gauze. If the lens tip is not thoroughly dried, the field of view may appear cloudy. After the procedure, the distal end (50 mm) of the instrument is soaked in povidone-iodine solution for 30 seconds, rinsed and dried, and laid on a sterile towel. Sterilization with the disinfecting solution is only used after every ten patients or between birds owned by different clients. A sterile glove is worn on the hand holding the tips of the instruments as they are inserted.

The surgical approach is always made on the patient's left side since most female avian species have only a left functional ovary. The male has two testes. The surgical site is located just anterior to the proximal one-third of the femur and behind the last rib. When palpated, this area forms an indented fossa. The overlying feathers are soaked with alcohol (a wetting agent) and plucked or separated; then the skin is aseptically prepared with povidone-iodine soap. A tape border is sometimes used to keep the area free from adjacent feathers (Fig. 25.2).

A 2- to 3-mm incision is made through the skin with a number 15 scalpel blade to facilitate placement of the trocar-cannula. Care must be taken not to incise the underlying muscle or cut

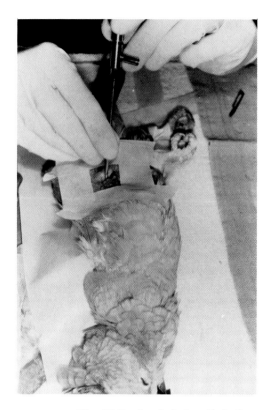

Fig. 25.2. Surgical site with feathers plucked and a taped border applied.

through a feather follicle, which can cause hemorrhage. If bleeding occurs, it should be controlled by direct pressure before proceeding.

The trocar-cannula is introduced through the skin incision perpendicular to the medium plane of the bird and angled slightly dorsally and cranially. The thumb and index finger of one hand holds the distal end of the cannula to provide support and prevent entering the abdomen with excessive force. The cannula is not used in patients weighing less than 200 g since it increases the puncture diameter. An attempt is made to penetrate between the sartorius and iliotibialis cranialis muscles; the sartorius is more often penetrated in the muscular species. With controlled, rotating pressure, the instrument is inserted into the abdominal cavity. A definite decrease in resistance is felt when the trocar perforates the abdominal wall and enters the posterior thoracic or abdominal air sac.

Following penetration, the trocar is withdrawn and the laparoscope is inserted through the cannula and its position verified visually. Internal viewing is enhanced by slowly withdrawing the laparoscope, which may be situated directly against the abdominal air sac or viscera. This also provides an enlarged field of view.

Occasionally it is possible to identify the gonad through an unpunctured abdominal air sac membrane if it is clear and transparent. Often the air sac membrane is opaque due to glare from reflected light, fat infiltration, airsacculitis, and hemorrhage. In such cases, the trocar is reinserted into the cannula and advanced cautiously, gently pushing the tip against the membrane to puncture it. The laparoscope can also be used to make a perforation, avoiding surface vessels and underlying organs. Penetration into the abdominal air sac is necessary to adequately visualize the abdominal contents (Fig. 25.3).

Following the examination, which usually takes about 1 minute, the laparoscope is withdrawn from the abdominal cavity. The skin incision is not sutured because the puncture diameter is small. Also, when the extended left leg is released it flexes anteriorly; the resulting nonalignment of the skin incision through the muscle seals the opening. If closure of the incision is indicated, absorbable suture material is chosen. Antibiotic therapy, either topical or systemic, is not given under normal circumstances.

Birds are tattooed according to their gender by injecting a bleb of black pigment subcutaneously on the inside of the wing web directly above the elbow. Males are marked on the right wing, females on the left. A vibrating, battery-operated tattoo machine can be used but is not very effective since avian dermis is thin. Examination of marked birds several years later still revealed the dye, although it had faded in some individuals.

Gonad Characteristics. The gonad is located in the anterior dorsal aspect of the left abdominal air sac adjacent to the cranial pole of the left kidney. Approaching from a caudal position through the patient's left side, the kidney is initially identified to the right as a large, lobulated, dark red or brown organ. It is followed anteriorly to its most cranial aspect, where the gonad and adrenal gland are found. These three organs form an easily identified triad. Anterior to this triad is the lung, which is pink. To the left and slightly posterior, the proventriculus, spleen, and intestines can be identified. The liver is not viewed from this approach. The adrenal gland is small, irregularly shaped, yellowish orange, and highly vascular. Normally, the gonad occurs to the left and slightly posterior to the adrenal gland, while the kidney is found to the right of both.

If there is any doubt about the sex of a bird, especially in an immature individual, visualization of a second gonad confirms it as a male. In an immature bird, the testes are usually very small and avascular (Plate 6). In a mature bird, the testes vary in size and enlarge during breeding season. The inexperienced operator can sometimes confuse a section of intestine with a testicle. A loop of gut, which can appear round and smooth and be off-white or yellow, may lie directly against the cranial pole of the kidney. In such cases, the laparoscope must be directed downward between the two organs to establish that the identified organ is the gonad and not a loop of gut.

The ovary of a mature bird has a grapelike cluster of prominent follicles, which is easy to identify (Fig. 25.4). Females ready to ovulate have several enlarged, yolk-colored ova protrud-

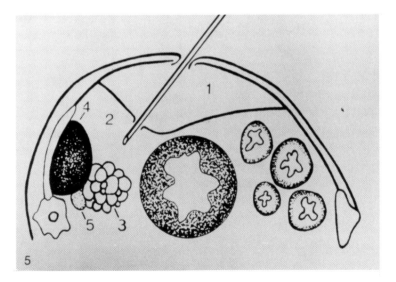

Fig. 25.3. Transverse section of a bird's abdomen showing the air sac membrane that must be punctured to allow visualization of the gonad with an endoscope: posterior thoracic air sac (*1*), abdominal air sac (*2*), ovary (*3*), kidney (*4*), adrenal gland (*5*). (*From Ingram 1980, by permission*)

ing from this cluster. The ovary is usually white but may be partially or totally pigmented. In the young, immature female bird, follicles are not present; this can make differentiation between ovary and testicle difficult. In these birds the ovary is flattened, contains smooth, brainlike grooves or folds (Fig. 25.5), and may resemble adipose tissue. The ovary of an older immature female has a fine granular surface that resembles cobblestone. Because of an ovary's irregular shape and variable size, it may hide the left adrenal gland from view.

Results and Complications. Since 1978, avian fatalities with this author have occurred at a rate of 0.4% (one death per 250 birds sexed). The most common cause of death has been cardiac arrest while under inhalation anesthesia (methoxyflurane). Significant pathological lesions (yolk peritonitis, hepatitis, aspergillosis) were found in several dead birds, but no abnormalities were seen in others, indicating that death was directly attributed to anesthesia. Other causes of death have included a bird ingesting the cotton bulb from the induction jar, inadvertent puncture of the proventriculus and kidney, internal hemorrhage, asphyxiation due to regurgitation of crop contents, and hypovolemic shock incurred from humeral fracture during restraint.

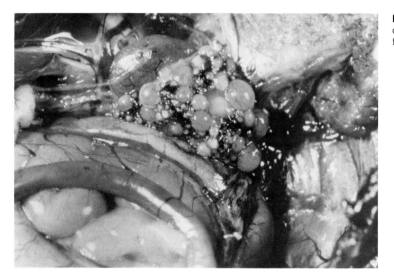

Fig. 25.4. Follicular development in a mature female.

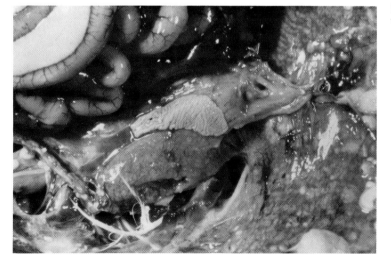

Fig. 25.5. Ovary in a very young female.

Hemorrhage frequently prevents adequate visualization of the gonad and is usually caused by trocar insertion through the muscle. When a small amount of blood obstructs the tip of the scope, it can be cleaned by blotting the lens against an intraabdominal organ or withdrawing the instrument and rinsing the tip with sterile water. The use of a device to deliver air internally to keep the lens tip clean is not necessary. In the presence of significant hemorrhage, as might occur with penetration of the kidney or laceration of the internal iliac vessel, the examination is terminated and the patient closely monitored during recovery.

Other conditions that may complicate the procedure include fat, tachypnea, and air sacculitis. Little can be done to resolve the problem of abdominal fat. Tachypnea may occur in excited birds manually restrained or occasionally in patients anesthetized with an inhalation agent. Excessive ventilation through the air sacs causes the loosely attached digestive organs to move back and forth, making it difficult to properly position the laparoscope. Hyperventilation can also produce "water bubbles" (condensation), which cloud the tip of the lens. Fluid in the air sacs as a result of airsacculitis will also prevent adequate viewing.

Minor postoperative emphysema has been observed at the insertion site; it usually subsides rapidly. Excessive amounts of trapped air can be evacuated with a needle and syringe.

In some species (columbiforms, galliforms, passeriforms), the testicle of an active mature male may be so large that only a small portion of it can be visualized. Inexperienced veterinarians may not even recognize it as a testicle and can become frustrated when they cannot find the gonad elsewhere. These large testicles are usually highly vascularized.

Occasionally, it is difficult to sex an active mature female because the greatly enlarged follicles fill a large portion of the abdominal air sac and not enough of the ovary is seen to identify it. Great care must be taken not to accidentally puncture the newly developing yolks, especially with the trocar when first entering the abdominal cavity.

Surgical Sexing by Laparotomy. If the veterinarian does not have access to a laparoscope, birds may be sexed with an otoscope through a laparotomy incision (Ingram 1980; Burr et al. 1981). A 1/3- to 1/2-in. skin incision is made dorsoventrally just anterior to the femur in the paralumbar fossa. The sartorius and iliotibialis cranialis muscles are identified, and hemostats are used to bluntly dissect between them. This greatly minimizes hemorrhage. The opening is enlarged enough to allow entry of an appropriate-size otoscope speculum. The underlying air sac membrane is punctured with a needle and the opening enlarged to allow penetration of the speculum into the abdominal air sac to clearly visualize the gonad. The skin is closed with absorbable sutures.

Entry between the last two ribs is recommended by some authors, especially when sexing birds weighing less than 200 g (Burr et al. 1981). With this approach, the skin incision is made over the last intercostal space. The sartorius muscle is identified and retracted posteriorly to expose the last intercostal space, which is then opened using blunt dissection.

Diagnostic Laparoscopy. The endoscope can be inserted into any body orifice or through the abdominal musculature in several sites for the purpose of visual examination, biopsy, or surgery. Information about the condition of organs or tissue can be ascertained with minimal surgical risk.

As well as an entry through the paralumbar fossa, the abdomen can also be examined through an incision made directly behind the sternum on the midline. This is the selected site if the liver is to be examined. For this procedure, the bird is anesthetized and positioned in dorsal recumbency with its legs extended caudally. Feathers are plucked to expose the abdomen and the posterior border of the sternum. The skin is incised with a number 15 scalpel blade. The trocar-cannula device is inserted through the musculature horizontally (with a very slight angle dorsally) toward the head (Fig. 25.6). If previous radiographs have indicated hepatomegaly, a slightly ventral angle of insertion may be necessary to avoid puncturing the liver. On penetration, the trocar is removed and the endoscope introduced.

The left and right lobes of the liver are initially visualized cranially and dorsally. The posterior border of the liver may be slightly caudal to the insertion site. As the endoscope is advanced further cranially, the heart is seen. On either side of the liver, air sac membranes are encountered, and if they are entered, the ventral border of the lung is easily viewed. A more thorough examination of the air sacs and lungs is possible from this approach than through the paralumbar fossa. Evaluation of the urogenital system and the spleen is not possible from this view.

An increasingly common diagnostic procedure is liver biopsy. Diseases such as avian tuberculosis (Fig. 25.7), viral or bacterial hepatitis, leukosis, amyloidosis, or toxicosis can be diagnosed without endangering the health of the

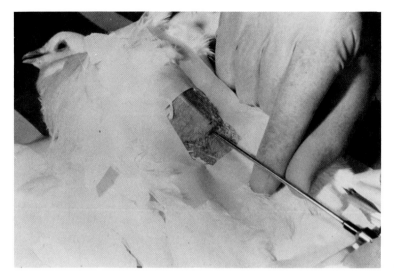

Fig. 25.6. Laparoscopy to examine the liver.

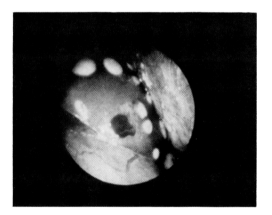

Fig. 25.7. Endoscopic view of avian tuberculosis lesions on the surface of the liver.

bird. Samples from other organs can be collected as well.

Several types of ancillary instruments have been developed that allow easy and safe biopsy of the liver (and other organs) under direct visualization in laparoscopy. The Cope Biopsy System has been developed for use with the Needlescope. The biopsy instrument, which passes down the cannula alongside the endoscope and appears directly in the center of the area visualized, may be a liver core aspiration needle or a microcupped biopsy instrument. Operation of this system is rapid and efficient.

An optical biopsy forcep system is available that consists of a LUMINA-SL telescope in connection with rigid, spoon-shaped biopsy forceps.

The jaws of the forceps, which can be opened or closed by manipulating the loop handle, appear in the field of view. This instrument is introduced into the abdominal cavity after initial puncture and withdrawal of the trocar.

Avian spoon-shaped biopsy forceps are less expensive but just as effective for obtaining tissue samples. This instrument is passed alongside the endoscope and positioned so that the jaws can be visualized as previously described. Hand-eye coordination with a second instrument is initially awkward, and practice is necessary to become proficient.

Esophagogastroscopy. The endoscope can be used to clearly visualize structures in the oral cavity and upper alimentary tract. With the bird properly restrained and its mouth held open, the endoscope (with or without a cannula) is slowly advanced into the oral cavity. Looking at the roof of the mouth, the palatal folds, choana, opening of the auditory canal, and pharynx can be thoroughly examined. Ventrally, the caudal aspect of the tongue, salivary duct, glottis, and laryngeal prominences can be seen. With the neck extended, the scope can be cautiously introduced into the esophagus and advanced into the crop. For this procedure, the bird is either placed in dorsal recumbency or held vertically with its head stretched upward.

The esophagus and crop often contain excess mucous and saliva, which can blur the field of view. The lumen of the esophagus is naturally collapsed, as well, increasing the amount of secretion contacting the lens tip. Therefore, the field of view is usually less obstructed when withdrawing the endoscope than when moving it forward. To minimize the problem of secretions, the esophagus can be swabbed with appropriate-sized cotton balls. Fasting the bird for up to 6 hours is also beneficial. Once the field of view becomes blurred after insertion, it may be possible to clean the lens tip by carefully blotting it against the wall of the esophagus or crop. If this is unsuccessful, the endoscope must be withdrawn and the tip cleaned with sterile water. If the endoscope is inserted with the cannula in place, the field of view may be enhanced by withdrawing the endoscope several millimeters within the cannula (preventing tissue from contacting the terminal lens). Lastly, insufflation of air through attachment sleeves in the cannula can increase internal viewing of these organs by increasing the space available in which to manipulate the scope. However, insufflated air tends to escape up the esophagus quickly.

The esophagus and crop can be examined for lesions of trichomoniasis and candidiasis or for bacterial infection. Identification and retrieval of foreign bodies is a common indication to examine the crop endoscopically, particularly in psittacines, which tend to be destructive. Wood chips used for bedding and subsequently swallowed by hand-raised baby birds are the most common foreign body encountered. Biopsy forceps can be passed alongside the endoscope to grasp the object.

With persistence, the endoscope can be passed beyond the crop into the proventriculus. In psittacines this is more easily accomplished in birds weighing over 500 g. It is usually not possible to enter the gizzard. In species such as raptors that do not have an expansive crop, the endoscope can easily be passed into the stomach. Visualization within the proventriculus is difficult in all species because of the glandular secretions from this organ.

Tracheoscopy. Endoscopic examination within the trachea is easily accomplished, limited only by the diameter of the tracheal lumen compared with the endoscope and by the length of the neck. In long-necked birds (cranes, herons, swans) only the proximal portion of the trachea can be viewed. In short-necked birds (e.g., parrots) the entire tracheal lumen including the bifurcation and proximal bronchi are easily visualized.

To examine the trachea, the bird is anesthetized and positioned with its neck extended. The endoscope, without cannula, is introduced through the glottis and slowly advanced down the windpipe (Fig. 25.8). Reflex coughing is common at first but usually subsides once the scope is in place. The lens tip is directed toward the center of the lumen (care must be taken not

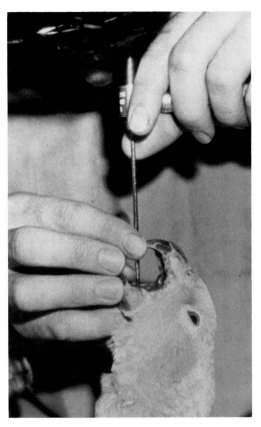

Fig. 25.8. Examining the trachea with an endoscope.

to scrape it against the tracheal wall, which can cause bleeding and stimulate coughing).

The windpipe can be examined for parasites (gapeworms, air sac mites), foreign bodies, and bacterial or fungal plaques. Caseated fungal plaques, such as those due to *Aspergillosis,* may cause partial or complete obstruction at the tracheal bifurcation or bronchi.

To remove a plaque for closer examination or culture, the tip of the endoscope can sometimes be used to free it from the tracheal wall. The tissue often adheres to the lens tip. Alternatively, biopsy forceps may be passed alongside the endoscope for sample collection. Placement of two instruments through the glottis at the same time may not be possible if the trachea is small or the lesion too far down the windpipe to reach.

Surgical removal of large caseated plugs from the bifurcation has been accomplished by entering the trachea through a longitudinal incision just cranial to the syrinx. The thoracic inlet is surgically opened to expose the trachea in this area. Small curettes or forceps are introduced through the incision while the surgery site is viewed through the endoscope, which has been passed down from the glottis. If the length of the trachea is too great, both instruments can enter the trachea through the incision site. Respirations are not impaired during this procedure because air is exchanged through the opened intraclavicular air sac that has been punctured to gain access to the syrinx. After the plug is removed, the trachea is sutured with chromic gut and the skin is closed. Follow-up medical therapy may be indicated.

References

Burr, E. W., F. W. Huchzermeyer, and A. E. Riley. 1981. Laparoscopic examination to determine sex in monomorphic avian species. *J. South African Vet. Assoc.* 1(March):45–47.

Harrison, G. J. 1978. Endoscopic examination of avian gonadal tissue. *Vet. Med. Small Anim. Clin.* 73:479–84.

Ingram, K. A. 1980. Otoscope technique for sexing birds. In *Current Veterinary Therapy VII,* ed. R. W. Kirk, pp. 656–58. Philadelphia: W. B. Saunders.

Satterfield, W. C. 1980. Diagnostic laparoscopy in birds. In *Current Veterinary Therapy VII,* ed. R. W. Kirk, pp. 659–61. Philadelphia: W. B. Saunders.

26

Cosmetic Surgery

CHRISTINE DAVIS

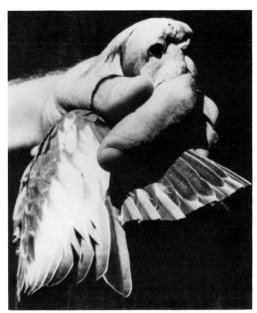

Fig. 26.1. One-wing clip.

IT IS IMPORTANT to the client that birds have a functional and esthetically pleasing appearance. Wing clipping and beak and nail trimming are integral parts of cosmetic surgery frequently performed by the veterinarian.

Several of the many different techniques used in cosmetic surgery are discussed below.

Clipping. The purpose of clipping is not to disable the bird totally but to allow limited flight (up to about 4 ft from the ground) that would cushion the bird if it falls and enable it to escape from possible danger yet not allow it to fly away if startled.

One-Wing Clip. Many people prefer clipping only one wing (Fig. 26.1). This gives an unbalanced appearance, which is esthetically unpleasing. Another disadvantage of the one-wing clip is that a bird has more power and thrust in the fully fledged wing than in the clipped one. With this limited, uneven control, a startled or frightened bird can fly into objects with great force, causing injuries. Yet another disadvantage of this type of clip is that owners sometimes do not notice when the clipped feathers regrow. A bird can attain almost full-flight capacity and, if outside and startled, can fly away.

Cosmetic Clip. The cosmetic clip is popular because it leaves the first two primary flight feathers intact; this is acceptable esthetically because these feathers are crossed on the bird's back. Large birds (macaws, cockatoos) have lengthy wingspans, which can cause injury to the bird and handler if the cosmetic clip is carried out. Large birds often break these feathers during handling due to thrashing about when

frightened. In small birds, especially, the wings can become caught in the cage wire as a direct result of the two long feathers. A bird can traumatize itself to death or can completely amputate a wing by thrashing about (or even by using its own beak) in order to gain freedom.

Secondary-Flight Clip. This is probably the most desirable clipping method and is very acceptable esthetically. The primary flight feathers are left intact, and only the secondaries are clipped. The main disadvantage of this method is that when a few of the clipped feathers grow out the bird may attain full flight.

Functional Clip. The functional clip consists of clipping the first six to eleven primary flight feathers, up to or just under the primary coverts. This leaves a neat scalloped edge and a balanced appearance. If the bird begins to grow feathers back it is quickly noticed. The number of feathers to clip depends on the species of the bird as well as the individual. A heavy-bodied bird often needs only the first six feathers clipped, while a lighter-bodied one may require the clipping of more feathers.

Trimming

Nail Trimming. Nail trimming is essential. If the nails of a bird become too long they may impair its stance, allow the bird to get caught in the cage bars (where it may injure itself in panic), and be painful when the owner holds the bird on one arm. (Clients should be instructed to avoid using sandpaper perch covers as a way of keeping the nails short because this common practice often results in foot injury and infection.)

Thick, black macaw nails are the most difficult to clip because it is not easy to determine the location of the vein. Shining a penlight against the back side of the nails can, in some birds, enable location of the vein. If this does not work, the difference in consistency of the nail pulp as it approaches the vein can indicate when enough has been cut. The nails usually have veins of comparable length with the exception of the rear inner nail, which often is short with a vein reaching almost to the end of the nail portion. *Do not clip the nails too short,* as the bird uses its nails for gripping and needs a certain amount of length to feel secure. Most birds coming from the wild need only the sharp points taken off. Caged birds require more aggressive clipping because they lack the natural wear that a bird in the wild gets. After the nails are clipped, the bird must stop bleeding and picking at them before it is sent home. A bird's feet may be sore for a couple of days after clipping, which may predispose it to disease or impair its desire to eat. The cage must be kept cleaner than usual during the healing period to prevent infection of the feet from fecal matter.

Beak Trimming. Beak trims are seldom necessary in the normal bird. If a parrot or other bird has enough wood or other materials to chew or rub its beak on, it should never require a beak trim. The slightly overgrown beaks of small and medium-sized birds can be trimmed with a nail file (Fig. 26.2).

Some birds, however, have overgrown beaks that result from injuries to the growth plate, hereditary factors, diseases (e.g., sinusitis), osteomyelitis involving the tissues surrounding the cere, mange (e.g., cnemodocoptic mange in Budgerigars), cancer of the cere and beak, endocrine disease in cockatoos, etc. Beaks have blood vessels and nervous tissue running their entire length, reaching surprisingly close to the end in many species. Care must be taken while trimming beaks with clippers. Some birds with newly trimmed beaks are in such pain following the procedure that they are unable to eat for a day or two. Thick macaw beaks may split longitudinally as the result of an overly aggressive beak trim. Sometimes beaks bleed after being trimmed and should be given prompt attention before the bird is sent home.

In small birds (Budgerigars, canaries, lovebirds, Cockatiels) the beak can be held shut and

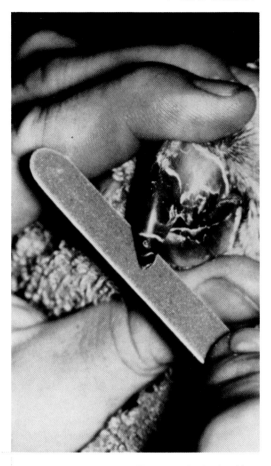

Fig. 26.2. Trimming the beak with a nail file.

a penlight directed through the top. By looking from underneath, the vascular tissue can be located and the beak trimmed accordingly. Dentists' tools work extremely well for beak trims, but care must be taken not to nick the tongue.

Feather Removal. Proper feather care leads to a healthier bird. Feather removal is often necessary because of injury or disease and/or to promote new feather growth. Broken blood feathers are removed by pulling, applying manual pressure, and cauterizing the follicle with a styptic such as ferric subsulfate liquid or powder. If many blood feathers are present, only a few are removed at a time and the rest clipped about ½ in. distal to the blood feather portion (Fig. 26.3). This lessens the chance of the bird banging the newly exposed, unprotected blood feather, causing bleeding. The feathers will have to be trimmed at a later date.

Sometimes during shipment a bird will

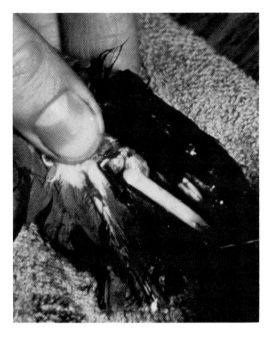

Fig. 26.3. Removing broken blood feathers.

damage all its tail feathers. For balanced regrowth, only half the tail feathers should be pulled (pulling every other one). When the first half have grown in, the remaining feathers are pulled.

Because of the body mass of a large bird, removal of too many tail feathers can make it extremely clumsy. It can even fall from a perch and injure itself. If the bird's primary flight feathers are splintered from disease or after capture in the wild, the splintered portions should be trimmed with scissors. If primary flight feathers must be pulled, care must be taken to grasp the thin metacarpal bones and pull each feather close to the base of the wing to avoid breaking the limb. If the primary covert feathers have been damaged or clipped as well, they can be pulled in the same manner as the tail in order to allow their regrowth.

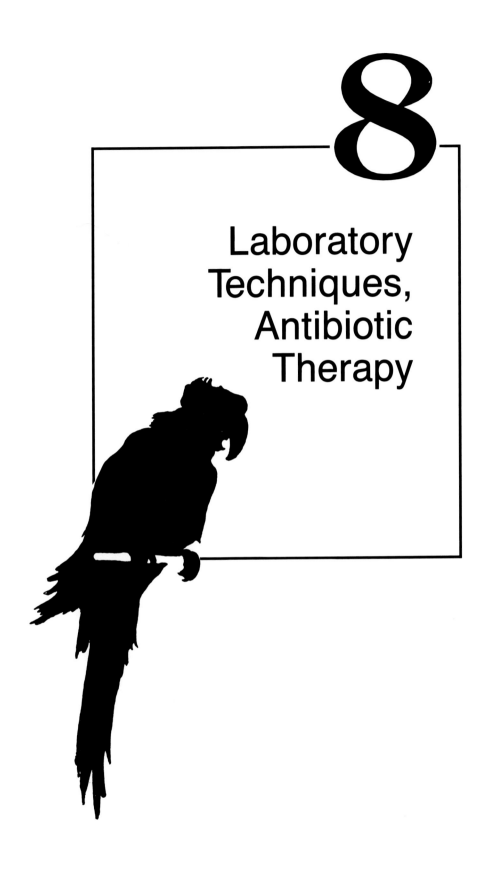

8

Laboratory
Techniques,
Antibiotic
Therapy

27

Clinical Pathology and Laboratory Diagnostic Tools

RICHARD W. WOERPEL
WALTER J. ROSSKOPF, JR.
MARILYN MONAHAN-BRENNAN

CAGED BIRDS possess the unique ability to compensate physiologically for organic dysfunction and maintain this compensatory state for a surprisingly long period of time. Sustained *subclinical* illness results. The problem of subclinical illness in caged birds makes diagnosis of illness difficult. Consequently, the avian veterinarian must rely heavily on the clinical pathology and laboratory tests to aid in disease diagnosis, as well as to aid in monitoring the clinical course of the avian patient (Rosskopf and Woerpel 1982).

This chapter details the diagnostic tests and methods available to the avian veterinarian and provides practical information regarding clinical applications.

Hematology and Blood Chemistry Evaluation

Laboratory Methodology. Filled microhematocrit tubes are clayed (one end only) and refrigerated prior to submission to the laboratory. Those tubes destined to be used for blood chemistry determination should be handled differently. Each of these tubes should be centrifuged for 5 minutes in a hematocrit centrifuge. The packed cell volume, plasma color and clarity, and magnitude of the buffy coat should be noted. The tubes are scored with a file and broken just above the packed cell–plasma interface. The plasma-containing half tubes are then reclayed on one end. These extra steps are necessary in order to avoid artifactual decrease in

blood glucose and sodium and artifactual increases in lactic dehydrogenase (LDH), total protein, and potassium.

Blood films (smears) are made in the standard fashion using bevel-edged microscope slides, or they are made on coverslips (Schalm 1975) to minimize damage to the avian leukocytes, which are more fragile than those of mammalian species. To minimize the potential for a stress hemogram, the blood films are made before any microhematocrit tubes are filled.

White blood cell (WBC) counts are either estimated by the laboratory or reported as a corrected value using an absolute heterophil count (Table 27.1). Red blood cell (RBC) counts are outlined in Table 27.2.

A Wright's-Giemsa (or modified Wright's) stain is used on all blood films because hemoparasites show up more clearly, polychromatic cells are more visible, and the stain allows easy differentiation between heterophils and eosinophils. The appearance of leukocytes can vary from species to species and with the type of stain used. The practitioner should experiment with a number of stains and stick with the one that works best. Several good ready-to-use Wright's-Giemsa stains are available commercially.

Table 27.1 details the methods used to perform the various cell counts. A discussion of the distinguishing features (morphology, color, etc.) of the various cell types noted on an avian blood film follows (Plates 7, 8, and 9).

Erythrocytes. Mature RBCs are oval to elliptical in shape and nucleated. The nucleus appears dark purple and possesses tightly packed chromatin. When a Wright's-Giemsa stain is used, the cytoplasm appears bluish pink, whereas a straight Wright's stain produces an orangish pink. Immature erythrocytes appear rounder. Their nuclei possess more loosely packed chromatin amid polychromatic cytoplasm.

Thrombocytes. On blood films, avian thrombocytes tend to clump together, which aids identification. They are smaller than erythrocytes. Their shape varies from oval to elliptical, the nucleus is very dark, and the cytoplasm reveals a transparent to slightly blue character. Most of the cytoplasm is positioned at each end of the nucleus, giving them a wispy appearance. A frequent mistake of technicians reading blood smears on high dry is to count thrombocytes as leukocytes (lymphocytes). This results in an artificially high estimated WBC count.

Heterophils. This is the major granulocyte in avian blood. The nucleus stains bluish to ma-

Table 27.1. Avian hematologic and blood chemistry methods currently in use

Test	Method
Hematologic tests	
RBC	Unopette #5851[a]
	Standard method using hemocytometer
Estimated WBC	Examine stained blood film at high dry (X40). Count all WBCs visible near feathered edge in 10 good fields, average all 10 counts, and multiply average by 2.0. Report estimate as range.[b]
Corrected WBC	Unopette #5877[a] (eosinophil enumeraton). Contents of Unopette will stain virtually all avian granulocytes. Using hemocytometer, make count from both sides of counting chamber. Multiply result by 1.1 (or add 10% to number). Multiply by 16 to get base granuloctye count. Corrected WBC = base granuloctye count/(% granulocytes in differential × 10).[c]
Differential	Standard method 100 cell count
PCV	Standard method
Plasma protein	Refractometer
Serum chemistries	
Total protein[d]	Biuret reaction
Glucose[d]	Modified Richterich and Dauwalder method
SGOT[d]	Modified Henry
LDH[d]	Modified Wacker
Uric acid[d]	Breakdown of uric acid and rate of oxidation of NADH
Creatinine[d]	Modified Jaffe
BUN[d]	Modified Talk and Schubert method
Calcium[d]	Modifed Connerty and Briggs
Phosphorus[d]	Modified Daly and Ertingshausen
T_4[e]	Enzymatic method: urea II enzyme
	Immunoassay for thyroxine

[a]Becton, Dickinson and Co., Rutherford, N.J.

[b]For example: If 10, 9, 8, 12, 14, 10, 11, 7, 12, and 10 WBCs are seen in 10 fields, the average is 10.3, the estimated WBC = 20.6 or 20,600/mm³, and the reported estimated WBC = 20,000–21,000/mm³.

[c]For example: If the granuloctye count from both sides of the counting chamber is 519, the base granulocyte count = 519 × 1.1 × 16 = 9134.4. The differential breakdown is heterophils 64%, lymphoctyes 21%, monocytes 5%, eosinophils 4%, and basophils 6%. Granulocytes = 74%. Corrected WBC = 9134.4/(74 × 10) = 12.3 × (10^3/mm³).

[d]Abbott A-Gent Reagents, Abbott Laboratories, No. Chicago, Ill.

[e]Organon Diagnostics, Division of Organon, Inc., West Orange, N.J.

genta and appears partially lobed. Typically, these leukocytes contain rod-shaped orange to pink granules within the cytoplasm. Sometimes, however, these granules appear round, making it difficult to distinguish the cell as a heterophil or an eosinophil. Heterophils stain differently in the various species. African Gray Parrots, ducks, and certain birds of prey are species that possess brighter-staining heterophilic granules. Amazon parrots often possess heterophilic gran-

ules, which have a ruddier or duller appearance. In some caged birds (e.g., macaws), the heterophilic granules stain more intensely at their ends, giving them the appearance of being multiple tiny, round granules, rather than rod-shaped.

Eosinophils. The nucleus of the eosinophil usually stains more intensely than the heterophil. The cytoplasm may appear invisible or may ex-

Table 27.2. Hematologic and blood chemistry normal values

	Species A	Species B	Species C	Species D
WBC ($\times$ 10³/mm³)	5-11	6-11	4-11	3-8
Differential				
Heterophils	45-75	30-75	40-70	45-70
Lymphocytes	20-50	20-65	20-50	20-45
Monocytes	0-3	0-3	0-2	0-5
Eosinophils	0-2	0-1	0-1	0-1
Basophils	0-5	0-5	0-5	0-5
PCV (%)	43-55	45-55	44-60	45-57
RBC ($\times$ 10⁶/mm³)	2.4-4.5	2.5-4.5	2.4-4.1	2.5-4.5
Total protein (g/dl)	3.0-5.0	3.0-5.0	2.6-5.0	2.5-4.5
Glucose (mg/dl)	190-350	220-350	180-300	200-400
Calcium (mg/dl)	8.0-13.0	8.0-13.0	10.0-15.0	
SGOT ((IU/L)	100-350	130-350	150-350	150-350
LDH (IU/L)	150-450	160-420	200-550	150-450
Creatinine (mg/dl)	0.1-0.4	0.1-0.4	0.1-0.3	0.1-0.4
Uric Acid (mg/dl)	4.0-10.0	2.0-10.0	4.0-12.0	4.0-14.0
Potassium (mEq/L)	2.6-4.2	3.0-4.5	3.0-4.5	
Sodium (mEq/L)	134-152	136-152	130-150	
T₄ (μg/dl)	0.3-2.0	.05-1.0	.20-1.1	2.5-4.4

	Species J	Species K	Species L	Species M
WBC ($\times$ 10³/mm³)	4.5-13.0	6-11	3-8	3-8
Differential				
Heterophils	30-70	40-75	20-65	40-75
Lymphocytes	20-65	20-50	20-65	20-55
Monocytes	0-3	0-2	0-1	0-2
Eosinophils	0-4	0-1	0-1	0-1
Basophils	0-5	0-5	0-5	0-6
PCV (%)	30-43	45-55	45-62	44-57
RBC ($\times$ 10⁶/mm³)	2.3-3.5	2.5-4.0	2.5-4.6	3.0-5.1
Total Protein (g/dl)	2.5-6.0	3.0-5.0	3.0-5.0	2.2-5.1
Glucose (mg/dl)	150-300	180-360	200-450	200-400
Calcium (mg/dl)	10.0-18.0	9.0-16.0		9.0-15.0
SGOT (IU/L)	5-100	130-350	150-350	100-350
LDH (IU/L)	150-800	200-400		100-350
Creatinine (mg/dl)	0.1-0.5	0.1-0.4		0.1-0.4
Uric Acid (mg/dl)	2.0-12.0	3.0-10.0	4.0-12.0	3.0-11.0
Potassium (mEq/L)	3.0-4.5			2.5-3.5
Sodium (mEq/L)	130-155			137-150
T₄ (μg/dl)	0.8-3.3	0.5-1.0		0.2-1.9

Note: A = African Gray parrots (*Psittacus erithacus erithacus* and *Psittacus erithacus timneh*), sample size: 108; B = amazon parrots (*Amazona* sp.), 640; C = Blue-headed Parrots (*Pionus menstruus*), 16; D = Budgerigars (*Melopsittacus undulatus*), 251; E = Gray-cheeked Parakeets (*Brotogeris pyrrhopterus*), 32, and Canary-winged Parakeets (*Brotogeris versicolorus*), 11; F = canaries (*Serinus canaria*), 62; G = Cockatiels (*Nymphicus hollandicus*), 364; H = cockatoos, 242; I = conures (*Aratinga* sp.), 85; J = domestic ducks, 31; K = Grand Eclectus Parrots

hibit a bluish cast. The eosinophils of most avian species possess uniform large, round granules that often stain pale blue.

Basophils. This particular granulocyte is easy to identify because of its dark-staining basophilic cytoplasmic granules. Frequently basophils are found in various stages of degranulation on a blood smear. Basophils of amazon parrots routinely possess larger and more prominent cy-

toplasmic granules than those of other caged birds. This tendency is most obvious with the basophils of the Mexican Red-headed Amazon (*Amazona viridigenalis*).

Lymphocytes. In basic morphology, avian lymphocytes resemble those of mammals. However, they exhibit a tremendous variation in size.

Monocytes. With the great variation in the size of

Species E	Species F	Species G	Species H	Species I
4.5–9.5	4–9	5–10	5–11	4–11
40–75	20–50	40–70	45–75	40–75
20–60	40–75	25–55	20–50	20–50
0–3	0–1	0–2	0–4	0–3
0–1	0–1	0–2	0–2	0–3
0–5	0–5	0–6	0–5	0–5
46–58	45–60	45–57	40–55	42–55
	2.5–4.5	2.5–4.7	2.2–4.5	2.5–4.5
2.5–4.5	3.0–5.0	2.2–5.0	2.5–5.0	2.5–4.5
200–350	200–450	200–450	190–350	200–350
		8.5–13.0	8.0–13.0	8.0–15.0
150–400	150–350	100–350	150–350	125–350
150–450		125–450	225–650	125–420
0.1–0.4		0.1–0.4	0.1–0.4	0.1–0.5
4.0–12.0	4.0–12.0	3.5–11.0	3.5–11.0	2.5–10.5
		2.5–4.5	2.5–4.5	3.4–5.0
		132–150	131–157	134–148
0.2–2.4	0.7–3.4	0.7–2.4	0.8–4.4	0.25–0.9

Species N	Species O	Species P	Species Q
6–13.5	6–11	4.5–11.5	4.0–10.0
45–70	25–65	35–70	35–65
20–50	20–60	20–60	25–50
0–3	0–3	0–5	0–4
0–2	0–3	0–0	0–4
0–5	0–7	0–5	0–5
45–55	44–55	45–55	45–60
2.5–4.5	2.4–4.0	2.4–5.0	2.5–4.5
3.0–5.0	2.3–4.5	3.0–5.0	3.0–5.0
200–350	190–350	190–350	220–350
9.0–13.0	9.0–13.0	10.0–16.0	10.0–19.0
100–280	130–350	130–350	130–330
75–425	600–1,000	130–425	200–400
0.1–0.5	0.1–0.6	0.1–0.4	0.1–0.4
2.5–11.5	4.0–10.0	4.0–10.0	4.0–14.0
2.5–4.5	3.0–5.1		
136–155	136–152		
1.0–4.0[a]	0.5–0.9	0.3–1.0	0.5–3.2

(*Eclectus roratos riedeli*), 9; L = finches, 21; M = lovebirds (*Agapornis* sp.), 78; N = macaws, 219; O = Greater Indian Hill Mynahs (*Gracula religiosa*), 35; P = Philippine Blue-naped Parrots (*Tanygnathus lucionensis*), 7; Q = toucans, 8.

[a]Value given for Blue-and-gold Macaw; T_3 and T_4 for others varies with species.

avian lymphocytes, larger size is not a good means of identification. Other properties of the monocytes must be relied on: a large amount of cytoplasm in relation to the nucleus, frequent vacuolization of the cytoplasm, eccentrically placed nucleus, very acute nuclear folds, etc.

Normal Pet Avian Hematology and Blood Chemistry Values. Several factors have been responsible for the difficulty in establishing criteria for "normality" in hematologic testing. The two factors are the difficulty in collecting significant quantities of blood from a bird and the lack of equipped veterinary laboratories capable of processing minute quantities of blood. Furthermore, determination of blood values is difficult to obtain among the numerous avian species. Normal hematologic and blood chemistry values for some of the common avian species are listed in Table 27.2. See Dolensek and Otis (1973),

Galvin (1978), Raphael (1981), Dein (1982a), and Hawkey et al. (1982).

Interpretation of Laboratory Results. The use of hematology and blood chemistry evaluation is vital to the establishment of a definite diagnosis in avian medicine. Serial laboratory testing monitors therapeutic changes rapidly, and sequential blood tests record a patient's clinical response. See Rosskopf and Woerpel (1982a), Rosskopf et al. (1982a), and Paster (1983a).

However, many amazon parrots with chronic disease (especially respiratory) exhibit apparently normal WBC counts and differentials. It can only be surmised that during the acute phase of the disease, the WBC count reflects a leukocytosis with changes in the differential (heterophilia, lymphopenia, basophilia). This finding is not as common among the other psittacine groups.

Interestingly, parenteral antibiotic treatment among these individuals usually results in a rapid leukocytosis that disappears as treatment progresses. Apparently the aggressive therapy directed toward a chronic disease process results in an acute inflammatory reaction that subsides as treatment is continued.

Stress hemograms may occur in extremely stressed or frightened caged birds. This phenomenon varies with the species and depends on whether the patient is heterophilic (cockatoos, macaws) or lymphocytic (many amazon parrots, most canaries and finches). The stress hemogram becomes more pronounced the longer the bird is restrained; therefore blood films should be made as soon as possible after catching a bird.

In stress hemograms in heterophilic birds, the absolute heterophil count increases, and in lymphocytic birds the absolute lymphocyte count increases.

In clinically ill heterophilic birds the heterophils rise, while in contrast, in sick lymphocytic birds the heterophils, not the lymphocytes, tend to increase. The exact mechanism of this phenomenon is unknown.

To achieve consistent results, the practitioner must handle blood samples properly. Hemolysis consistently produces elevations in LDH, SGOT (serum glutamic oxaloacetic transaminase, also called SAST), total protein, and artifacts. Proper refrigeration of the laboratory sample is vital. Plasma samples may be preserved indefinitely by freezing. Plasma that remains in contact with erythrocytes (even when centrifuged) yields lower glucose and sodium readings.

The following laboratory tests are commonly performed on birds.

White Blood Cell Count. Increases in the WBC count (leukocytosis) can be caused by inflammatory processes (bacterial, chlamydial, fungal, mycobacterial), tissue trauma, stress reaction, corticosteroid usage, or response to sudden blood loss.

Decreases in the WBC count (leukopenia) can be caused by overwhelming infections (especially in the smaller caged birds such as Budgerigars and Cockatiels), viremias, bone marrow hypoplasia, or aplasia (e.g., toxemias).

Differential. Certain caged birds may exhibit rather unusual differential patterns. Many clinically healthy amazon parrots exhibit consistently high relative and absolute lymphocyte counts that are considered a normal physiological lymphocytosis. Canaries and finches also appear lymphocytic. The value of knowing the individual caged bird's normal values cannot be overemphasized.

1. *Neutrophils.* Neutrophils have been reported in birds but are extremely rare.
2. *Heterophils.* The heterophil is the one leukocyte that often shows increases with acute or chronic inflammation and with stress. This leukocyte is the equivalent of the mammalian neutrophil. Evaluation of serial absolute heterophil counts is an excellent method of monitoring a patient's progress. Convalescence is usually indicated by a drop in this value and an increase in the absolute lymphocyte count. Band heterophils are rarely observed but may be found in large numbers in cases of chlamydiosis (Rosskopf et al. 1981a) and in other conditions involving severe, acute inflammatory reactions (e.g., egg-yolk peritonitis). Metamyelocytes have also been noted in a substantial number of acute chlamydiosis cases.
3. *Lymphocytes.* Lymphocytoses may be seen with stress reactions in lymphocytic amazon parrots, canaries, and finches and in viral conditions (e.g., herpes virus hepatitis) (Rosskopf et al. 1981b) and other chronic diseases, especially in Cockatiels and African Gray Parrots (immune stimulation). Absolute lymphopenias are usually observed during the acute phase of severe inflammatory processes and following corticosteroid injections.
4. *Eosinophils.* The eosinophil is the least often seen of the granulocytes. Eosinophilias may be associated with internal parasitism (cestodes in African Gray Parrots and cockatoos, trematodes in cockatoos [Kock and Duhamel 1982], giardia in Budgerigars and Cockatiels, ascarids in amazon parrots and Australian Grass Parakeets), external parasitism

(cnemidocoptic mange in Budgerigars, finches, etc., sarcoptiform mite infestation in Gray-cheeked Parakeets), respiratory parasites (air sac mites in Lady Gouldian Finches and canaries), hemoparasites (*Plasmodium, Haemoproteus,* microfilariasis [Rosskopf et al. 1981c; Burr 1983]), and allergic conditions and conditions involving marked tissue damage, especially in Cockatiels.

5. *Monocytes.* The monocyte is the rarest of the mononuclear leukocytes. Monocytosis may be observed with chronic illness (bacterial, fungal) and is especially prominent in cases of chlamydiosis.

6. *Basophils.* Basophilias are often noted with respiratory disease and in association with the eosinophilias of respiratory parasitism (e.g., air sac mites) of canaries and finches. Any condition characterized by marked tissue damage may exhibit a basophilia.

7. *Smudge cells.* Smudge cells are often seen in avian blood smears. They are the smeared out free nuclei of damaged leukocytes (often lymphocytes). The presence of these cells is usually the result of excess pressure applied to the blood as a smear is being made. The use of a coverslip eliminates this problem.

8. *Toxic cells.* In severe disease states (often acute), toxic-appearing heterophils, lymphocytes, etc., may be noted. As in mammals, the presence of these cells is a poor prognostic sign and dictates urgency of treatment.

Thrombocytes. These cells are the equivalent of mammalian platelets. They are difficult to enumerate and are usually reported as "present" or "normal," "decreased" or "increased." Thrombocytopenias result most often from severe septicemias (disseminated intravascular coagulation may occur in all birds [Galvin 1984]) or hematopoietic neoplasia. Increased thrombocyte counts may occur in cases of acute septicemias and overwhelming parasitemias.

Hemoparasites. The frequency of blood parasites is variable among the exotic bird species commonly kept as pets (Rosskopf et al. 1981c; Burr 1983). Concurrent disease associated with immune suppression is thought to influence the magnitude of the parasitemia (Clubb 1982). Anemia and increased SGOT and LDH values in caged birds parasitized with hemoparasites may be seen. (See the section on parasitology later in this chapter for further information.)

Packed Cell Volume (PCV). The PCV (hematocrit) is a reliable subjective index of RBC numbers. Values higher than normal may reflect dehydra-

tion or polycythemia (especially with Cockatiels and some Budgerigars). An occasional high value is seen as an individual idiosyncrasy.

Low values may be associated with acute or chronic disease (chlamydiosis, septicemias, hemorrhagic problems, endocrinopathies, neoplasia, egg-yolk peritonitis, toxicities [notably heavy metal], hemoparasitism, malnutrition). Cockatoos have the lowest normal PCV range of any of the psittacine species studied. See Rosskopf et al. (1981b, 1981d, 1982b, 1982c), Fudge (1982), Rosskopf and Woerpel (1982b, 1983), Woerpel and Rosskopf (1982a,b), and Paster (1983a).

Red Blood Cell Count. The RBC count is a more involved technique than the PCV. It is not used on a routine basis, but is a useful test for calculating anemia indices (mean corpuscular volume, hemoglobin, and hemoglobin concentration). Correlation of the PCV and RBC can be confusing. In many situations a PCV value is not accompanied by a correspondingly proportionate RBC. The reason for this phenomenon is not known.

Polychromasia. This index, which refers to the appearance of erythrocytic series cells, characterizes the degree of basophilic and hemoglobin coloration in the cytoplasm. Polychromasia is reported as occasional, slight, moderate, or heavy. Most normal caged birds exhibit occasional to moderate polychromasia due to the short life span of avian RBCs (approximately half that of the dog) and the fact that they regenerate more quickly than do mammalian erythrocytes.

The clinician is provided with a reliable measure of RBC regeneration by using this index. Moderate to heavy polychromasia is often recorded in cases of regenerative anemias.

Anisocytosis. This index, which refers to erythrocyte size variation, is reported using the polychromasia subjective scale. Most normal caged birds exhibit slight anisocytosis.

Basophilic Red Blood Counts. Basophilic RBCs (reticulocytes) provide a measure of the erythrocyte regenerative capacity of the patient. This test utilizes the new methylene blue stain (1–5% is normal; 10–15% is expected with regenerative anemias).

Plasma Color and Clarity. Plasma color, which varies from species to species, is influenced by the type of food and vitamin supplements being consumed. A common error is to misinterpret the normal yellow-colored plasma or serum of certain species (notably the Cockatiel) as icteric. Truly icteric plasma is rarely encountered even when hepatopathies are known. It is most commonly seen in macaws with liver disease (e.g., chlamydiosis).

Hemoglobinemia is also rarely encountered. Plumbism (Woerpel and Rosskopf 1982a,b) or iatrogenic hemolysis secondary to improper handling of blood samples is the most common cause of hemoglobinemia in caged birds.

Lipemic plasma or serum may be seen in postprandial situations and in birds on high-fat diets or with liver disease or hypothyroidism (Rosskopf et al. 1982c; Rosskopf and Woerpel 1983). Egg-yolk peritonitis may occasionally produce yolk emboli in the blood, which may turn the plasma a thick, creamy orange color and mimic lipemia.

Table 27.3 shows the results of a survey conducted on normal plasma color for different avian species.

Total (Plasma) Protein. Hyperproteinemia (high total protein) values may be associated with dehydration, hyperglobulinemias (increased antibody production associated with chronic disease), and lipemia. Uncentrifuged, slightly hemolyzed blood results in an artifactual elevation with this test.

Hypoproteinemia (low total protein) values may be secondary to malnutrition, inanition, hepatopathies, chronic disease associated with malabsorption, chronic parasitism, and acute hemorrhage.

Cockatiels and cockatoos appear to have the lowest normal total protein values (as low as 1.1 g/dl in clinically ill birds). These values often

Table 27.3. Normal plasma color for common pet avian species (with normal blood panels)

Species	Normal Predominant Color	No.	Variables
African and Timneh Gray parrots	Clear colorless to light clear yellow	18	Clear colorless (18) Light clear yellow (11)
Amazon parrot	Clear colorless to light clear yellow	43	Clear colorless (15) Light clear yellow (28)
Australian Grass Parakeet	Clear yellow	4	Clear yellow (4)
Birds of prey	Clear colorless	5	Clear colorless (5)
Brotogeris parrots (Gray-cheek and Canary-wing)	Clear colorless to light clear yellow	14	Clear colorless (5) Light clear yellow (7) Carrot color (2)
Budgerigar	Clear yellow to amber	35	Clear yellow or amber (33) Clear colorless (2)
Canary	Clear yellow	8	Clear yellow (7) Clear colorless (1)
Cockatiel	Clear yellow to amber	47	Clear yellow to amber (45) Clear colorless (1) Carrot color (1)
Cockatoo	Clear colorless to light clear yellow	19	Clear colorless (12) Light clear yellow (7)
Crows and ravens	Clear colorless to clear yellow	3	Clear colorless (1) Clear light yellow (1) Clear yellow (1)
Conure	Clear colorless to light clear yellow	15	Clear colorless (7) Light clear yellow (8)
Dove and pigeon	Clear colorless to clear yellow	5	Clear colorless (4) Clear yellow (1)
Duck	Light clear yellow	2	Light clear yellow (2)
Finch	Clear yellow	2	Clear yellow (2)
Lory	Clear straw yellow	2	Clear straw yellow (2)
Lovebird	Clear colorless to clear straw yellow	4	Clear colorless (2) Clear straw yellow (2)
Macaw	Clear colorless to light clear yellow	27	Clear colorless (15) Light clear yellow (12)
Mynah	Clear colorless to clear straw yellow	7	Clear colorless (3) Clear light yellow (1) Clear straw yellow (2) Clear yellow (1)
Indian Ring-necked Parakeet	Clear yellow	2	Clear yellow (2)

Source: Richard Biss, veterinary student, University of Illinois; a 2-week survey completed at the Animal Medical Centre of Lawndale, 1982.

increase to normal with convalescence of the patient.

Serum Proteins and Protein Electrophoresis. Galvin (1978) reports that albumin is the largest individual protein fraction in avian serum. The lowering of plasma protein in disease states is usually due to a decrease in the albumin level rather than to the globulin fraction. He states that in some diseased avian patients, the globulin increase can offset the albumin decrease, resulting in a normal protein level. A low albumin level that fails to increase with treatment is a poor prognostic sign.

Changes in the various components of plasma proteins suggest trends in the avian patient but are not specifically diagnostic. The most common cause of increased globulins is infection. The alpha globulins include the glycoproteins, haptoglobins, ceruloplasmin, and the alpha-2 macroglobulin. Increases in the alpha globulin fraction can be seen in many situations involving tissue damage (inflammation, infection, surgery, and trauma). Alpha globulins can be lowered with liver disease, malabsorption, or malnutrition.

The major components of the beta fraction include transferin and beta lipoprotein. A beta elevation is usually due to an increase in the beta lipoprotein component.

The gamma fraction consists primarily of circulating antibodies, and increases usually reflect chronic inflammation or infection. Antibodies can migrate in the beta or gamma range in birds. The IgM migrates mostly in the beta range. Disease states may result in alterations of more than one fraction. The beta and/or gamma globulins are most often elevated with infectious diseases, and alpha is less often elevated. In some cases, gamma, beta, and alpha are all elevated.

Glucose. Hyperglycemia (values up to 450–600 mg/dl) may be noted in pet birds undergoing marked stress. Diabetes mellitus is confirmed, most commonly in Budgerigars (Spira 1981) and Cockatiels (Rosskopf and Woerpel 1982b) but is also seen in amazon parrots, Scarlet Macaws (Pitts 1984), Umbrella Cockatoos (Shackelford 1984), and toucans (Douglass 1981). The range of reported blood glucose values has been 800–1500 mg/dl. Recent research suggests several types of diabetes mellitus in caged birds, including insulin-responsive and insulin-nonresponsive (glucagon excess) types as well as others. Three cases of renal adenocarcinomas were seen in Budgerigars possessing glucose readings greater than 1200 mg/dl. None of these birds had any gross or histopathologic pancreatic lesions. Serum amylase elevations and pancreatic pathology are seldom seen with hyperglycemia. Instead, hepatic fat infiltration and fibrosis are the main findings; this may have resulted from a prolonged obesity state (Schultz and Rich 1984). High blood glucose values occur, associated with "deranged carbohydrate metabolism" secondary to renal failure (Galvin 1978). Temporary high glucose levels have also been noted in some cases of egg-yolk peritonitis. These values fall as the inflammation of the pancreas subsides.

Low blood glucose values usually result from inanition, malnourishment, hepatopathies (Dein 1982a), septicemia, and endocrinopathies (Rosskopf et al. 1981b, 1981d, 1982b). Low blood glucose values may occur following prolonged avian anesthesia (Paster 1983a). Borderline hypoglycemia is common in cockatoos. Low blood glucose values do not result in convulsions in pet avian species, as occur in mammals (dogs, seals) and in certain reptiles (alligators) (Wallach et al. 1967). An exception to this occurs in birds of prey. Hypoglycemia-induced convulsions may be seen in accipiters, especially goshawks and Cooper's Hawks. Transient hypoglycemia is seen in some egg-yolk peritonitis cases and may be the result of adrenal involvement. Hypoglycemia secondary to adrenal insufficiency is most commonly seen in cockatoos and ducks (Rosskopf et al. 1982b,c).

Low blood glucose values will rise with appropriate treatment (dexamethasone in adrenal insufficiency, antibiotics in bacterial hepatitis) of the patient. Blood samples must be centrifuged immediately following collection and the plasma separated from the packed cells to avoid artifactual hypoglycemia (rapid RBC metabolism of glucose).

Calcium. High calcium levels are occasionally reported (Rosskopf et al. 1983a) and may result from contamination of the blood with mineral particles from clipped toenails (Lapinski 1984), but attempts to reproduce the artifact have failed. Borderline high calcium levels are seen in early nutritional secondary hyperparathyroidism associated with increased parathyroid activity approximately 2 weeks prior to egg-laying in Cockatiels (Paster 1983). Excessive vitamin D_3 in the diet can result in hypercalcemia (Galvin 1978). Low calcium levels may be seen in advanced nutritional hyperparathyroidism (with early hyperparathyroidism, the serum calcium may remain normal because calcium is reabsorbed from the bone), parathyroiditis, renal failure, and idiopathic hypocalcemic syndrome of the African Gray Parrot (which may be a species-specific manifestation of inadequate calcium absorption [Rosskopf et al. 1983a]). Blood calcium levels less than 6.0 mg/dl usually result in convulsions in psittacines, and levels between 6.0 and 8.0 mg/dl may result in weakness.

Serum Glutamic Oxaloacetic Transaminase (SGOT). This enzyme, more recently named serum aspartate aminotransferase, is not liver specific in the bird and has been found in a variety of tissues (myocardium, liver, brain, lung, striated muscle) (Ivins et al. 1978). In the parrot, low levels of SGOT are found in bone and RBCs; moderate levels in spleen and lung; high levels in intestines, kidneys, and skeletal muscle; and the highest levels in heart and liver (Galvin 1978). The distribution of SGOT in different avian tissues varies from one genus to another. In ducks, for example, the highest concentration of SGOT is found in skeletal muscle, followed by heart, kidney, brain, and liver. In contrast, in the turkey the order of decreasing SGOT concentrations is heart, liver, kidney, brain, and skeletal muscle. Two- to fourfold elevations of SGOT have been reported in raptors with soft tissue injuries (Ivins et al. 1978).

High SGOT values are commonly seen with clinically ill birds, regardless of presenting symptoms. Birds tend to be septicemic and frequently suffer from multisystem disease, which results in elevation of plasma SGOT.

When elevated SGOT values occur, liver disease and septicemia should be considered in the differential diagnosis (Rosskopf and Woerpel 1982d). Infectious, stress, traumatic, toxic, metabolic, and neoplastic etiologies commonly result in SGOT elevations. Certain antibiotics, such as the tetracyclines, cefotaxime, and ticarcillin, as well as corticosteroid injections may cause increased SGOT values in certain species or in certain individuals. In psittacines, macaws exhibit the lowest normal SGOT range, Gray-cheeked Parakeets the highest.

Lactic Dehydrogenase (LDH). Elevated LDH values are not specific for any particular organ dysfunction. High LDH values may result from hemolysis, hepatopathies, trauma, neoplasia, and damage to a host of organs.

This enzyme is probably the most labile of the chemistries studied. With liver disease, the LDH rises quickly and falls relatively quickly in response to appropriate treatment while the SGOT tends to increase and decrease more slowly.

High LDH values may result from vigorously "milking" blood from a toe during blood collection or from failure to centrifuge whole blood following collection to separate the plasma portion from the packed cells, or to refriger-

ate the sample properly prior to submission to the laboratory.

Alkaline Phosphatase. This chemistry increases with hepatic and bone diseases, as in mammals (Altman 1979). It is found in high levels in skeletal muscle, spleen, intestine, kidney, and red blood cells. It may increase due to nutritional secondary hyperparathyroidism and corticosteroid usage. See Altman (1977) and Galvin (1978).

Creatinine Phosphokinase (CPK). CPK increases are reported with lead intoxication, septicemias, liver disease, cardiac disease, and abnormalities involving skeletal muscle. Concurrent elevations of SGOT and LDH are not uncommon. Intramuscular injections do not elevate CPK levels unless substantial hemorrhage or necrosis occurs. Second-degree heart block (ECG diagnosis) and a concurrent CPK rise were seen in a cockatoo, which decreased as the patient reverted to a normal rhythm. See Galvin (1978).

Creatinine. This test was once considered a good indicator of renal integrity. However, recently investigators have reported cross-reactions with other enzyme increases, which make this test unreliable (Dein 1982a).

High values have been noted in clinically normal psittacines fed diets proportionately high in animal protein (monkey chow, dog and cat kibble). High creatinine readings may also result if instruments are not cleaned after every usage. Birds of prey and psittacines on diets high in mammalian protein exhibit high creatinine values, whereas birds of prey on avian protein (e.g., baby chicks) exhibit lower values.

Creatinine levels are useful if normal values are established for the laboratory. High values may also be secondary to primary renal disease (Yanoff 1981), egg-yolk peritonitis (Rosskopf and Woerpel 1982c), septicemia (e.g., chlamydiosis), prerenal azotemia, renal trauma (Rosskopf and Woerpel 1982e), and the use of potentially nephrotoxic drugs (e.g., aminoglycosides such as gentamycin, and less severely with tobramycin, amikacin, and spectinomycin).

Blood Urea Nitrogen (BUN). This is a questionable chemistry for determining renal integrity. Increases may occur with renal disease, renal trauma, renal failure, gout, prerenal azotemia (dehydration), and in response to the use of nephrotoxic drugs. Values are low (1–6 mg/kl) for most psittacines. Low values may result from liver disease.

Uric Acid. Elevated uric acid values are most

commonly associated with renal disease (primary or secondary) and gout. Visceral gout is a common cause of secondary renal disease in avian species (Ward and Slaughter 1968; Altman 1977; Rosskopf et al. 1982b). Potential nephrotoxic drugs may also cause elevations in this chemistry. Galvin (1978) reported decreased uric acid levels during ovulation.

Small amounts of urate contamination on the toe or toenail may create uric acid increases. Consequently, the nail clipping technique for blood collection in the avian patient requires prior cleansing of the nail.

Phosphorus. Increases in phosphorus may occur with renal disease, as occurs in mammals. Advanced nutritional hyperparathyroidism may exhibit increased phosphorus and decreased calcium levels (Fowler 1978). Galvin (1978) describes many cases of renal failure in psittacines without concomitant increased phosphorus levels.

Potassium. Increased potassium levels may accompany renal disease, severe dehydration, and adrenal disease (Rosskopf et al. 1981c, 1982b; Richkind et al. 1982). Hyperkalemia resulting from adrenal insufficiency is most commonly seen in cockatoos and the African Gray Parrot. Hyperkalemia is a frequently encountered artifact of blood chemistry analysis in uncentrifuged blood. It may also be seen from diuretic therapy (rarely utilized in avian medicine).

Sodium. Hyponatremia is seen with adrenal insufficiency (Rosskopf et al. 1981b,d, 1982b) and can be anticipated with renal disease and prolonged diarrhea. Artifactual hyponatremia results from failure to centrifuge whole blood samples and separate plasma from packed cells immediately after blood collection.

Hypernatremia may result when a caged bird is allowed to consume unlimited quantities of salt (salted nuts, crackers) and is not allowed free access to water.

Thyroxine (T₄). Determinations of thyroxine levels are useful in the diagnosis of thyroid-related problems (Rosskopf et al. 1982c, 1983a, 1983b; Rosskopf and Woerpel 1983). Normal values vary widely from species to species and may vary seasonally (with sexual cycles). The TSH response test is the most accurate method of measuring thyroid function, since resting thyroid levels may vary and be influenced by other factors. One IU of TSH is given intramuscularly and a baseline thyroxine level taken. Another value is taken 4–6 hours later. A thyroxine in-

crease of twofold or more is considered normal. This test cannot measure TSH deficiency or disease characterized by inability to utilize thyroxine (Zenoble and Kemppainen 1984).

Decreased T_4 values may be seen with hypothyroidism, thyroiditis, iodine deficiency, and tyrosine deficiency. Hypothyroidism is a surprisingly common condition among caged birds. See Richkind (1982), Richkind et al. (1982), Rosskopf (1982c), and Rosskopf and Woerpel (1983a).

Cockatoos possess the highest normal thyroxine readings of the psittacines.

Corticosterone. This hormone has been found to be the main adrenal hormone of avian species. An ACTH stimulation test has been reported using 16–25 IU ACTH and then collecting baseline corticosterone samples and stimulated corticosterone samples 1–2 hours later. Normal increases of 4 to 13 times resting levels occur (Zenoble and Kemppainen 1984).

Cholesterol. This chemistry is often elevated in cases of avian hypothyroidism (lipemic plasma is common). Some nonhypothyroid birds fed high-fat diets (e.g., excess quantities of sunflower seeds or oats) may have high plasma cholesterol levels and fatty livers. Liver disease can result in low plasma cholesterol levels.

Microbiology

Bacteriology. Of the diagnostic modalities available, bacteriology is one of the most important in avian medicine. All experts agreed that gram-positive bacteria (cocci, bacilli) predominate in the psittacine gastrointestinal and respiratory systems. The same is also true of the skin and feather follicle flora. Gram-negative bacteria are considered abnormal in caged birds and, when isolated, are considered to be potentially pathogenic. Gram-negative bacteria are most often the cause of bird diseases. This fact, coupled with the septicemic nature of birds, makes the techniques of Gram staining and culturing with antibiotic sensitivity testing extremely useful in avian diagnostic medicine. See Dolphin and Olsen (1977), Bowman and Jacobsen (1980), Olsen and Dolphin (1980), Fudge (1981), McDonald and Watts (1981), and Rosskopf et al. (1983b).

Samples are collected by first moistening the culture swab in its transport medium to reduce friction with the mucosal surface and then rolling the swab on a sterile microscope slide before placing it into the culture medium. Collection sites include the choanal slit, pharynx, and cloaca, as well as fresh feces, abdominal fluid, nasal-ocular discharges, abscesses (pus), crop contents, feather pulp (blood feathers), and necropsy specimens. Fecal Gram stains work well if the feces are fresh but may yield fewer organisms than cloacal collections.

Gram-positive bacterial isolates are first classified according to their Gram stain reaction and then separated according to their morphology (cocci, bacilli, yeast). Gram-negative bacteria are primarily separated by their ability or inability to ferment glucose. Gram stains, cultures, and antibiotic sensitivity testing should be included as diagnostic aids in the therapy of clinically ill birds.

Certain gram-positive bacterial agents are predominant in caged birds. *Staphylococcus aureus* seems to be an infrequent isolate from most psittacines; amazon parrots that are infected, however, may exhibit clinical symptoms. *Bacillus* spp., normal in the gut of most psittacines, can occasionally be a pathogen in African Gray Parrots. Certain *Staphyloccus* spp. and *Streptococcus* spp. may create clinical illnesses in psittacines under certain circumstances (especially in Budgerigars and Cockatiels).

Gram-negative bacteria are most often classified as bacilli or coccobacilli (very tiny rods that resemble cocci). If a direct Gram stain reveals gram-negative coccobacilli, they most often turn out to be *Pasteurella* spp. (often pleomorphic), *Acinetobacter* spp. (mostly diplococcal, sometimes bacillary), or *Actinobacillus* spp. (cocci to coccobacilli).

The presence of gram-negative bacteria on a direct Gram stain (depending on the source) may also represent anaerobic bacteria. Gram-negative anaerobes will not grow under usual aerobic conditions. However, many aerobic bacteria are facultative anaerobes.

Fungal and Yeast Problems. Respiratory disease that has been refractory to antibiotic therapy and exhibits a high white count with heterophilia (occasionally monocytosis) is typical of a fungal infection. Certain species of birds seem to be more susceptible to fungal disease (African Gray Parrots, birds of prey, penguins). Besides the WBC count, other diagnostic aids for fungal infections (e.g., aspergillosis) include radiography, serology (unreliable), laparoscopy, tracheal cytology, and culture. A small number of systemic fungal infections caused by other agents, most notably *Mucor* spp., are recorded.

Yeasts encountered in avian practice include *Candida albicans* (causing candidiasis or moniliasis) and *Cryptococcus neoformans* (causing cryptococcosis).

Most fungal infections grow rapidly (within 2–4 days) at room temperature or above (up to 45°C) on Sabouraud's dextrose agar or blood agar. The diagnosis of *Candida albicans* is made by Gram staining wet mounts from the lesions and feces, or by culturing the same. Colonies of *Cryptococcus neoformans* usually appear within several days when grown at 37°C on Sabouraud's dextrose agar or blood agar. The diagnosis of cryptococcosis is most often made at the time of necropsy. Indian ink preparations (impression smears) of infected tissues or the gelatinous material in the areas of lesions may yield encapsulated yeast forms. Furthermore, periodic acid–Schiff stains may reveal organisms within the tissues.

Further information on taking fungal samples and disease descriptions can be found in Chapter 16.

***Mycoplasma* spp.** Mycoplasmal infections and problems have been studied for years in poultry (Hofstad 1978). Mycoplasmal infections have been described in Budgerigars and Cockatiels and sporadic reports occur in other psittacines (Gaskin and Jacobsen 1979). Microaerophilic techniques have been developed to allow routine culture of specific *Mycoplasma* spp. in caged birds. Serological titers cannot be routinely used until pathogens can be differentiated from commensals. Intracytoplasmic inclusion bodies, characteristic of mycoplasmal infections, are frequently found in Giemsa-stained impression smears of infected organs (Fudge 1981). Rhinitis and air sacculitis typical of mycoplasmal infections can mimic the symptoms of bacterial and chlamydial infections (Hitchner 1980).

***Campylobacter* spp.** New techniques have been developed to grow campylobacter organisms. This disease has been found to be much more prevalent in avian species than previously thought.

Cytology

Impression Smears. Impression smears of tissues from live birds can be stained and examined cytologically for evidence of neoplasia or infection. At necropsy, impression smears should be made from the pericardial sac, liver, spleen, and air sac. Many laboratories provide this service for avian practitioners. Antemortem diagnosis of psittacosis can be enhanced by examination of Machiavello-stained nasal exudates for elementary bodies, although the technique is not widely used. The Giemsa stain is also frequently used in the diagnosis of mycoplasmosis.

Other Uses of Cytology. Tracheal washes, fluid collected via abdominocentesis, fluid aspirated from cysts, etc., may be examined cytologically. The physical aspects of the sample (specific gravity, quantity of protein, glucose) are routinely analyzed in avian practice.

Fluid collected from the swollen abdomen of a geriatric bird examined in this manner often aids in the diagnosis of neoplasia, hemorrhage, liver failure, congestive heart failure, or infection (peritonitis).

Urinalysis.
Urinalysis is a useful but infrequently used diagnostic tool. Collection of the specimen is usually not a problem with avian patients. The bird must be at least slightly polyuric to obtain a suitable sample (polyuria is most commonly encountered in a bird presented with "loose droppings"). When conditions require urinalysis, a sample is taken via aspiration by syringe off waxed paper, aluminum foil, or a metal surface. If urinalysis is desired in a nonpolyuric bird, the patient may be given water by crop tube, which results in a transient polyuria 5–30 minutes postadministration.

Normal Values. Use of dipsticks designed for mammals (humans, dogs, cats) works well with avian patients. The sediment analysis is executed in the usual manner. Studies of the results of urinalyses from sources of clinically abnormal and normal birds led to the following generalizations.

Color. Urine color varies with the specific gravity, the concurrent ingestion of water-soluble vitamin products (e.g., B-complex produces yellow urine), the normal color of the bird's plasma, the amount of uric acid and feces mixed with the urine/urates, and the concurrent existence of certain diseases (e.g., plumbism may produce hemoglobinuria, resulting in mahogany-colored urine and urates, mainly in amazon parrots; psittacosis frequently results in chartreuse-colored urine/urates, thought to be the result of increased excretion of biliverdin). Normal colors range from clear to various shades of yellow, straw, orange, light green, and greenish white. Nonpolyuric birds produce only a very small quantity of urine and a variable quantity of uric acid (urates) admixed with the feces. In healthy birds, the urates should be pure white, pale yellow, or light shades of beige. Liver disease consistently produces urates that are yellow or mustard color.

Appearance. Bird urine is usually described as opaque, cloudy, or flocculent in appearance.

Specific Gravity. The specific gravity, as in mammals, varies with the state of hydration of the individual and with certain disease states. The nonpolyuric bird excretes a semisolid uric acid waste product with a nonreadable specific gravity. In polyuric birds, values vary from 1.002 to 1.033. Most values fall within the 1.005–1.020 range.

pH. The pH of pet bird urine falls in the 6.0–8.0 range. A caged bird with a pH value as low as 5.0 would be considered acidotic (Galvin 1978).

Protein. Protein values vary from 0 to 3 +; 90% of normal bird urine yields a trace protein reading. Nephropathies can be expected to produce significant proteinuria.

Glucose. Glucose readings are usually negative or zero, but many trace glucose readings are encountered in normal avian urine. The renal threshold for glucosuria varies with the species (e.g., the urine from many cockatoos and amazon parrots yields trace readings with blood glucose levels as low as 270 mg/dl, while the urine from many of the Red-tailed Hawks and Cockatiels yields trace readings with simultaneous blood glucose values of 350 mg/dl and higher). Once the renal threshold is reached, increases in urine glucose are rapid. The urine from most birds will yield maximum glucose values when their blood glucose levels exceed 600 mg/dl. Birds suffering from diabetes mellitus routinely possess blood glucose values above 800 mg/dl. However, a persistent glucosuria without elevation of blood sugar levels could indicate renal tubular disease. In mild cases, blood uric acid levels stay within normal limits. Normal range in granivorous birds is 2–10 mg/ml. Care should be exercised when interpreting postprandial uric acid levels in carnivorous and fish-eating birds; values up to 60 mg/ml have been recorded (Schultz and Rich 1984). Periodic subjective measurements of the reduction in the degree of polyuria during the initial treatment of diabetic patients can be useful.

Ketones. Ketonuria is occasionally noted in severely diabetic or ketoacidotic patients. Galvin (1978) reported ketoacidosis in the avian patient resulting from catabolic processes such as severe hepatitis (liver disease, low blood glucose, mobilization of fat for energy, ketoacidosis) or diabetes mellitus.

Blood. Values from +1 to +3 have been associated with either frank hematuria or hemorrhage from the intestines, reproductive tract, or cloaca. A positive reading for blood on a uric dipstick does not automatically indicate hematuria.

Bilirubin. Bilirubin readings are usually zero, although occasionally birds with severe liver disease and yellow urates exhibit strong "bilirubinuria." Biliverdin has been reported as the major bile pigment of birds that does not react with the bilirubin portion of the uric dipstick (Galvin 1978). Occasionally patients with frank hematuria have 1+ bilirubin readings.

Urobilinogen. Urobilinogen readings are usually 0–0.1 in normal birds.

White Blood Cells/Red Blood Cells. WBCs and RBCs in small numbers (zero to three per high power field) are not uncommon in avian urine; four to six (or more) WBCs or RBCs per high power field should be viewed with concern, especially if the patient is exhibiting signs of disease. Any cells noted within the urine sediment may have origins within the urinary, reproductive, or gastrointestinal tracts or from within the cloaca itself.

Casts. Casts are commonly seen in avian kidney disease. They may contain white or red cells, be waxy or hyaline in nature, or consist of the epithelial lining that has sloughed following kidney damage. The presence of casts is a valuable tool in diagnosing subclinical kidney disease. All polyuric birds should be checked for casts. Casts may be present while blood chemistry readings are normal.

Epithelial Cells. Epithelial cells are an infrequent finding in the urinary sediment of caged birds. Any epithelial cells in the urinary sediment should be viewed with suspicion by the clinician.

Crystals. Most normal avian urine samples contain many amorphous urates. Sulfonamide, tyrosine, and other crystals may be seen.

Bacteria. Bacteria (gram-positive rods and cocci) are commonly seen in the urinary sediment if fecal contamination of the sample has occurred (as is common). Reports of bacteria too numerous to count (TNTC) or numerous cocci and rods in reasonably clean urine samples should be viewed with suspicion.

Parasitology. Caged bird parasites and their treatment are discussed in Chapters 20, 21, and 22. Isolation techniques are carried out using the following methods.

External Parasites. Visual inspection (with or without magnification) and the examination of skin scrapings are the two most common methods used for diagnosing ectoparasites of caged birds.

Visual inspection of the ventral surfaces of the primary and secondary feathers may reveal lice and/or their nits, ticks, mites, and other insects. Magnification is usually required to visualize the tiny feather mites (*Dermanyssus gallinae* and *Ornithonyssus sylviarum*). Lesions of cnemidocoptic mange (most often affecting the nonfeathered portions of the bird: cere, face, eyelids, legs and feet, vent, and rarely the wing tips) are pathognomonic. Mite infestation is easily confirmed by examining a skin scraping of the lesions.

Internal Parasites

Blood Films. Examination of blood films may reveal the presence of hemoparasites (microfilaria, *Haemoproteus* spp., *Plasmodium* spp., trypanosomes) or may suggest the presence of other internal parasites. Air sac mites of Lady Gouldian Finches and canaries often cause chronic respiratory disease that is unresponsive to antibiotics. Differentials on these birds may reveal eosinophilia and/or basophilia. The definite diagnosis is made at necropsy (gross visualization of the mites) or by histopathology (presence of mites within the tissues). Blood films are made thin, rapidly air-dried, fixed in 100% methanol or ethanol, and stained in a Romanowsky-based stain. Best and most permanent results are obtained following the protocols of Bennett (1970) using a commercial grade of Giemsa stain mixed with buffered (pH = 7.2) water at a ratio of 1:9; the smears should be stained for 30–35 minutes. Although a variety of fast stains are commercially available, these stains tend to fade rapidly and the smear cannot be used as a permanent record. Examinations of smears should be carried out using the × 100 objective and × 10 oculars, under oil immersion.

Fecal Flotations. Standard fecal flotations and direct smears are useful in caged bird medicine. Ova from nematodes (*Ascaridia* spp., *Capillaria* spp.), trematodes (causing a rarely diagnosed hepatic disease of certain cockatoos [Kock and Duhamel 1985]), and acanthocephalans (gizzard worms in macaws) may be identified.

Cestode ova are rarely seen on fecal flotations. Tapeworm infections are usually confirmed by identification of proglottida, either in the droppings or hanging from the vent of an infected bird. Cockatoos and African Gray Parrots are the psittacines most often infected with these parasites. A significant rise in eosinophils in these species may indicate a tapeworm infection. Treatment with Droncit often causes passage of tapeworm and a normal eosinophil count. Finches are also commonly plagued with tapeworms.

Internal protozoa are common in psittacines, especially *Giardia* spp. in young Budgerigars and Cockatiels. These parasites are best seen in saline wet mounts under low light. Repeat wet mounts may be necessary to establish a diagnosis. Occasionally, coccidial oocysts, schistosomes, cryptosporidia, histomonas, and hexamita are found on wet mounts of fecal flotations. Polyvinyl alcohol may be used to preserve feces for later protozoal examination using a trichrome staining technique.

Trichomoniasis is a fairly common disease in many species. A diagnosis is made by examining saline wet mounts containing material from lesions within the oral cavity, pharynx, or crop.

Direct observation (antemortem or postmortem) can also reveal the presence of internal parasites. Lesions (sarcocysts) of *Sarcocystis* spp. or *Leucocytozoon* spp. may be noted within skeletal muscle and even be visible through the skin of a living bird. Adult filarid nematodes may be noted within air sacs or fascial planes during necropsy (especially in cockatoos). These parasites are occasionally found when a cyst or mass with an external location is lanced (Paster 1983b). Direct observation of the avian patient may also reveal lesions containing larvae or maggots of several insect species.

Necropsy. The postmortem examination can be extremely useful in confirming the diagnosis suspected antemortem or upon death. Gross and histopathologic findings combined with clinical and laboratory tests make necropsy an excellent diagnostic tool.

Clients should be encouraged to submit specimens for necropsy as soon after death as possible. The body should be immersed in icy water for about 30 minutes to facilitate heat loss and delay autolysis (especially important with small caged birds). If any delay in presenting the specimen is anticipated, it should be refrigerated immediately but *not* frozen (freezing produces significant cytologic artifacts and interferes with histopathologic interpretation of the submitted tissues).

The clinician should take great care in submission of specimens. Ten percent neutral buffered formalin is used for tissue specimens destined for histopathology. Very tiny organs (thyroids/parathyroids, adrenals, pituitary gland, ultimobranchial bodies) should be submitted in individual containers so that they will not be lost during processing.

Diagnostic Tests Available

Chlamydial Isolation. Currently, chlamydial isolation is offered by many laboratories. Isolation is carried out in chick embryos (which requires a minimum of 10–14 days) or in cell culture (which requires a minimum of 48 hours postinoculation). Specimens used for these isolation techniques include cloacal swabs, feces, or tissue samples.

Chlamydial isolation carried out in chick embryos is disappointing. The time required to receive results is unacceptable when this test is being used to diagnose psittacosis and dictate therapy. Furthermore, shedding of chlamydiae may be intermittent, especially in apparently healthy birds. A suspect bird should receive a cloacal swab daily for 5–7 days. The swab is introduced into the transport medium immediately after being removed from the patient and is mixed with the medium. The transport medium is refrigerated between sample collections. This test, although no more than 40% reliable, is the only one presently available to detect the asymptomatic shedder.

Chlamydial isolation in cell culture is the diagnostic test of choice. The greatest advantage of this method is the reduced amount of time required to receive results. Intermittent shedding and false negative results are the disadvantages.

Once the patient begins to receive treatment (tetracyclines, chloramphenicol), the chances of receiving a positive result from chlamydial isolation are greatly diminished.

Serology

Chlamydia. Results can be obtained within 5–7 days using the direct complement fixation test. The titer results are evaluated along with data from the history, physical exam, and clinical pathology. The results are interpreted as follows: $<1:8$ = negative, $1:8$–$1:16$ = equivocal or suspicious, $>1:16$ = positive. When possible, more than one sample should be tested to detect a rising titer, signifying active disease. Titers usually remain elevated for an extended period (42–83 days) after treatment. Recent research has shown that some avian species do not develop high antibody titers, notably the Budgerigar and Cockatiel. Also doxycycline therapy may shorten the time necessary to develop an immune response and therefore interfere with antibody levels. Grimes (1984) has shown that clinical signs and hematology plus a fourfold or more increase in the titer over a 25- to 40-day period may be the only way to confirm the disease in a live bird.

Aspergillosis. An aspergillosis precipitin test is available, called the Fungal Immunodiffusion Kit. This test detects precipitating antibodies in the patient's serum. Unfortunately, it is unreliable in avian species, and false negatives are extremely common.

Pacheco's Disease. Tests are currently under study for the identification of Pacheco's herpesvirus carriers.

Glucose Tolerance Test. If the blood sugar is elevated, a glucose tolerance test is performed (Schultz and Rich 1984). The subject is fasted for 2–4 hours and a blood sample is taken to determine fasting glucose level. An oral dose of a 40% w/v D-glucose solution is then administered at the rate of 2 g glucose/kg body weight. Blood samples are taken 0.175 hours and 1.5 hours after administration, and glucose determination is made on the plasma.

The three glucose values derived from the test are converted into factors of the fasting level by dividing each value by the fasting level (this procedure yields a factor of 1 for the fasting level). These factors are then compared for any radical departure from normal. Absolute glucose values are used due to the variance in fasting glucose levels and hence the test levels. The truly diabetic bird is unable to alter its blood sugar on administration of glucose and will fail the glucose tolerance test. This test may be useful in questionable cases with glucose readings of 600–800. If stress glucose readings are suspected, repeating the test at a later time should differentiate them.

Galactose Tolerance Test. The galactose tolerance test is used as a measure of the liver's ability to convert galactose to glucose via the galactokinase-transferase pathway (Schultz and Rich 1984). The principle of the test is to administer an oral dose of a 40% w/v D-galactose solution, at the rate of 2 g galactose/kg body weight, to a 2-hour fasted subject.

Blood samples are withdrawn at 0.5-hour intervals up to 2 hours from the time of administration. No initial sample is required, as the circulating level of galactose is insignificant. Galactose determination on the plasma of those samples will yield the peak time and magnitude for the subject (0.5–1 hour and 14–19 mmol/l respectively, depending on body weight). The elimination rate is calculated by the regression analysis of log galactose versus time, using the peak value as zero time. The half-time of galactose in the subject's plasma can then be determined. Elevated values are a distinct measure of liver malfunction. Samples drawn at 1- and 2-

hour intervals may be more practical for the avian practitioner. The calculations remain the same; however, the peak time and magnitude values, which are useful in assessing gastrointestinal tract status, may be obscured.

A third version is to sample only at 2 hours and compare the galactose value to the expected values. This third procedure may lead to false negatives when malabsorption of galactose induces low peak values.

Anaerobic Microbiology. Very little is known about the role that anaerobic microbes play as possible constituents of the normal flora or as pathogens in avian species. Very few laboratories are equipped to handle anaerobic microbiology and do not receive pressure to research this area.

Virology. Virus isolation is costly and requires special methods but is being carried out in many academic institutions and veterinary laboratories. Furthermore, electron microscopy is revealing a myriad of new disease entities. The role of viruses in pet bird disease is, undoubtedly, extremely significant. Viral agents such as those of Newcastle disease and herpesvirus are of tremendous economic importance to both poultry and pet bird industries. Virus isolation procedures for these diseases are routinely performed by diagnostic laboratories because of the constant threat they pose to the poultry industry.

A number of viruses are currently being studied, including the avian poxviruses, beak and feather disease of cockatoos, herpesviruses, patchy skin disease of cockatoos and macaws, paramyxoviruses (Seune 1983), avian influenza viruses (Seune 1983), adenovirus of lovebirds, and papovavirus of Budgerigars (Bernier et al. 1981). There is little doubt that viruses play a significant role in the pathogenesis of disease in the avian patient, but a tremendous amount of research (virus isolation, electron microscopy) remains to be done. A viral etiology may one day be discovered for the macaw wasting syndrome (Gallerstein and Ridgway 1983; Woerpel and Rosskopf 1983) and the hemorrhagic conure syndrome (involving erythemic myelosis and related conditions).

References

Altman, R. B. 1977. Diseases of the avian urinary system. In *Current Veterinary Therapy VI,* ed. R. Kirk, pp. 703–5. Philadelphia: W. B. Saunders.
―――. 1979. Avian clinical pathology, radiology, para-

sitic and infectious diseases. In *Proceedings of the 46th Annual Meeting of the American Animal Hospital Association*, pp. 15–27.

Bennett, G. F. 1970. Simple techniques for making avian blood smears. *Can. J. Zool.* 39:17–23.

Bernier, G., M. Morin, and G. Marsolais. 1981. A generalized inclusion body disease in the Budgerigar (*Melopsittacus undulatus*) caused by a papovavirus-like agent. *Avian Dis.* 25(4):1083–92.

Bowman, J. A., and E. R. Jacobsen. 1980. Cloacal flora of clinically normal captive psittacine birds. *J. Zoo Anim. Med.* 11:81–85.

Burr, E. W. 1983. Parasites of psittacine blood. *Mod. Vet. Pract.* 64(4):333–36.

Clubb, S. 1982. Parasitic diseases of pet avian species. In *Proceedings of the 1982 Annual Meeting of the Association of Avian Veterinarians*, pp. 102–7.

Dein, F. J. 1982a. IME 278. *Assoc. Avian Vet. Newsl.* 3(4):86.

_____. 1982b. Avian clinical hematology. In *Proceedings of the 1982 Annual Meeting of the Association of Avian Veterinarians*, pp. 5–29.

Dolensek, E. P., and V. Otis. 1973. Clinical pathology in avian species. *Vet. Clin. N. Am.* 3(2):159.

Dolphin, R. E., and D. E. Olsen. 1977. Fecal monitoring of caged birds. *Vet. Med. Small Anim. Clin.* 72:1081–85.

Douglass, E. M. 1981. Diabetes mellitus in a toucan. *Mod. Vet. Pract.* 62(4):293–95.

Fudge, A. 1981. Antimicrobial therapy in avian medicine. *Calif. Vet.* 35(10):25–29.

_____. 1982. Clinical findings in an amazon parrot with suspected lead toxicosis. *Calif. Vet.* 36(5):23–25.

Gallerstein, G. A., and R. A. Ridgway. 1983. Proventricular dilatation syndrome. *Proceedings of the 1983 Annual Meeting of the Association of Avian Veterinarians*, pp. 228–33.

Galvin, C. 1978. *Laboratory Diagnostic Aids in Pet Bird Practice.* Wildlife Rehabilitation Council, Walnut Creek, Calif.

_____. 1984. Personal communication (Veterinary Hospital of Ignacio, Calif.).

Gaskin, J. M., and E. R. Jacobsen. 1979. A mycoplasma-associated epornitic in Severe Macaws. *Annual Proceedings of the American Association of Zoo Veterinarians*, pp. 56–59.

Grimes, J. E. 1984. Serological and microbiological detection of *Chlamydia psittaci* infections in psittacine birds. *Avian/Exot. Pract.* 1(4):6–12.

Hawkey, C. M., M. G. Hart, J. A. Knight, J. H. Samour, and D. M. Jones. 1982. Haematologic findings in healthy and sick African Grey Parrots. *Vet. Rec.* 18(25):280–82.

Hitchner, S. B. 1980. *Isolation and Identification of Avian Pathogens.* American Association of Avian Pathologists Handbook.

Hofstad, M. S., ed. 1978. *Diseases of Poultry.* Ames: Iowa State University Press.

Ivins, G. K., G. D. Weddle, and W. H. Halliwell. 1978. Hematology and serum chemistries in birds of prey. In *Zoo and Wild Animal Medicine,* ed. M. E. Fowler, pp. 286–90. Philadelphia: W. B. Saunders.

Kock, M. D., and G. E. Duhamel. 1982. Hepatic distomiasis in a Sulphur-crested Cockatoo. *J. Am. Vet. Med. Assoc.* 181(11):1388–92.

Lapinski, A. 1984. Personal communication.

McDonald, S. E., and G. Watts. 1981. Aerobic bacterial flora in the choana of clinically normal captive psittacine birds. In *Annual Proceedings of the American Association of Zoo Veterinarians,* pp. 38–42.

Olsen, D. E., and R. E. Dolphin. 1980. Update of fecal culture techniques for companion birds. *Calif. Vet.* 34(11):27–28.

Paster, M. B. 1983a. Common avian diagnostic laboratory tests. *Bird World* 6(1):22–49.

_____. 1983b. Filarial worms in the foot of a Nanday Conure. *Bird World* 6(2):18–22.

Pitts, C. 1984. Personal communication.

Raphael, B. L. 1981. Hematology and blood chemistries of macaws. In *Annual Proceedings of the American Association of Zoo Veterinarians,* pp. 97–98.

Richkind, M. 1982. Hormonal influences on normal and abnormal feathering and moult. *Bird World* 5:42–47, 56.

Richkind, M., A. P. Gendron, E. M. Howard, W. J. Rosskopf, Jr., and R. W. Woerpel. 1982. Pseudomonas septicemia associated with auto-immune endocrinopathy in a Red-vented Cockatoo. *Vet. Med. Small Anim. Clin.* 77(1):1548–54.

Rosskopf, W. J., Jr., and R. W. Woerpel. 1982a. The use of hematologic testing procedures in caged bird medicine: An introduction. *Calif. Vet.* 36(3):19–22.

_____. 1982b. Pancreatic adenocarcinoma in a mynah bird. *Mod. Vet. Pract.* 63(7):573–74.

_____. 1982c. Egg-yolk peritonitis in a Cockatiel. *Mod. Vet. Pract.* 63(5):420.

_____. 1982d. Liver disease in a parrot. *Mod. Vet. Pract.* 63(10):824.

_____. 1982e. Egg-binding in an Amboina King Parrot. *Vet. Med. Small Anim. Clin.* 77(2):231–32.

_____. 1983. Lipomatous growth responsive to L-thyroxine therapy in a Budgerigar. *Vet. Med. Small Anim. Clin.* 78(10):1415–18.

Rosskopf, W. J., Jr., R. W. Woerpel, H. J. Holshuh, E. M. Howard, and G. Matsumoto. 1981a. Psittacosis in a parakeet. *Mod. Vet. Pract.* 62(6):540–42.

Rosskopf, W. J., Jr., R. W. Woerpel, H. J. Holshuh, and E. M. Howard. 1981b. Chronic endocrine disorder associated with inclusion body hepatitis in a Lesser Sulphur-crested Cockatoo. *J. Am. Vet. Med. Assoc.* 179(11):1273–76.

Rosskopf, W. J., Jr., R. W. Woerpel, and G. Rosskopf. 1981c. Blood parasite in caged birds. *Vet. Med. Small Anim. Clin.* 12(76):1763–65.

Rosskopf, W. J., Jr., R. W. Woerpel, M. Richkind, and E. M. Howard. 1981d. Adrenal insufficiency in psittacine birds: Pathogenesis, diagnosis, and management. *Proc. 30th W. Poult. Dist. Conf. 15th Poult. Health Symp.,* pp. 76–79.

Rosskopf, W. J., Jr., R. W. Woerpel, G. Rosskopf, and D. Van De Water. 1982a. Hematologic and blood chemistry values for common pet avian species. *Vet. Med. Small Anim. Clin.* 77(8):1233–39.

Rosskopf, W. J., Jr., R. W. Woerpel, M. Richkind, and E. M. Howard. 1982b. Pathogenesis, diagnosis and treatment of adrenal insufficiency in psittacine birds. *Calif. Vet.* 36(5):26–30.

Rosskopf, W. J., Jr., R. W. Woerpel, and G. Rosskopf. 1982c. Normal thyroid values for common pet birds. *Vet. Med. Small Anim. Clin.* 77(3):409–12.

Rosskopf, W. J., Jr., R. W. Woerpel, and M. Monahan-Brennan. 1983a. Seizures induced by hypo-calcemia in an African Gray Parrot associated with an adrenalopathy and parathyroid hyperplasia. In

Proceedings of the 1983 Annual Meeting of the Association of Avian Veterinarians, pp. 267–71.

Rosskopf, W. J., Jr., R. W. Woerpel, M. L. Sievers, and C. Pater. 1983b. Bacterial feather folliculitis in a lovebird. *Mod. Vet. Pract.* 64(1):45.

Schalm, O. W., et al. 1975. *Veterinary Hematology.* 3d ed. Philadelphia: Lea and Febiger.

Schultz, D. J., and B. G. Rich. 1984. Unpublished data.

Seune, D. A. 1983. IME 312. National Veterinary Services Laboratory data. *Assoc. Avian Vet. Newsl.* 4(1).

Shackelford, R. 1984. Personal communication.

Spira, A. 1981. Clinical aspects of diabetes mellitus in Budgerigars. In *Scientific Proceedings of the 48th Annual Meeting of the American Animal Hospital Association.*

Wallach, J. D., C. Hoessle, and J. Bennett. 1967. Hypoglycemic shock in captive alligators. *J. Am. Vet. Med. Assoc.* 151:893.

Ward, F. P., and L. J. Slaughter. 1968. Visceral gout in a captive Cooper's Hawk. *Bull. Wildl. Dis. Assoc.* 4:91.

Woerpel, R. W., and W. J. Rosskopf, Jr. 1982a. Heavy metal intoxication in caged birds. Part I. *Compend. Contin. Educ. Pract. Vet.* 9:729–38.

———. 1982b. Heavy metal intoxication in caged birds. Part II. *Compend. Contin. Educ. Pract. Vet.* 10:801–6.

———. 1983. IME 323. New macaw syndrome? *Assoc. Avian Vet. Newsl.* 4(1):22.

Yanoff, S. R. 1981. Renal disease in a lovebird. *Assoc. Avian Vet. Newsl.* 2(2).

Zenoble, R. D., and R. J. Kemppainen. 1984. The influence of ACTH on plasma corticosterone and cortisol and influence of TSH on plasma T_4 and T_3. In *International Conference on Avian Medicine, Toronto, Annual Proceedings of the Association of Avian Veterinarians,* pp. 103–11.

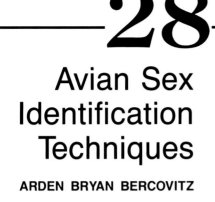

28

Avian Sex Identification Techniques

ARDEN BRYAN BERCOVITZ

AVIAN SEX identification techniques have become a necessary component of health care services for captive birds as interest has increased in providing a safe and reliable means of sex identification for companion species lacking any discernible phenotypic secondary sexual characteristics. Males and females of monomorphic species can be similar in size, weight, coloration, and sexual behaviors. Accurate sexing/pairing of birds is essential for successful captive breeding.

Published documentation of sexual differences for all extant avian species remains incomplete. Archivists at the Smithsonian Institution, Washington, D.C., have estimated that 20–30% of 9,019 total avian species are not sexually distinct as adults (this approximation would exceed 50% if immature birds were also considered).

How practical, safe, and reliable are current methods? What equipment or training is required to perform these tests? What are the comparative risks and benefits? Genetic sexing (cytogenetics), excretory sex steroid analysis, and other noninvasive endocrine sexing methods are explained in this chapter (a discussion of surgical sexing methods can be found in Chapter 25). Only an abbreviated procedure is described for each sexing method; specific details can be found in the cited references.

Variables Used in Sex Identification.

There is no single best way of sexing monomorphic species, except by verification through successful reproduction. Categorically speaking, genetic, behavioral, and physiologic sex constitute independent test variables as well as complementary reproductive factors. Accur-

ate sex identification will not guarantee captive reproduction; however, it is an absolute prerequisite.

Anatomical Aspects. Sexual distinction of cloacal anatomy (the visual or palpable presence of a rudimentary male copulatory organ) continues to be commercially reliable as a sexing method in domesticated fowl, other galliforms, waterfowl, and ratites (Bercovitz et al. 1983). The vast majority of bird species, however, are monomorphic; neither chicks nor adults possess cloacal structural distinctions. To human eyes, avian sexual differences range from the obvious to the obscure.

In many species, there is much to learn about measurable sexually dimorphic changes in body size, structural proportion, vocalization, ritualistic behavior, and/or coloration of eyes, skin, or feathering. Despite striking examples of sexual dimorphism in Grand Eclectus Parrots (Plate 10), other psittacines can be devoid of external secondary sexual characteristics, such as the Grand Cayman Island Parrots.

Behavioral Aspects. Sexually distinct reproductive behavior during courtship, breeding, nesting, and rearing can be reliably used to sex participating adults. However, a study of captive bird breeding in the United States indicated that more than one-third of all species surveyed were not breeding and two-thirds were not breeding enough to maintain a self-sustaining captive population (Muller 1983). Sex identification based solely on isolated reproductive behaviors can be confounded by numerous factors: (1) imposition of captive conditions that disrupt or prevent completion of sequential sexual behaviors, (2) shared behaviors that complicate recognition of sexual distinction, and (3) abnormal behaviors induced by suboptimal environmental, nutritional, social, and/or microclimatic conditions.

Genetic Sexing Methods

Historical and General Procedures. Many highly mitotic tissue types have been utilized for avian cytogenetics: feather pulp, blood leukocytes, bone marrow, and fibroblast cultures. Somatic cells, however, particularly dermal and fibroblast cells, have been of only theoretical value to avian cytogenetics because of their poor culture growth with current in vitro techniques (Biederman 1983). All cells contain the full genetic complement, even nonmitotic erythrocytes.

Historically, several major problems have affected avian cytogenetics. Incomplete or unevenly stained chromosomal preparations were commonplace. Microchromosomes, barely differentiated under light microscopy, were too numerous to evaluate. Variable results were produced by different laboratories using similar techniques (Toone 1981). Misidentification resulted from artifactual and natural rearrangements in autosome and sex chromosome morphology (Bloom 1974).

The diploid (2N) chromosome number in birds is species specific and ranges from 52 to 92. Based on gross morphology, chromosome nomenclature is classified according to linear measurement, shape, centromeric position, and specific staining qualities attributed to each chromosome.

Unlike mammalian sex chromosome nomenclature (XX for a female, XY for a male), avian species are defined by the ZW method. Female birds are the heterogametic sex (ZW) and males homogametic (ZZ). Avian W chromosomes are smaller than the Z's; this discrepancy between size of ZZ and ZW paired sex chromosomes remains one distinctive measure utilized for sex identification. However, variations in gross morphology of W's between species and artifacts from various methods can preclude their accurate identification (Mengden and Stock 1976). Specific methods for detecting W chromosomes, analogous to the mammalian Y, are described later in the chapter in the section on advanced cytologic techniques.

Karyotype Evaluation Techniques. Karyotype evaluation is generally accomplished by three basic methods of sex chromosome detection: (1) squash preparations using pinfeather pulp cells, (2) culture of peripheral blood leukocytes, and (3) culture of feather pump cells. The end result of all methods is a highly mitotic, late prophase or metaphase-arrested preparation of condensed and complete pairs of all chromosomes, from which sex chromosomes are identifiable.

Squash Preparations. The simplest and earliest preparation technique for avian chromosomes were the 2-week pinfeather pulp cells. Although less favored than cultured blood cells, this method continues to be improved and remains the only validated noninvasive avian genetic technique (Ivins 1975; Rasch and Kurtin 1976; Toone 1981). In brief the procedure involves collecting the feather shaft, cleaning and treating it with a mild hypotonic solution, fixing it in methanol/acetic acid, dissecting the pulp and manually squashing it with a coverslip on a glass slide, and evaluating it microscopically. Difficulties can arise: (1) a low mitotic index ($<3\%$ metaphases/total cells) can result in laborious microscopic searches for the few metaphase nuclei present, (2) inferior or incomplete chromosomal morphology can result from damage or loss caused by the trauma of squashing, and (3) relatively poor staining characteristics can result from nonmitotic contaminants. Obvious advantages are the noninvasive nature of sample collections, particularly suited to rare animal studies, and the potential for long-term storage of pulp material prior to squashing. However, specific staining procedures may be more successful with fresh preparations.

Blood Leukocyte Culture. This remains the traditional and generally recommended technique for avian cytogenic studies. Detailed descriptions of avian blood culture methodology are readily available; these methods are labor intensive and require personnel experienced in culture work (Hungerford et al. 1966; Shoffner et al. 1967; Zartman 1973; Biederman and Lin 1982). The procedure of Biederman and Lin is routinely utilized for bird of prey karyotyping at the San Diego Zoo. In brief, the technique requires a minimum of 2–4 cc heparinized blood, gradient separation of a leukocyte-rich fraction, centrifugation, and resuspension in a complete culture medium with the addition of homologous avian serum. Mitosis is stimulated by phytohemaglutinin, cell growth is synchronized in part by fresh medium exchanges, incubation occurs at avian physiological conditions (100–106°F, or 38–41°C), and culture proceeds for 72 hours. A 30-hour culture technique is being utilized by the San Diego Zoo in California Condor sex testings. Cell growth in all cultures is arrested by Colcemid addition, followed by centrifugation and harvest of leukocyte metaphase nuclei (including resuspension in a mild hypotonic solution, fixation, and drop or spread slide preparations). Gross chromosomal morphology can be determined with Giemsa staining, although other staining and banding techniques can be utilized for specific applications.

Feather Pulp Cultures. Recently revised, the culture of pulp cells combines the best of the above two methods (van Tuinen and Valentine 1982). Feather collection is the same as for squash preparations. Gelatinous pulp tissue is separated from the shaft, with care not to include any dark-pigmented lining; minced pulp is treated with collagenase, transferred to a complete culture medium, agitated, and then centrifuged; the pulp is resuspended in a flask with fresh medium, flushed with carbon dioxide, and incubated (fresh medium after a 24-hour incubation flushes out contaminating erythrocytes that interfere with culture growth). Subculturing and harvesting techniques are similar to those of leukocyte preparations. The crucial factors in pulp culture cells concern the use of collagenase, low-volume changes of medium, and relatively short times for mitotic arrest with Colcemid. Same-day collections and cultures are preferred for banded preparations. The principal advantages are the quantity of metaphase cells obtained and their superior banding and staining characteristics from squash preparations.

Advanced Cytologic Techniques

Specific Banding and Staining Procedures.

Unique fluorescent surface patterns can be produced, evaluated, and documented by chromosome maps produced according to specific chemical constituents. Nomenclature for banding and staining techniques has been standardized according to a three-letter code, the first letter denoting the type of banding, the second letter the general technique, and the third letter the type of stain used (Bergsma 1971/1975). The most common preparations used for avian cytogenetics are QFQ (indicating Q-bands by fluorescence using quinacrine), GTG (indicating G-bands by trypsin using Giemsa), CBG (indicating C-bands by barium hydroxide using Giemsa), and RBA (indicating R-bands by BUdR using acridine orange). The genetic significance of comparative banding and staining characteristics for specific chromosomes remains undefined. C-banding is mentioned later because of its specificity for heterochromatin, repetitive DNA, and the specific identification of W chromosomes.

Specific W Chromosome Identification.

The W chromosome in birds and snakes is composed almost totally of constitutive heterochromatin, as are the centromeres of all chromosomes. Heterochromatin can be identified after treatment with quinacrine, C-banded or Q-banded. Heterochromatic composition of W chromosomes is uniform, which enhances their identity from other macrochromosomes with large nonfluorescing areas. Comparative studies about repetitive DNA as well as a more accurate sex identification method is under investigation. Specific methodology, which requires cytogenic expertise, can be obtained from Mendgen and Stock (1976) and Biederman et al. (1980).

Genome Size Differentiation.

The DNA content of erythrocytes has been evaluated, and the weight difference between ZZ and ZW chromosomes has been proposed as a possible avian sexing technique (Rasch and Kurtin 1976). A scanning cytophotometer was used to measure picogram weight differences, with preliminary data in cranes demonstrating a 4–6% chromosome weight difference between males and females. However, recent studies utilizing fluorescent cytophotometry with improved sensitivity report no significant sex difference in DNA content, based on genome size determinations (Biederman et al. 1982; Biederman 1983). Additional work is needed to verify this technique.

H-Y (H-W) Antigen. Originally investigated for its role in sex determination, H-Y antigen was isolated many years ago from male rodents. Within the last several years it has been demonstrated to induce exclusive immunologic absorption to tissues with a heterogametic karyotype, such as from male mammals, turtles, and amphibians and female birds and snakes (Willys and Wachtel 1977; Short 1979). There has been some controversy about H-Y-positive identification of animals with intersex characteristics or chromosomal abnormalities; however, H-Y (H-W) antigen has generally been positive for sex-reversed male quail with ovotestis (Muller et al. 1980; Zaborski et al. 1981). The W chromosome and its H-Y antigen characteristics are female-determining and ovary-organizing; the mammalian Y chromosome and its H-Y activity are male-determining and testis-organizing (McCarrey et al. 1981).

Sexing based on identification of heterochromatin with an H-Y antigen test has been successful in turtles and amphibians (Engel and Schmid 1981; Engel et al. 1981). Further investigation is needed to validate the utility of this sexing method in birds.

Molecular Genetic Techniques. Bkm, a minor fraction of satellite DNA with a specific sequence of nucleotides, was uniquely and quantitatively located on the W chromosome in banded krait snakes and only detected in females (Singh et al. 1979). Jones et al. (1983) described the universality of the Bkm nucleotide sequence and its apparent conservation in the heterogametic sex from a wide variety of eukaryotic species.

This aspect of molecular genetics, exploring specific DNA sequence homologies, is being investigated as a gene control mechanism (for sex determination) and as a probe for identifying heterochromatic sex chromosomes (Biederman 1983). Purified satellite DNA is isolated for the Bkm fraction from tissues of the unsexed animal; these two fractions are hybridized; the hybrid Bkm is exposed to isotope-labeled (P^{32}) Bkm; the pattern of hybridization and detection of the Bkm probe is isolated by agarose gel electrophoresis (Jones et al. 1983). At present, this sexing method is experimental, requires expertise with molecular genetic techniques, and is labor intensive. Future developments may improve its utility, particularly with selected endangered species.

Hormonal Sexing Methods

Historical Aspects of Excretory Endocrinology.
Endocrinologists have documented that hormonal metabolites, some with biologic activity, are discharged from the body through various routes (salivation, perspiration, urination, defecation).

Sex steroid hormones produced by the gonads and adrenal glands can be traced, as a common thread, through the complex process of reproduction. Estrogenlike substances are ubiquitous across phylogeny. All egg-laying vertebrates, even primitive cyclostomes, utilize gonadal estrogens to control the deposition of yolk in developing oocytes (Chester-Jones et al. 1972). The basic pattern of mammalian steroidogenesis supports an assumption that three major gonadal estrogens predominate: estradiol (E_2), estrone (E_1), and estriol (E_3) (see the excellent review of the fowl by Ozon [1972]).

Evidence relating urinary estrogens to specific physiologic events has not been well established because investigators have centered on monitoring hormones in circulation or on mechanistic studies with specific steroidogenic tissues. The onset of sexual maturity/initial and impending ovulations in mature birds represents physiologic correlations to elevated excretion of E_1/E_2 and elevated 24-hour ratios of E_1/E_2 from mixed colon and urinary excrement (Ozon 1972). Current radioimmunoassay (RIA) methods of hormone analysis have been greatly improved; sensitive to picogram (10^{-12} g) changes in concentrations, they are now 6 times more perceptive than methods employed 30 years ago.

Fecal Steroid Analysis.
A need for precise determination of sex, without stress of trauma, in captive monomorphic birds led to the development of a technique comparing relative amounts of excreted sex hormones. Avian fecal steroid analysis was proposed to measure total immunoreactive estrogen (E) and testosterone (T); females produced and excreted more E; males produced and excreted more T. Sex identification was enhanced when fecal steroids were evaluated as a simple ratio of excretory E/T. Mature females were identified by their high E/T ratio (>2.5), mature males by their lower ratio (<1.4).

Czekala and Lasley (1977) modified and adapted a human urinalysis procedure used for human pregnancy testing (De Vane 1975). The basic fecal steroid analysis procedure involved five steps: (1) fresh droppings were mixed with phosphate buffered saline (PBS), (2) buffered feces supernates were enzymatically hydrolyzed, (3) hydrolysates were diethyl ether extracted, evaporated, and reconstituted with PBS, (4) RIAs of the total immunoreactive T fraction and total E fraction were measured from the same sample, and (5) E/T values from unknown birds were compared with values from known-sex birds. Erb et al. (1982) further developed a combination technique for detecting and measuring estrogenic compounds in urine, feces, and plasma by using high-performance liquid chromatography.

Bercovitz et al. (1978) reported that E/T measurements in male parrots were distinguishable by an average E/T value of 0.64 ± 0.13, and females by an average of 2.78 ± 0.58 (P <0.001). Similar results have been reported from nonpsittacine species. Excretory hormones analyzed from cloacal samples taken during autopsy confirmed that histologic evidence for steroidogenesis was the basis for sex-distinct changes in hormonal discharge.

The initial application for fecal steroid analysis is dependent on functional differences between testicular and ovarian tissues; immature or inactive (in seasonal reproductive quiescence) birds with marginal gonadal function are not consistently sexable.

A data base of E/T values from a wide variety of known-sex birds is necessary to properly interpret results from any unsexed animals. This has been a key factor preventing the casual use of the techniques. Another difficulty has been the variability of reported guidelines for interpretation among laboratories, which was due to different estrogen antiserum used in various RIA systems. A nonspecific antiserum has been recommended to measure the total immunoreactivity of all estrogens present; separate guidelines for interpreting the normal range of E/T values for males and females must be established with new assay systems in each laboratory (Czekala and Lasley 1977; Stavy et al. 1979).

Changes in reproductive condition during the onset of sexual maturity or the period of seasonal reproductive activity in adult birds has not been readily detectable in captive birds. Broad generalizations and circumstantial evidence have been the norm for anticipating a 2- to 7-year span of time for sexual development in captive amazon parrots.

Fecal steroid analysis of sequential monthly E/T ratio evaluation can therefore be used to assess seasonal variations in sex hormone excretion (Bercovitz et al. 1982, 1983). This noninvasive endocrine monitoring technique has several potential applications: (1) as a screening method to identify birds with active gonads and maximum reproductive function, (2) as a method to identify and cull birds with little steroidogenic function, and (3) as a research tool for investigating the developmental and seasonal changes in reproductive condition from various species, especially rare or endangered species.

Egg-Waste Estrogen Analysis. The first artificially incubated California Condor chicks were hatched in captivity in 1983 (Fig. 28.1). Their sex was confirmed, one male and three females, by chromosome analysis (leukocyte culture) and an experimental endocrine sexing method was also tested, based on egg-waste estrogen analysis.

Sex hormones have been measured from steroidogenically active embryonic gonads from domesticated fowl (Tanabe et al. 1979). Elevated concentrations of E_2 in blood plasma and adrenal and gonadal tissues were indicative of female chicken embryos (Guichard et al. 1979; Woods and Brazzill 1981). Mixed urine and feces collected at hatching from egg-waste material (allantoic sac and cloacal contents) were analyzed for estrogen activity, similar to avian fecal steroid analysis procedures (Czekala and Lasley 1977; Bercovitz et al. 1978). Neonatal egg-waste samples were homogenized with PBS, hydrolyzed, extracted, and prepared for separation by high-performance liquid chromatography (HPLC) and/or direct measurement by estrogen RIA. Estradiol fractions were chromatographically isolated from the total array of immunoreactive estrogens. Egg-waste estradiol measurements from one Andean and three California Condor chicks presented a striking sexual difference; both female California Condors had estradiol levels 8 to 10 times higher than those from an Andean or a Californian Condor male.

HPLC was used to isolate the estradiol fraction; nonchromatographic methods of E_2 assessment were being tested. This sexing technique was particularly attractive for captive hatched birds. Egg-waste estrogens research has concentrated on birds of prey, parrot, and crane species, which represent a variety of monomorphic species and unfortunately include a large number of endangered species.

Safety and Application. The primary reason for developing better methods of sexing birds is to enhance captive breeding and survival. Rare or endangered species (California Condors, Puerto Rican Parrots) are not recommended candidates for any sexing method that jeopardizes their survival (i.e., surgical sexing). Therefore nonintrusive sexing methods such as fecal steroid analysis are essential. Zero mortality with fecal steroid analysis has been an important factor with all methods discussed in this section. At the San Diego Zoo, fecal steroid methods resulted in only one serious case of trauma and wing contusions (during initial attempts to confine a 90-lb Emperor Penguin in a 30-gal waste container). The reliability of genetic sexing methods has been good, with greater than 95% accuracy (Bercovitz et al. 1978; Stavy et al. 1979; Biederman and Lin 1982).

Although the need to sex birds of unknown

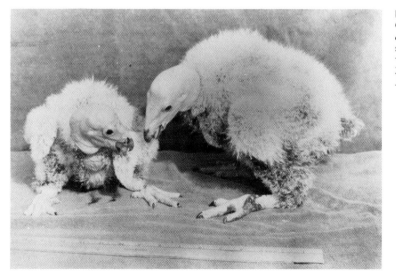

Fig. 28.1. California Condor (*Gymnogyps californianus*) chicks successfully hatched from wild eggs at the San Diego Zoo. (*Courtesy of the San Diego Zoological Society*)

age and breeding condition has frequently accounted for 20–40% of all birds tested (Bercovitz et al. 1978; Stavy et al. 1979; Bercovitz 1981), the functional nature of this particular test is a moot point for those birds with little or no measurable gonadal activity. The reliability of egg-waste estradiol measurement may prove more consistent because the samples are uniformly limited to a period of known gonadal activity at the time of hatching.

Sex identification from karyotype representations or fecal steroid evaluations are all subject to interpretation based upon initial guidelines established with known-sex individuals. Comparative data for E/T ratios are predictable over a designated range for males and females and subject to continual revision. No single guideline for evaluation of reproductive condition is appropriate for all avian species. Raptors have consistently presented sex-distinct male E/T values that were 2 to 3 times higher than parrot male values, and male turacos have characteristically presented E/T values 6 times smaller than those of male parrots.

Surgical sexing techniques (see Chapter 25) continue to be the most available and most routinely applied of all methods. However, specific anatomical attributes do not define functional capacity or genetic potential. The immediate results and minor risks of surgical sexing make this the recommended method for sexing birds not considered endangered or valuable.

Genetic and endocrine sexing methods are highly specialized and still experimental because of the expertise and special equipment required for laboratory analysis. Genetic methods offer the distinct advantage of invariance due to age or breeding condition of the unsexed animal, although little has been done to define avian chromosomal reproductive abnormalities. Endocrine evaluations offer the most direct assessment of functional reproductive activity. Excretory hormone analysis has been developed so that rare and endangered species can be sampled throughout the year.

References

Bercovitz, A. B. 1981. Fecal steroid analysis: A noninvasive approach to bird sexing. *Proc. Am. Fed. Avicult. Vet. Med. Semin., San Diego.*

Bercovitz, A. B., N. M. Czekala, and B. L. Lasley. 1978. A new method of sex determination in monomorphic birds. *J. Zoo Anim. Med.* 9(4):114–24.

Bercovitz, A. B., J. Collins, P. Price, and D. Tuttle. 1982. Noninvasive assessment of seasonal hormone profiles in captive bald eagles (*Haliaeetus leucocephalus*). *Zoo Biol.* 1:111–17.

Bercovitz, A. B., J. Baine, and F. Fryne, Jr. 1983. Applications of fecal steroid analysis (waste not, want

not). *Proc. Jean Delacour/Int. Fdn. Conserv. Birds. Symposium on Breeding Birds in Captivity,* ed. G. Schulman, pp. 513–23. N. Hollywood, Calif.: IFCB.

Bergsma, D. 1971/1975. Standardization in Human Cytogenetics. Paris Conference (1971) and Supplement (1975). Basel: S. Karger; New York: National Foundation for the March-of-Dimes.

Biederman, B. M. 1983. Personal communication (San Diego Zoological Society).

Biederman, B. M., and C. C. Lin. 1982. A leukocyte culture and chromosome preparation technique for avian species. *In Vitro* 18:415–18.

Biederman, B. M., D. Florence, and C. C. Lin. 1980. Cytogenetic analysis of great horned owls (*Bubo virginianus*). *Cytogenet. Cell Genet.* 28:79–86.

Biederman, B. M., C. C. Lin, E. Kuyt, and R. C. Drewien. 1982. Genome of the whooping crane. *J. Hered.* 73:145.

Bloom, S. E. 1974. Current knowledge about the avian W chromosome. *BioScience* 24:340–44.

Chester-Jones, I., D. Bellamy, D. K. O. Chan, B. K. Follett, E. W. Henderson, J. G. Phillips, and R. S. Smart. 1972. In *Steroids in Nonmammalian Vertebrates,* ed. D. R. Idler, pp. 415–99. New York: Academic.

Czekala, N. M., and B. L. Lasley. 1977. A technical note on sex determination in monomorphic birds using fecal steroid analysis. *Int. Zoo Yearb.* 17:209–11.

De Vane, G. W. 1975. Circulating gonadotrophins, estrogens and androgens in polycystic ovarian disease. *Am. J. Obstet. Gynecol.* 121:496–500.

Engel, W., and M. Schmid. 1981. H-Y antigen as a tool for the determination of sex in amphibia. *Cytogenet. Cell Genet.* 30:130–36.

Engel, W., B. Klemme, and M. Schmid. 1981. H-Y antigen and sex determination in turtles. *Differentiation* 20:152–56.

Erb, L., B. L. Lasley, N. M. Czekala, S. L. Monfort, and A. B. Bercovitz. 1982. A dual radioimmunoassay and cytosol receptor binding assay for the measurement of estrogenic compounds applied to urine fecal and plasma samples. *Steroids* 29(1):33–46.

Guichard, A., L. Cedard, Th.-M. Mignot, D. Scheib, and K. Haffen. 1979. Radioimmunoassay of steroids produced by chick embryo gonads cultured in the presence of some exogenous steroid precursors. *Gen. Comp. Endocrinol.* 39:9–19.

Hungerford, D. A., R. L. Snyder, and J. A. Griswold. 1966. Chromosome analysis and identification in the management and conservation of birds. *J. Wildl. Manage.* 30:701–12.

Ivins, G. K. 1975. Sex determination in raptorial birds: A study of chromatin bodies. *J. Zoo Anim. Med.* 6(3):9–11.

Jones, K. W., L. Singh, and C. Phillips. 1983. Conserved nucleotide sequence on sex chromosomes. In *Genetic Rearrangement,* ed. K. F. Chater et al., pp. 265–87. Sunderland, Mass.: Sinauer.

McCarrey, J. R., H. Abplanalp, and U. K. Abbott. 1981. Studies on the H-W (H-Y) antigen in chickens. *J. Hered.* 72:169–71.

Masui, K. 1967. The rudimentary copulatory organ of the male domesticated fowl with reference to the sexual differentiation of chickens. In *Sex Determination and Sexual Differentiation in the Fowl,* ed. K. Masui, pp. 3–15. Ames: Iowa State University Press.

Mengden, G. A., and A. D. Stock. 1976. A preliminary report on the application of current cytological techniques to sexing birds. *Int. Zoo Yearb.* 16:138–41.

Muller, K. A. 1983. Observations on the bird breeding survey as a management tool. *Proc. Jean Delacoure/ Int. Fdn. Conserv. Birds. Symposium on Breeding Birds in Captivity,* ed. G. L. Schulman, pp. 533–50. N. Hollywood, Calif.: IFCB.

Muller, U., A. Guichard, M. Reyss-Brion, and D. Scheib. 1980. Induction of H-Y antigen in the gonads of mail quail embryos by diethylstilbestrol. *Differentiation* 16:129–33.

Ozon, R. 1972. Estrogens in fishes, amphibians, reptiles and birds. In *Steroids in Nonmammalian Vertebrates,* ed. D. R. Idler, pp. 390–441. New York: Academic.

Rasch, E. M., and P. J. Kurtin. 1976. Sex identification in Sandhill Cranes by karyotype analysis. *Proc. Int. Crane Workshop* 1:309–16.

Shoffner, R. N., A. Krishan, G. J. Haiden, R. K. Bammi, and J. S. Otis. 1967. Avian chromosome methodology. *Poult. Sci.* 46(2):334–44.

Short, R. V. 1979. Sex determination and differentiation. *Br. Med. Bull.* 35(2):121–27.

Singh, L., I. P. Purdom, and K. W. Jones. 1979. Behavior of sex chromosome-associated satellite DNAs in somatic and germ cells in snakes. *Chromosoma* 79:167–81.

Stavy, M., D. Gilbert, and R. D. Martin. 1979. Routine determination of sex in monomorphic bird species using fecal steroid analysis. *Int. Zoo Yearb.* 19:209–14.

Tanabe, Y., T. Nakamura, K. Fujioka, and O. Doi. 1979. Production and secretion of sex steroid hormones by testes, the ovary and the adrenal glands of embryonic and young chickens. *Gen. Comp. Endocrinol.* 39:26–33.

Toone, W. D. 1981. Improvements in cytogenetic techniques for gross karyotype and morphological studies of avian chromosomes. *Proc. Am. Fed. Avicult. Vet. Med. Semin., San Diego.*

van Tuinen, P., and M. Valentine. 1982. A non-invasive technique of avian tissue culture (feather pump) for banded chromosome preparations. *Mamm. Chromosome Newsl.* 23(4):182–86.

Willys, K. S., and S. S. Wachtel. 1977. H-Y antigen: Behavior and function. *Science* 195:956–60.

Woods, J. E., and D. M. Brazzill. 1981. Plasma 17 beta-estradiol levels in the chick embryo. *Gen. Comp. Endocrinol.* 36:360–70.

Zaborski, P. A., A. Guichard, and D. Scheib. 1981. Transient expression of H-Y antigen in quail ovotestis following diethylstilbestrol (DES) treatment. *Biol. Cell* 41:113–23.

Zartman, D. L. A. 1973. A microculture technique for chick leukocytes. *Cytogenet. Cell Genet.* 12:136–42.

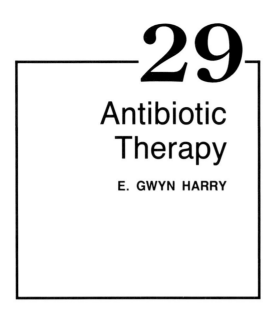

29

Antibiotic Therapy

E. GWYN HARRY

EVER SINCE bacteria were found to be the cause, or exacerbating factor, in certain diseases, a need has been felt for specific antibacterial substances that could be administered orally or parenterally without adverse effect on body cells. The first antimicrobial agent of this nature, sulfanilamide, was discovered in the early 1930s. This was to be the parent compound of a series of derivatives, the sulfonamides, that are still widely used for the treatment of certain diseases. Other chemotherapeutic compounds that have subsequently come into use are the nitrofurans and the compound trimethoprim, which

is often used as a sulfonamide potentiator.

The most versatile of the chemotherapeutic agents, and consequently the most widely used, are the antibiotics. Penicillin was the first of these to be used, in the 1940s. The antibiotics differ from the other chemotherapeutic agents in being produced naturally by certain species of fungi, actinomycetes, and bacteria. Once their molecular structure was elucidated, further antibiotics were produced by chemical modification. In some cases (e.g., tetracyclines), they were produced entirely by synthesis, based on the molecular structure of the natural product. The term "antibiotic" has now been extended to include all these compounds (Table 29.1).

The antibiotics, collectively, constitute various groups (Table 29.2); each of these groups share certain modes of action related to their similarities in chemical structure. Some, as indicated, are effective against groups of microbes other than bacteria, such as mycoplasmas, chlamydiae, and fungi. Because of the similarity in application of those chemotherapeutic agents (e.g., sulfonamides) not derived from or based directly or indirectly on compounds originating from natural sources, it is convenient to discuss all these compounds under the general description "antibiotics."

When to Use Antibiotics

Therapeutic Use. The therapeutic role of antibiotics for the treatment of infectious diseases is well established. Treatment should be

Table 29.1. Some common antibiotics and dosages (if available)

Antibiotic	Route	Dosage	Source[a]
Amikacin	IM	10 mg/kg	3
Amoxicillin	IM	50–100 mg/kg	1
	oral	100–150 mg/kg	1
	SC	30–70 mg/kg	5
Amphotericin/neomycin/thiostrepton			
Amphotericin B	oral	1 mg/kg	1
	IV	0.75 mg/kg	5
Ampicillin	IM	50–100 mg/kg	1
	oral	100–150 mg/kg	1
	IM or oral	110 mg/kg	4
	IM or oral	50–100 mg/kg	3
	IM	100–250 mg/kg	2
	oral	250 mg/kg	2
Benethamine penicillin			
Benzathine penicillin			
Benzylpenicillin (penicillin G)			
Carbenicillin	IM	100–200 mg/kg	3
Cefotaxime	IM	100 mg/kg	3
Cephalexin	oral	40 mg/kg	3
Cephoxazole			
Chloramphenicol	IM or oral	100–200 mg/k	3
Chlortetracycline	IM	50–250 mg/kg	1
	oral	20–40 mg/kg	1

Table 29.1. (*Continued*)

Antibiotic	Route	Dosage	Source[a]
Cloxacillin	IM	100–250 mg/kg	2
	oral	250 mg/kg	2
Co-trimazine-sulfadiazine/trimethoprim	oral	1 ml/4 lb	3
Co-trimoxazole-sulfamethoxazole/ trimethoprim			
Cycloserine	oral		
Doxycycline	oral	20 mg/kg	3
Erythromycin	oral	250 mg/kg	1
	SC	25 mg/kg	5
	oral	50 mg/kg	4
Framycetin			
Furaltadone			
Furazolidone	IM or oral	50 mg/kg	4
Gentamicin	IM	2 mg/kg	3
	SC	10–20 mg/kg	5
Griseofulvin	oral	125 mg/kg	1
Kanamycin	IM	50–100 mg/kg	1
	oral	100–150 mg/kg	1
Lincomycin	oral	250 mg/kg	1
	oral	<50 mg/kg	2
Methicillin			
Miconazole			
Nafcillin			
Nalidixic acid			
Neomycin	oral	15 mg/kg	2,4
Nitrofurantoin	oral	8–10 mg/kg	4
Nitrofurazone			
Novobiocin			
Nystatin (3000 units/mg)	oral	10–100 mg/kg	3
Oxytetracycline			
Phenoxymethylpenicillin (penicillin V)			
Penicillin/streptomycin	IM	50 mg/kg	1
Phthalylsulfacetamide/neomycin			
Polymyxin			
Rifampicin			
Spectinomycin	IM	50–100 mg/kg	1
	oral	100–150 mg/k	1
Spiramycin	IM	20 mg/kg	2
	oral	250 mg/g	2
Streptomycin	oral	15 mg/kg	2
	IM	50 mg/kg[b]	4
Sulfonamides (various)	oral	500 mg/kg	1,2,3
Tetracycline hydrochloride	IM	8–10 mg/kg	1
	oral	350 mg/kg	1
	oral	250 mg/kg	2
Tobramycin	IM	11 mg/kg	3
Tylosin	oral	200 mg/kg	3
	IM	10–25 mg/kg	3
	IM	15 mg/kg	1
	oral	150–200 mg/kg	1
	IM	15 mg/kg	2
	IM	15 mg/kg	4
Vancomycin			

[a]Dosage regimes, come from the following:
1. Burr, E. W. 1982. *Diseases of Parrots*. Neptune, N.J.: T.F.H. Publications.
2. Cooper, J. E. 1978. *Veterinary Aspects of Captive Birds of Prey*. Saul, Gloucestershire, Engl.: Standfast Press.
3. Emanuelson, Sandra. 1983. Oral lesions in raptors: Their diagnosis and treatment. *Wildl. Rehabil. Counc. J.*, spring, pp. 7–10.
4. Galvin, C. 1978. *Avian Drugs and Dosages*. Walnut Creek, Calif.: Wildlife Rehabilitation Council.
5. Schultz, D. J. 1984. Unpublished data (Veterinary surgeon, 30 Belair Road, Hawthorn, S. Australia 5062, Australia).
[b]Maximum safe dose is 150 mg/kg.

Table 29.2. Classification of antibiotics and other antimicrobial agents used in veterinary medicine

Penicillins			**Sulfonamides**	
+	Phenoxymethylpenicillin[a] (penicillin V)		+ −	Sulfanilamide
+	Benzylpenicillin[a] (penicillin G)		+ −	Sulfadimidine[a] (sulfamezathine)
+	Benethamine penicillin		+ −	Sulfanylamido chlorpyridazine
+	Benzathine penicillin		+ −	Sulfamethoxy pyridazine
+ −	Ampicillin[a]		+ −	Sulfapyridine
+ pr	Nafcillin		+ −	Sulfamethyl phenazole
+ −	Carbenicillin[a]		+ −	Sulfadiazine[a]
+ pr	Cloxacillin[a]		+ −	Phthalylsulfacetamide
+ pr,M	Methicillin			
+ −	Amoxicillin[a]		**Tetracyclines**	
			+ −	Tetracycline[a]
Aminoglycosides			+ − M	Chlortetracycline[a]
+ − T	Streptomycin[a]		+ − M	Oxytetracycline[a]
+ −	Tobramycin[a]		+ −	Methacycline
+ − T	Kanamycin[a]		+ −	Doxycycline[a]
+ − T	Neomycin[a]			
+ − T	Framycetin		**Nitrofurans**	
+ − T	Gentamicin[a]		+ −	Furazolidone[a]
			+ −	Furaltadone
Macrolides			+ −	Nitrofurantoin
+ M	Erythromycin[a]		+ −	Nitrofurazone[a]
+ M	Spiramycin[a]			
+ M	Tylosin[a]		**Miscellaneous synthetic**	
			and semisynthetic compounds	
Polypeptides			+ −	Amikacin[a]
+ −	Thiostrepton[a]		+ T	Rifampicin
+	Bacitracin[a]		+ − M	Chloramphenicol[a]
− P	Polymyxin		+	Vancomycin
			T	Cycloserine
Polyenes			F	Griseofulvin[a]
F	Nystatin[a]		− M	Spectinomycin[a]
F	Amphotericin[a]		+	Lincomycin[a]
			+ −	Trimethoprim[a]
Cephalosporins			+ (−)	Novobiocin
+ −	Cefotaxime[a]		−	Nalidixic acid
+ −	Cephalexin[a]		+ F	Miconazole[a]
+ −	Cephoxazole		(−)	Clavulanate

Note: + = active mainly against G+ bacteria; − = active primarily against G− bacteria; pr = penicillinase-resistant penicillins; + − = active against many G+ and G− bacteria; T = particularly active against *M. tuberculosis;* P = particularly active against *P. aeruginosa;* M = particularly active against *Mycoplasma* spp.; f = particularly active against fungi.

[a]Previous use in cage birds recorded.

commenced as soon as possible after clinical signs of disease are noticed and the nature of the infection diagnosed. An exception to this occurs when the nature of the disease makes the destruction of the infected bird preferable to treatment (psittacosis, pseudotuberculosis).

Prophylactic Use

Application Following Exposure to Infection. Although the prophylactic use of antibiotics is not as well defined as their use in the treatment of established cases of disease, they can play an important role in the prevention of disease in a number of situations. One of these is the prevention of spread of an infection within birds in an aviary. This situation may arise when a contagious disease such as erysipelas is contracted by

a particularly susceptible bird in the aviary. It can also arise if a symptomless carrier of an infection is brought into the aviary from an outside source.

Application Following Subjection to Stress. There is a greater risk of transfer of infection if exposure occurs at a time when birds are subjected to various physiological or psychological stressors (nutritional deficiencies, abnormal temperatures, social disturbances). Stress may also predispose birds to infection by lowering their resistance to potentially pathogenic commensal organisms.

Application in Viral Infections. Although, apart from certain of the larger viruses, antibiotics are ineffective antiviral agents, they can prevent suprainfection with potentially pathogenic bacteria normally present in the birds or their environment. Their use is particularly valuable with respiratory tract infections; without antibiotics, chronic disease syndromes involving bacteria (e.g., certain strains of *Escherichia coli*) can complicate an otherwise transient viral infection.

Application in Surgical Procedures. Prophylaxis can also be of value when applied to individual birds prior to surgery to reduce the risk of or to control a subsequent bacteremia. In operations on the gut, for example, an orally administered antibiotic with a low rate of absorption from the alimentary tract can be given 2 days before operating to reduce the bacterial population at the site of operation. Neomycin or the poorly absorbed sulfonamides (sulfathiazole, phthalylsulfacetamide) are suitable for this purpose.

Limitations of Prophylaxis. The nature of a disease must be considered when attempting to control its spread. For example, because of the likely persistence of symptomless carriers, prophylactic medication alone is unlikely to eradicate the presence of salmonella in a colony of birds in which salmonellosis has occurred. Its use at intervals, however, may prevent the activation of latent infection.

Misuse of Antibiotics. Antibiotics should not be administered in prophylactic doses as a substitute for maintaining proper standards of hygiene and husbandry. The administration of low doses of an antibiotic over a prolonged period can be disadvantageous. Apart from other undesirable effects, such as the possibility of immunosuppression, the prevalence of mutant strains of bacteria resistant to this antibiotic may be increased. This would result in the future use of the antibiotic being ineffective in that aviary. Therapeutic treatments should be continued only long enough to prevent recurrence of the disease after discontinuation of the antibiotic. This is usually not less than 2 days after cessation of clinical signs, or in some diseases, such as pasteurella or salmonella infections, until the pathogen concerned is absent from the feces.

Selecting Antibiotics

Selection Based on Bacterial Identity. When bacteria are the main or contributory cause of a disease condition, the choice of antibiotic for treatment is fundamentally based on the species of bacteria involved. Of particular importance is whether the bacteria are gram-positive or gram-negative or of a species particularly sensitive to certain antibiotics (Table 29.2). Antibiotics usually preferred for use in various diseases are shown in Table 29.3; when some contraindication to their use exists (e.g., the involvement of strains with acquired resistance to the antibiotic indicated), an alternative should be selected.

Selection Based on Strain Sensitivity Pattern. The widespread use of antimicrobial compounds has resulted in the prevalence of mutant strains resistant to those compounds most frequently used. For this reason, in addition to identifying the species of the bacteria involved, an antibiotic sensitivity test should be made on the isolated strain to determine whether or not it is resistant to an otherwise appropriate antibiotic. For example, if *Staphylococcus aureus* is the cause of disease, treatment with an antibiotic of the penicillin group would be appropriate. These antibiotics attain bactericidal levels in the blood shortly after administration, which is desirable when, as with this organism, a septicemic condition may develop. If the isolated strain possesses a beta-lactamase enzyme such as penicillinase, a sensitivity test would show it to be resistant to the types of penicillin usually used (penicillin G or V, ampicillin). The strain would, however, be sensitive to these penicillins if they were used in combination with potassium clavulanate, as this compound can inhibit beta-lactamases. A similar effect is obtained if these penicillins are used in combination with an antibiotic resistant to beta-lactamases, such as cephoxazole. Both of these combinations are available commercially. But certain forms of penicillin are penicillinase-resistant, such as cloxacillin, nafcillin, and methicillin. These, however (in particular, methicillin), are less active on a weight-for-weight basis than is penicillin G so their use is advantageous only in special circumstances.

As a general rule, strains of bacteria resistant to one antibiotic are resistant also to other antibiotics of that particular group. In this case they are likely to be sensitive to antibiotics of other groups. Fortunately, strains possessing multiple resistance are relatively uncommon, with the possible exception of members of the Enterobacteriaceae group. The likelihood of encountering strains resistant to a particular antibiotic in a given environment is increased with its frequency of use. For this reason, in aviaries where there is a frequent necessity to use antibiotics, it is advantageous to use one of a number of antibiotics of different groups in rotation.

Selection Based on Mode of Action. As well as the results of the Gram and sensitivity

Table 29.3. Applications of antibiotics in various disease conditions

Disease or Disease Agent	Antibiotic	Route
Mycoplasmosis	Erythromycin	Injection
	Tetracyclines	Oral/injection
	Spectinomycin	Oral/injection
	Spiramycin	Oral/injection
	Tylosin	Oral/injection
Ornithosis, psittacosis	Tetracyclines	Oral/injection
	Tylosin	Oral/injection
	Spectinomycin	Injection
	Doxycycline	Oral
E. coli septicemia	Spectinomycin or ampicillin	Injection
	Tetracyclines	Oral
	Furazolidon	Oral
	Sulfonamides	Oral
Salmonellosis	Spectinomycin	Injection
	Oxytetracycline	Oral/injection
	Furazolidone or nitrofurazone	Oral
	Chloramphenicol	Oral/injection
	Sulfadimidine	Oral
	Sulfadiazine + trimethoprim	Oral
Pasteurellosis	Spectinomycin	Oral/injection
	Sulfonamides	Oral
Erysipelas	Penicillins	Oral/injection
	Tetracyclines	Oral
Streptococcal infection, staphylococcosis	Penicillins	Oral/injection
	Furazolidone	Oral
	Tetracyclines	Oral
Pseudomonas infections	Gentamicin or polymyxin	Oral/injection
	Tobramycin	Oral/injection
Pseudotuberculosis	Tetracyclines	Oral/injection
Candidiasis	Nystatin	Oral
Aspergillosis	Amphotericin or miconazole	Oral/injection
Favus	Griseofulvin or miconazole	Topical
Skin mycoses	Griseofulvin powder	Topical
	Miconazole powder	Topical
Septicemia	Spectinomycin and other similarly acting antibiotics	Injection
Upper respiratory tract infection	Spectinomycin + lincomycin	Oral
	Tetracyclines	Oral
Intestinal tract infection	Sulfadimidine	Oral
	Sulfadiazine + trimethoprim	Oral
	Lincomycin	Oral
	Chloramphenicol	Oral
Urinary tract infection	Tetracyclines	Oral
Wound infection	Oxytetracycline	Topical
	Bacitracin spray powder	Topical
Eye infection	Oxytetracycline aqueous drops	Topical

tests, other factors determine the selection of an appropriate antibiotic. One of these factors is the mode of action of the antibiotic, that is, whether it is bacteriostatic or bactericidal. In the treatment of an acute infection, such as a septicemia, the use of bactericidal antibiotics such as the penicillins, cephalosporins (e.g., cephoxazole), or aminoglycosides are indicated. For subacute or chronic conditions, antibiotics that are mainly bacteriostatic (chloramphenicol, tetracyclines, macrolides, sulfonamides) can be given. In the treatment of most infections of this kind, inhibition of growth alone is sufficient, as once bacteriostasis is achieved, the infecting organisms will be removed by the body's normal bacterial defense mechanisms.

Selection Based on Suitability for Oral Administration. Another factor influencing the choice of antibiotic is the proposed route of administration. Oral dosage is advantageous when parenteral administration is likely to be hazardous and not justifiable (e.g., with the smaller varieties of cage birds). It also can provide a convenient means of continuing treatment following initial parenteral medication. Oral administration is also indicated when treating infections of the alimentary tract. To be effective when given orally, the antibiotic must be water soluble but, like penicillin V and cloxacillin, not inactivated by the low pH encountered in the upper part of the alimentary tract. Inactivation may also result from the presence of ingested foodstuffs, as in the case of cloxacillin, and it is for this reason generally advisable to medicate before feeding. When oral administration is carried out by medicating the drinking water, the antibiotic should be sufficiently stable to remain active for at least 12 hours before replacement. Penicillin, for example, shows a considerable loss of activity in solution form (in 1 day at room temperature).

The degree to which the antibiotic is absorbed into the circulatory system after ingestion also must be considered. Antibiotics used in the treatment of systemic infections should be a readily absorbed type. These include certain of the penicillins, such as penicillin V, ampicillin, and in particular, amoxycillin, which gives higher blood levels than the same dose of ampicillin. The tetracyclines, spectinomycin, lincomycin, and certain of the sulfonamides, such as sulfadimidine and sulfadiazine combined with trimethoprim, are also readily absorbed. Long-acting sulfonamides are also available, such as sulfadimethoxine and sulfamethoxypyridazine; with these a dose needs to be given only at long intervals (once a day or even once a week). To treat infections of the alimentary tract, anti-biotics must be a type not absorbed from the alimentary tract (amphotericin, nystatin, thiostrepton, streptomycin, neomycin, and the poorly absorbed sulfonamides, such as succinyl-sulfathiazole or phthalylsulfacetamide). For this reason, amphotericin, thiostrepton, and nystatin are also suitable for the treatment of mycotic diarrhea and crop mycosis involving *Candida albicans*.

Selection Based on Suitability for Parenteral Administration. When it is necessary to produce bactericidal tissue levels as quickly as possible, antibiotics may be administered by subcutaneous, intramuscular, or intravenous injection. Most antibiotics are available in forms suitable for parenteral use. Sulfonamides are, however, mainly administered only orally, apart from sulfamethoxypyridazine. Bactericidal levels of antibiotic are obtained more rapidly with injection of water-based solutions than with oral administration, which is advantageous in treating acute infections such as a septicemia. Subsequently it may be better to continue treatment with an antibiotic that is absorbed at a slower rate (benzathine, benethamine penicillin), which requires less-frequent injections because of the lower blood levels necessary.

Selection Based on Spectrum of Activity. Despite the advantages of delaying antibiotic selection until both the identity and sensitivity of the bacteria involved in an infection have been established, in practice this is not always possible. Infected tissues or exudates may not be available for culture, or the acuteness of a disease may justify immediate treatment. At times, immediate prophylactic medication may be necessary, as in the case of birds that have been stressed or in contact with birds from an outside source. Clinical signs of an infection may be inadequate to allow a diagnosis. In such cases it is advisable to administer a broad-spectrum-type antibiotic that is effective against both gram-positive and gram-negative bacteria, preferably one with bactericidal activity (ampicillin, amoxycillin). Alternatively, a combination of antibiotics differing in modes of action may be used; for example, an antibiotic such as penicillin can be combined with cephoxazole or streptomycin. The spectrum of such a combination may also be broadened to include fungi such as *C. albicans* (e.g., combining neomycin with thiostrepton and amphotericin). A preparation of this nature is available for oral administration in the treatment of a mixed infection causing diarrhea. For a condition primarily of fungal origin, the administration of miconazole would be more effective.

In addition to broadening the antimicrobial spectrum, combinations involving antibiotics of different groups are also effective against strains resistant to one of the component antibiotics. In some cases, such as a combination of a sulfonamide and trimethoprim (co-trimazine, co-trimoxazole), a potentiating effect is also obtained when a sequential blocking of bacterial synthesis of an essential nutrient, folinic acid, is achieved by inactivating two different enzyme systems. Such a combination has a level of activity much greater than either compound alone, reducing the risk of bacterial resistance. A similar effect is achieved when amoxycillin, which is inactivated by bacterial penicillinase, is combined with clavulanate or cephoxazole, both of which inactivate this enzyme.

Antibiotics, however, should not be combined indiscriminately, as some compounds can inactivate others. For example, penicillin, which acts only on rapidly dividing cells, is inactivated when combined with compounds having a bacteriostatic action, such as the tetracyclines or sulfonamides.

When antibiotics are administered on an empirical basis in the absence of a sensitivity test or when the diagnosis of the disease is in doubt, it is particularly important to note the response to the treatment. No apparent benefit after a few days may indicate the need for an alternative treatment.

Selection Based on Possible Toxicity or Side Effects. As well as obvious side effects, such as allergy and hypersensitivity reactions, certain antimicrobial compounds can produce nonlethal toxic effects that are not immediately apparent. These reactions are more likely to occur following prolonged administration and can affect the liver, kidneys, or nervous system (Table 29.4). The severity of these side effects varies with different species of birds and the age and condition of individual birds treated. In allergies, particularly, the severity of the reaction is influenced by previous exposure to sensitizing doses, in some cases even as little as a trace contact (for this reason, persons handling penicillin should avoid unnecessary skin contact and wash their hands after its use). In some individual cases, injected penicillin can cause an acute anaphylactic reaction. As a precaution against a fatal reaction of this type, adrenaline should be available at the time of injection (Cooper 1978). Procaine penicillin is particularly likely to produce anaphylaxis when injected and should not be used in the treatment of cage birds.

Certain adverse reactions are specifically associated with orally administered antibiotics.

Table 29.4. Adverse reactions associated with misuse of antibiotics

Antibiotic	Reactions
Penicillins	Allergy and hypersensitivity; risk of toxicity if test doses not given when injecting cloxacillin; procaine penicillin too toxic for injection in birds
Aminoglycosides	Allergy and hypersensitivity; neurotoxicity; nephrotoxicity; apnea. Treatments should be limited to 4–7 days. Orally usually safe. (Streptomycin in particular may cause shock in psittacines when injected, particularly in acutely sick birds.)
Tetracyclines	Hepatoxic; apnea; injections may be painful
Polypeptides	Allergy and hypersensitivity; nephrotoxicity
Sulfonamides	Nephrotoxicity (less-soluble forms); hypersensitivity; risk of toxicity when treatment is continuous and prolonged
Chloramphenicol	Hepatoxicity; risk of aplastic anemia
Lincomycin	Apnea
Cephalosporins	Allergy, nausea, vomiting, and diarrhea
Macrolides	Painful injections with some preparations

Note: For further general information see Martindale, 1982, *The Extra Pharmacopoeia*, 28th ed., ed. E. L. Reynolds, London, The Pharmaceutical Press. For information specifically related to birds, consult manufacturers.

Irritation of the intestinal mucosa can follow ingestion of ampicillin, lincomycin, and the tetracyclines, as well as most antibiotics, when given in large doses. Growth supression of certain bacterial species capable of synthesis of B group vitamins can also occur in the gut following oral administration of large doses of neomycin and other broad-spectrum antibiotics. When such antibiotics are administered orally, therefore, it is advisable to supplement the diet with extra vitamin B, particularly B_{12}. These vitamins can be conveniently provided in the form of vitamin-impregnated dehusked seeds or by subcutaneous injection of a vitamin B complex preparation. Changes in the gut flora produced by broad-spectrum antibiotics can also often result in the suppression of the bacteria that stabilize pH at a level inimical to potential pathogens such as pseudomonads, *Proteus* spp., and fungi (e.g., *C. albicans*). This can cause inflammation of the cloacal membranes or diarrhea.

In some cases the toxicity of individual antibiotics can be lowered by the use of synergistic combinations (sulfadimidine plus trimethoprim, penicillin plus streptomycin). With such combinations the effective dose rate of the component antibiotics can be lowered. In the case of the sulfonamides, the risk of crystalluria and resultant kidney damage can be reduced by the combination of three sulfonamides, such as sulfathiazole, sulfadiazine, and sulfamerazine. The presence of one of these sulfonamides in the urine does not reduce the solubility of the others. A lesser amount of each compound can thus be used without loss of therapeutic activity of the combined product.

How to Use Antibiotics

Dosage. Relatively few of the many antibiotics used in the treatment of human diseases have been used in treating birds. The reasons for this are the difficulty of estimating a suitable dose for much smaller animals and the possibility of differences in species susceptibility to any toxic side effects. The method of determining an appropriate dose empirically by giving a dose well below toxic level and increasing the dose until a therapeutic effect is obtained can be ineffective, as it may initiate the development of resistant strains. Appropriate first estimates of doses and dosage regimes for birds is provided by the dose/body weight relationship described by Kirkwood (1983a). Calculated dosages require subsequent adjustment following clinical observations. Dose rates of a number of the commonly used antibiotics that are suitable for birds are given in Table 29.1. Consideration must also be given to the age and condition of the bird being treated, especially in the case of antibiotics known to have undesirable side effects and particularly when administered parenterally. The antibiotic should be administered at sufficiently regular intervals to maintain therapeutic blood levels, and medication should be continued for some time after acute symptoms have abated.

Administration

Parenteral Administration. The administration of antibiotics by injection has the advantage of greater control of the dosage rate. In addition, a high level of antibiotic can be attained in a short time, which is desirable in acute infections, particularly in the early stages of treatment. For an ailing or comatose bird, injection may be the only means of administration available.

Inoculation Techniques. Injections are usually made by subcutaneous or intramuscular routes. They should be made using a microliter, tuberculin, or multiple milliliter syringe, depending on the medication. Needles of 24 to 26 gauge are suitable for parrots and 27 gauge for small birds such as canaries. Needles 2.5 cm long are suitable for subcutaneous injections, 6.25 mm long for intramuscular injections.

Intravenous Injections. These can be given by injecting the jugular vein in small birds but can be hazardous in very small fragile birds. In larger birds, such as parrots, the brachial vein can be used.

Subcutaneous Injections. The favored sites for subcutaneous injection are the dorsal surface of the neck, the ventral surface of the wing, or the medial or lateral aspect of the leg. Due to the thinness and relative inelasticity of the skin of birds, administering a calculated dose can be difficult because of the likelihood of leakage of fluid from the injection site. The volume of fluid retained depends on the size of the bird; the maximum amount in 20-g birds is usually not more than 1 ml at any one site.

Intramuscular Injections. The optimal site for injection is the thigh or pectoral muscle. In both cases it is advisable to withdraw the plunger of the syringe before giving the injection to ensure that the tip of the needle is not situated in a blood vessel. This risk can also be minimized by making the injection close to the keel; this also avoids the pectoral sinus present in some birds. As repeated handling of birds during parenteral administration can cause distress, especially in the case of intramuscular injections, consideration should be given to the use of a slow-release form of the antibiotic, if available. For example, in the case of acute infections, benzathine or benethamine penicillin are suitable following the initial use of one of the readily absorbed forms of penicillin. The use of the relatively insoluble procaine penicillin is not, however, recommended for use with birds because of its toxicity, especially to raptors (Cooper 1978). There is also a risk of tissue damage following the injection of oil-based antibiotics.

Oral Administration. The oral administration of antibiotics has the advantage of avoiding frequent handling. It is, as well, a convenient way of continuing medication after the infection has been brought under control by parenteral administration. Antibiotics can be administered orally in the drinking water or food, or when a bird is disinclined to eat or drink in a normal fashion, by direct introduction into the esophagus. It is also possible to administer the antibiotic to larger birds in the form of tablets or capsules.

One of the disadvantages of food or water medication is the lack of control of intake, as the rate of intake may be abnormal in sick birds, making accurate dosage impossible. Oral administration also requires an antibiotic that is absorbed from the alimentary tract, has a subsequent low rate of excretion, is relatively tasteless and preferably colorless, and has a low toxicity.

Water Administration. Although suitable for species such as canaries that have a relatively high intake of water, water medication is less suitable for fruit-eating species, such as the mynahs and lorikeets. Water medication has a further disadvantage in that some antibiotics are relatively unstable in aqueous solution, particularly at room temperatures. Medication by the drinking water is considered suitable, usually in conjunction with parenteral medication, for tetracycline, lincomycin, tylosin, erythromycin, chloramphenicol, ampicillin, kanamycin, and spectinomycin (Dolphin and Olsen 1977). Tetracycline is frequently administered prophylactically against psittacosis in quarantine stations. The amount of the antibiotic added to the drinking water each day is based on the calculated dose to be administered, taking into account the daily water consumption and the volume of water in the drinking container.

Food Administration. This has the advantage that antibiotics are more stable in a dry form. The antibiotic can be incorporated in ground foodstuffs, such as soybean meal, which can be subsequently presented in the form of crumbs. Furazolidone is frequently administered in this form. Initially a loading dose is given, which is later halved to provide a maintenance dose. Alternatively, in treating seed-eating birds, the seeds can be impregnated with antibiotics such as the tetracyclines, penicillins, chloramphenicol, or one of the sulfonamides (Graham-Jones 1961). Seeds should be dehusked before they are medicated because some species of birds, such as Budgerigars, dehusk seeds before eating them. Medicated seeds should be fed to the exclusion of other foods. As with other forms of indirect medication, however, the amount ingested cannot be accurately determined because of unaccountable loss from spillage.

Direct Oral Administration. This method, which has the advantage of more accurate dosage, is suitable for use with a bird sufficiently robust to withstand the handling involved. A solution or suspension of the antibiotic can be introduced into the mouth using a medicine dropper. The antibiotic can be more accurately administered by means of a calibrated syringe connected to a fine flexible cannula, which is inserted into the esophagus. To minimize the risk of the antibiotic being inactivated after administration, this should be carried out when the crop is empty of food.

Topical Application. For the treatment of localized infections, antibiotics can be applied by brushing on the antibiotic in the form of solution or powder. Ointments tend to mat the feathers so that in birds it is preferable, for example, to treat eye infections with oxytetracycline in the form of an aqueous solution. For the prevention of aspergillosis, nystatin can be applied to feathers by means of an aerosol spray (Burr 1982).

Antibiotic Resistance. Although some species of bacteria are naturally resistant to certain antibiotics (e.g., the resistance of gram-negative bacteria to certain members of the penicillin group), many species normally sensitive to a particular antibiotic can become resistant as a result of the natural process of mutation. For example, a small proportion of a population of *S. aureus* strains can develop the beta-lactamase enzyme penicillinase, which makes them resistant to the growth-inhibiting action of penicillin. Other changes may occur in the permeability of the cell wall. Both of these types of change may also be conferred by plasmids, as in the case of transmissible resistance. The frequent or prolonged use of antibiotics, particularly at the low levels used for prophylaxis, exerts a selection pressure favoring the predominance of these mutant strains, resulting in the loss of activity of these antibiotics when applied for therapeutic use.

Cross-resistance. Strains resistant to one antibiotic may also be resistant to other members of the same group having a similar chemical structure or mode of action. For example, strains resistant to tetracycline will show cross-resistance to chlortetracycline and oxytetracycline. Similarly, strains resistant to streptomycin will show cross-resistance to kanamycin. Strains of *S. aureus* that, by mutation, possess a penicillinase enzyme and thus a resistance to penicillin, may still remain sensitive to cloxacillin, methicillin, and nafcillin because these antibiotics differ structurally in a way that makes them resistant to this enzyme. Strains that develop resistance to these particular penicillins, however, are then resistant to the penicillin group as a whole.

Multiple Resistance. Strains of bacteria that have acquired resistance to one group of antibiotics, as described above, may also become resistant to one or more other groups following prolonged exposure to antibiotics of these other groups. The normal antibiotic-sensitive strains also present in their environment will, however, regain their former predominance gradually when exposure to the antibiotic is removed; the change in selection pressure, in consequence, then operates in their favor. This is the reason why, as mentioned previously, antibiotics belonging to different groups should be used in rotation for disease control in each particular aviary.

Transferrable Resistance. In species of Enterobacteriaceae, *Pasteurella, Proteus, Pseudomonas,* and *Vibrio,* antibiotic resistance can be transferred from resistant to sensitive strains through contact by means of conjugation or transduction. In the case of conjugation, a resistance transfer factor (RTF) is involved. This consists of a fragment of genetic material (termed a "plasmid" or "episome") that may code for both resistance and the transfer mechanism. Conditions for conjugation are optimal in the intestinal tract and are favored by the oral administration of low levels of an antibiotic to which the RTF-possessing strains are resistant, which exerts a selection pressure aiding their proliferation. Strains possessing RTF are capable of transferring, on contact, resistance that may be multiple in nature, usually to other strains of the same species. As the transfer factor itself can also be included in the genetic material transferred, bacterial cells infected in this way can become capable of conferring transmissible resistance to other cells in turn. By this mechanism it is possible, in some cases, for strains of nonpathogenic species to confer multiple resistance to pathogenic species that have never been exposed to the antibiotics concerned. Transduction is another mechanism whereby transfer of genetic material, coded for antibiotic resistance, can be made from resistant to sensitive strains. Transfer in this case is mediated by bacteriophage. Transferable resistance can present a problem when low levels of antibiotics are orally administered over a prolonged period. The problem can be solved by withholding for several weeks the antibiotics to which resistance has been acquired.

Antibiotic Sensitivity Testing. The methods for antibiotic sensitivity testing have been described by Garrod et al. (1981). The popular test consists of spreading pure cultures of the organism or organisms causing or contributing to the disease over the surface of an agar-based medium. Paper disks impregnated with various antibiotics are placed on the surface. The inoculated plates of media are then incubated, usually at 37°C for 12–24 hours, and the size of the clear zone of inhibited growth around each disk is recorded, sensitivity being directly related to zone size. The medium used for this test is especially prepared to support the growth of a wide range of pathogens and also to give clearly defined zones of inhibition with organisms sensitive to antibiotics and sulfonamides and other antimicrobial compounds. It is also free from substances inhibitory to antibiotics and antimicrobial compounds. This, in the case of sulfonamides, can be ensured by the inclusion of 5–10% lysed blood.

The density of the inoculum should be such as to produce discrete colonies. Usually, approximately 0.1 ml of a 1-to-10 dilution of a 24-hour broth culture of the strain to be tested is satisfactory when spread evenly over the surface of a standard, 9-cm-diameter plate of culture medium. A heavier inoculation may give a false suggestion of resistance.

The antibiotic sensitivity disks are usually applied in the form of filter paper disks with six or eight projecting arms, the tips of which are impregnated with different antibiotics. These are available commercially with different ranges and concentrations of antibiotics and antimicrobial compounds.

References

Burr, E. W. 1982. *Diseases of Parrots.* Neptune, N.J.: T.F.H. Publications.

Cooper, J. E. 1978. *Veterinary Aspects of Captive Birds of Prey.* Saul, Gloucestershire, Engl.: Standfast Press.

Dolphin, R. E., and D. E. Olsen. 1977. Antibiotic therapy in cage birds for pathogenic bacteria detected by fecal culture technique. *Vet. Med. Small Anim. Clin.* 72:1504–7.

Garrod, L. P., H. P. Lambert, and F. O'Grady. 1981. *Antibiotics and Chemotherapy.* 5th ed. London: Churchill, Livingstone.

Graham-Jones, O. 1961. Administering medicine to small birds. *Vet. Rec.* 73:331–32.

Kirkwood, J. K. 1983a. Dosing exotic species. *Vet. Rec.* 112:486–87.

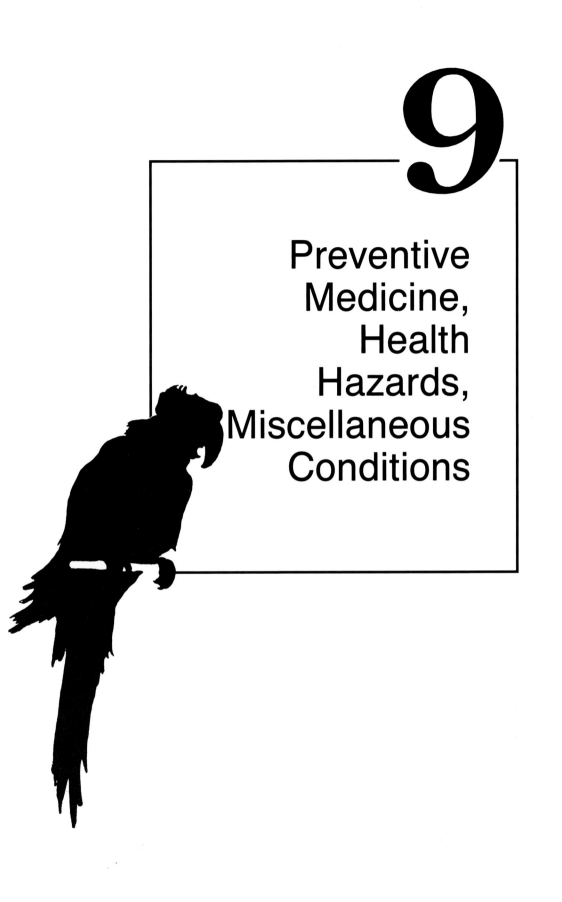

9

Preventive Medicine, Health Hazards, Miscellaneous Conditions

30

Quarantine and Isolation

PAUL T. GILCHRIST

THE CLASSIC CONCEPT of 40 days isolation for prevention of human disease such as plague gave the form of isolation called "quarantine" its name (from the Italian "quarantina" or the French "quarante," meaning "forty"). If a bird is in the incubation stage of a disease, keeping it in isolation for 2–3 weeks allows clinical symptoms to develop. A quarantine of 40 days is ideal but is probably unnecessarily long.

When new birds are brought into an established cage or aviary, there is always a danger of the introduction of undesirable genes or infectious disease agents. A quarantine system should be able to provide, at a reasonable cost, a facility that will exclude the most important diseases and also reduce the risk of other diseases although quarantine is never foolproof. Some methods of implementing quarantine are described in this chapter.

Planning

Location. Quarantine planning begins with choosing the location of the unit. Isolation and security of a unit by distance improves the chance of disease freedom.

Transmission. Quarantine facilities should always have wire or slatted floors because separation of birds from their feces minimizes disease transmission.

In planning the conditions of isolation or the precautions to be taken with the introduction of birds (or eggs), consideration must be given to two types of transmitted conditions:

1. Vertically transmitted conditions
   a. Undesirable genes
   b. Infectious agents carried inside the egg
2. Horizontally (or laterally) transmitted conditions
   a. Eggshell contamination
   b. Contamination of the environment with infected exudates, feces, or expired air
   c. Direct contact with infected birds

Isolation. Planning involves isolation between age groups, different sources, and different species. Isolation may be achieved by physical barriers such as birdproofing, ventilation control, air filtration, and distance or by separation time. Separation time may be associated with procedures for checking clinical signs, laboratory tests, and/or transmission tests.

Risk. A decision about the acceptable level of risk (cost-benefit evaluation) is based on the value of the stock, the severity of potential diseases, and the cost of precautions.

Following are the three disease classifications for quarantine purposes:

1. Those diseases expected to produce clinical signs in the species of bird being introduced
2. Those diseases that produce no signs in the introduced species but, if carried, could be dangerous to other species
3. "Unknown" diseases

Treatment. Quarantine planning should take into account the possibility of eliminating disease by vaccination or medication.

Principles of Quarantine. There are four main principles of quarantining birds:

1. Import healthy birds from a clean source. Provide clean handling, transport, and quarantine facilities.
2. Check for diseases. Carry out a clinical examination and tests on feces, serum, etc.
3. Provide a surveillance period at the source and quarantine at the destination.
4. Give preference to transferring eggs. The second choice is very young birds that have been reared in isolation, the third choice, older adults that may have developed immunity.

The ideal duration of surveillance at the source and in quarantine is hard to define, but most authorities agree that 21 days is the minimum, with 30 days desirable. Separate facilities, utensils, and personnel, if possible, should be used for each shipment.

A clear policy on action to be taken in the event of discovery of a disease must be established in advance to avoid the need for decision making under crisis.

Conditions for Introduction.

It is not possible to prescribe conditions for every type of introduction, but several isolation and quarantine considerations are discussed in this section.

Household Pets. Isolated pet birds are more likely to be free from disease but may have a low immunity due to lack of exposure to local pathogens. Introduced birds, especially if from a large flock or a pet shop, are more likely to be infected and infectious. Birds from a small breeder may be inbred and more susceptible to disease. Professional advice is helpful in determining the feasibility of importing new birds.

Avicultural Hobbyists. These clients usually have birds of great sentimental and/or financial value. Part of the attraction of the hobby is the acquisition of new varieties and species of birds. When new birds are introduced, disease problems are inevitable. Built-in quarantine facilities for isolation of sick birds is essential to the conduct of a successful enterprise.

Aviculture Industry. The industry is built around dealing in birds. A dealer who is conscious of health problems can minimize risk of infection by reducing the frequency of contact between groups of birds. Arranging a direct supply of birds is the best method of reducing contact but is often impractical due to housing requirements and distribution. The dealer can reduce disease risk, however, by separating species, age groups, and birds from different sources.

National Quarantine. The main objective of a national quarantine for imported birds is to prevent the spread of infectious diseases to the poultry industry, rather than the protection of pet birds. For this reason, as well as the high cost of effective quarantine procedures, there is a strong incentive for smuggling. Unfortunately such unscrupulous conduct can be disastrous for both poultry and pet birds, for example, by introducing diseases such as Newcastle disease and avian influenza. Any country that has remained free from or has gained control over certain diseases strives to prevent disease introduction. However, an attempt on the part of quarantine authorities to prevent the introduction of a long list of diseases is less likely to succeed; the only alternative may then be to prohibit introduction of all birds.

When calculating the potential benefit from the cost or risk involved, many considerations must be taken into account. What is the danger of smuggling? How severe would an outbreak of imported disease be? What are the natural means of disease spread? What degree of risk is acceptable? How many diseases are to be excluded?

The authorities must prepare a set of acceptable conditions for the following factors:

1. An acceptable source
   a. Reliability of veterinary services of the country of origin
   b. Disease status of the country or region of origin
   c. Disease status of the aviary or flock of origin
   d. Availability of isolation facilities and test procedures
2. Acceptable transport arrangements
   a. Secure transport
   b. Protection from infection during transit
3. Quarantine at destination
   a. Isolation (mechanical or by distance)
   b. Testing
   c. Duration of quarantine period
   d. Size of facility
   e. Frequency of importation

Clinical Examination. A physical and fecal examination is a minimum requirement in a clinical examination. A repeat examination by the veterinarian at the end of the isolation period is also recommended. Some diseases are apparent on clinical examination, others are likely to become apparent only after a few weeks in quarantine, and still others with a lengthy incubation period may show up after a long time or be latent until the bird suffers from stress. Carrier birds can also pose a risk to exposed birds and aviaries.

Individual Pets. Isolation of an introduced pet must be tailored to individual circumstances. Separate air space is needed; adjoining rooms are not good enough. A detached shed or garage is usually adequate. Protecting the existing flock is the objective in designing a quarantine plan. Prevailing winds and the work-flow pattern of the owner should determine the movements from the existing aviary to the quarantine area. The client must be instructed to feed and care for the new bird after caring for the resident birds. Hands and implements should be cleaned immediately so the following day's care is started clean.

The veterinarian must be aware of the disease status of the client's flock so that local diseases transmitted to the quarantine area and diseases imported with the bird are determined.

Multiple Birds. Large quarantine stations are designed with the assumption that birds and eggs may be infected with disease. In such large units, negative pressure is used to ensure that leakage of air will not push imported organisms into the external atmosphere. Negative pressure ventilation and filters are required on both the inlet (to prevent local infections getting in) and the outlet (to keep imported organisms within the unit). Such a facility is expensive, especially if high-tolerance filtration is required. The quality of the facility depends on an evaluation of the risk of infection passing the barrier. The minimum requirement for a commercial quarantine station is a filtered-air, positive-pressure house.

Positive-pressure ventilation means that the internal pressure is higher than the outside atmospheric pressure, thus making it unlikely that a disease would gain entry but not stopping the escape of disease agents. If a low level of filtration is accepted, the location of the facility remote from possible disease in commercial or wild birds should be considered.

Secondary Quarantine. Suggestions are sometimes made to keep birds or their progeny in isolated situations after recommended quarantine times. Quarantine provisions should be designed to give as much security as needed and not be an unnecessary burden to the bird owner.

Frequency and Number of Imports. A well-isolated country might be able to require a very strict quarantine: small numbers of birds imported into a high-security facility and held for a long duration, with many tests carried out.

But when the number of importations is large and the risk of smuggling high, practical circumstances may limit quarantine conditions to an elementary level. Extensive land borders and a preexisting liberal policy on quarantine are other factors that favor minimal quarantine conditions. Such a country might require 30 days holding in an owner-operated quarantine facility subject to government surveillance. Clinical observation or serological testing for Newcastle disease is a minimum condition.

Policy for Action. The veterinarian should prepare in advance a policy recommendation for the client that specifies the action to be taken in the event of an occurrence of any particular disease. Examples of such policy options follow:

1. Kill the birds in quarantine (for birds with Newcastle disease, avian influenza, Pache-co's parrot disease, or chlamydiosis)
2. Return affected birds to source (for cripples and birds with tumors, injuries, or other noninfectious conditions)
3. Treat the birds in quarantine (for birds with parasites, pox, or enteritis)
4. Extend the quarantine period (for birds with depression or nasal or ocular discharges or for any suspicious circumstances not ascribed to a definite cause)

Treatment in Quarantine. Medication or vaccination while in quarantine is common.

The principal reason for a quarantine period in isolation is to prohibit disease, particularly from new or imported birds. Although this period is not primarily an opportunity to treat diseases, treatment can be undertaken at the same time. Because of the public health hazard of chlamydial infection, prophylactic treatment is carried out in quarantine. A 45-day course of oral tetracyclines is essential in quarantine stations to inhibit chlamydial infection in psittacines. Treatment starts at the beginning of the quarantine period and continues until the bird is introduced to its new premises. Care must be taken, because a treatment such as a broad-spectrum antibiotic (to control chlamydiosis) could mask the symptoms of salmonellal, pasteurellal, mycoplasmal, or other infections.

All parasitic infections should be treated in quarantine. A preventive regime of medication should span at least one life cycle. A period of 21–28 days covers most worms, mites, and insects, but a shorter period of 7–10 days may be all that is necessary for protozoa.

Tests. The duration of quarantine and type of tests required varies with the country, number of birds, species, significant diseases, and degrees of risk. All imported birds ideally should be serologically tested by the hemagglutination inhibition test for both Newcastle disease and avian influenza during the observation period at the source and again during quarantine.

Adults can be tested, kept 21–30 days for observation, and released after obtaining satisfactory results. If it is specified in the original conditions, birds that test positive can be rejected or killed.

Young birds do not develop normal immune mechanisms until 3 weeks of age. Tests can be carried out at 9 weeks of age and the birds observed for 3 weeks and released at 12 weeks of age. Testing at 9 weeks of age allows for an adequate safety margin for most imported diseases.

Source

Local Birds. A professional contract between the seller and buyer of pet birds helps both parties to find, solve, and prevent disease problems. Regular inspection of the premises and the birds helps establish disease patterns and the normal flock mortality rate. Salmonella, yersinia, and pasteurella infections and Newcastle disease, chlamydiosis, and Pacheco's parrot disease outbreaks should be known to the veterinarian in the area.

The source flock or aviary can be rated by the veterinarian on a number of points:

1. The degree of physical isolation from other aviaries and the physical and operational isolation within the aviary between various species and age groups
2. The stocking rate or population density (as crowding tends to encourage disease)
3. The general health and fitness of the whole aviary

Ideally, a number of individual birds should be caught and examined carefully. External parasites are likely to be found, but exudates from nostrils or eyes, mouth or foot lesions, physical deformities, and diarrhea must be noted. Body weight can be assessed or (preferably) the birds weighed.

Autopsy of any dead or sick birds is desirable.

Imported Birds. Ideally, the country or place of origin should be free from Newcastle disease and avian influenza for 12 months before shipment. For aviary birds, this condition is often difficult to meet as many desirable species come from high-risk countries. The establishment of enclosed, isolated facilities for preshipment observation and testing is a possibility in commercial importations.

Transport. The parents of the eggs or birds to be shipped should be housed in a filtered-air building during testing and isolation. Eggs for shipment should be fumigated with formalin vapor or other approved shell sanitizer as soon as possible after laying. A suitable fumigation procedure is described at the end of this chapter.

Disposable Isolation Unit. Birds for shipment should be housed in normal shipment containers, which are placed inside an impervious solid container with a slatted or perforated opening designed to hold a pad of filter material. This permits passive transmission of air and limits the chance of organisms gaining entry during shipment. Careful design is required to minimize the chance of puncture of the filter pad and occlusion of the airway. On arrival at the destination, the eggs or birds are removed from the shipping crate inside the quarantine facility.

The United States Department of Agriculture used the units in Fig. 30.1 during the 1972 Newcastle disease outbreak in Southern California to house chickens used in transmission experiments. This unit can be adapted for bird transport by using more durable materials. One adult hen or six chicks were housed in these units for up to 10 days.

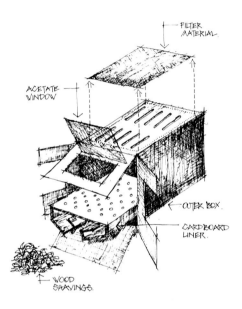
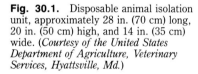

Fig. 30.1. Disposable animal isolation unit, approximately 28 in. (70 cm) long, 20 in. (50 cm) high, and 14 in. (35 cm) wide. (*Courtesy of the United States Department of Agriculture, Veterinary Services, Hyattsville, Md.*)

The filter material is the normal virus-proof type used in high-security virus containment laboratories. Masking tape secures all openings and edges. The filter material is also taped onto the top of the box over the ventilation holes.

Gravity-fed waterers and feeders with a small-area feeding aperture are needed. If birds are trained to drink from a suspended drop waterer, chances of survival are greater.

The design can be improved by using two buffers, as in chick transport boxes, to prevent material being placed over the filter and occluding the airway.

Fumigation of Eggs. Bacteria that are present on the eggshell can penetrate the egg as it cools. To reduce penetration, it is advisable to fumigate eggs as soon as they are collected, while they are still warm. The eggs should be collected in wire baskets or placed in plastic trays that will permit the fumigant to contact as much of the shell surface as possible.

To avoid recontamination of the eggs after fumigation, the eggs should be packed in fumigated trays and cases as soon as possible. Placing the trays of eggs in polyethylene bags provides the maximum protection from contamination.

Following are requirements for a fumigation cabinet:

1. Large enough to fumigate each collection of eggs while they are still warm
2. Slatted shelves to permit good air circulation
3. A heater to hold temperature at 75–100°F (23–38°C)
4. Two fans, one to circulate the fumigant in the cabinet and the other to expel the gas after fumigation
5. Water pans or other equipment to obtain a wet bulb reading of 68°F (20°C) or higher
6. A timer to ring an alarm after fumigation is complete and to activate the exhaust fan

The eggs should be fumigated for 20 minutes with a concentration of 1.5 ml formalin mixed with 1 g potassium permanganate/ft³ (0.1 m³) of space.

Egg trays and cases can be fumigated along with the eggs. If molded fiber trays are used for packing the eggs, they should be loosely packed in the fumigation cabinet so that the fumigant is in contact with the maximum amount of the tray surface.

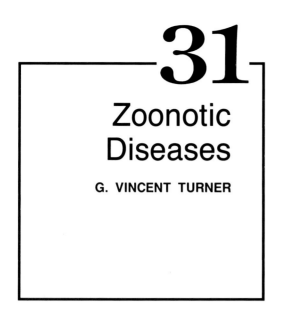

31

Zoonotic Diseases

G. VINCENT TURNER

MORE THAN 150 infections or diseases of domestic and wild avian species are potential threats to human health. Birds play an important role in many infectious and parasitic diseases of humans, acting as hosts or direct or intermediate vectors, or contaminating the environment with causative agents of diseases. A number of emerging zoonoses have added a new dimension to the study of the interrelationship of diseases and health in humans and birds. For example, *Campylobacter fetus* ssp. *jejuni* has only recently been recognized as an important cause of gastroenteritis in humans. As the extent of the occurrence of *C. fetus* ssp. *jejuni* in the intestines of animals became known, the problem was seen to rival and probably to exceed salmonellosis in terms of zoonotic implications (Doyle 1981; Prescott and Munroe 1982).

Although some zoonotic infections may have only minor clinical manifestations in humans, they are nevertheless of particular concern to the affected person. In certain instances zoonotic infections may be life-threatening and may even assume epidemic proportions. Disseminated, systemic zoonotic conditions are being diagnosed with increased frequency in people who have been rendered immunologically incompetent. With expanded knowledge of immune deficiency–type disorders, it is likely that certain zoonoses, especially the opportunistic infections, will be considered to be of greater public health importance. For example, since the medical community was alerted to the existence of an acquired immunodeficiency syndrome (AIDS) there has been an alarming increase in the number of cases documented (Anderson et al. 1983). The syndrome is often associated with severe, life-threatening, oppor-

tunistic zoonotic infections that in the past were associated only with obvious clinical disease in animals. Recently there has been a growing awareness of public health problems in birds, such as campylobacter, salmonella, and chlamydia infections (Bell and Palmer 1983).

Public education regarding the significance of zoonotic diseases is a responsibility of the veterinary profession. This chapter emphasizes the veterinary aspects of zoonotic diseases encountered in cage and aviary birds. Detailed descriptions of most of these diseases are found elsewhere in this book and in standard avian disease and zoonotic texts.

Epidemiology. The increased frequency with which pet birds are encountered in private practice makes it necessary for the practitioner to possess adequate knowledge of the diseases and conditions that may have zoonotic implications. Recent advances in epidemiological methods and diagnostic technology have contributed to the increased awareness of the potential zoonotic hazards in owning and caring for pet birds. Zoonoses may be acquired from association with pet birds or by working with infected birds in zoos, private aviaries, and breeding establishments. Rarely will a zoo patron or visitor to an aviary contract a disease (Fowler 1978). The zoonotic diseases manifest themselves in various ways in both birds and people. In general a client should be concerned if a new bird dies, other birds become sick, or a family member and a bird show similar signs of illness.

As the majority of the human population are urban dwellers, most people have little direct contact with animals other than pets. Most families keep one or more companion animals in their homes, 90% of them dogs, cats, or caged birds (English 1982). There are an estimated 40 million cage and aviary birds in the United States. It is generally accepted in Western society that companion animals make a significant contribution to improving the physical, mental, and emotional well-being of humans. The scientific credibility of the significance and beneficial effects of human-animal interrelations has received attention from health professionals only within the last decade. In particular, the human–companion animal bond and pet-facilitated therapy has been stimulating public and professional awareness and interest. The therapeutic use of companion animals in homes for the aged and in institutions such as prisons and facilities for the handicapped and mentally ill is gaining in importance. In this respect cage birds will play an increasingly important role in the future.

One of the major problems in diagnosing and implicating the source of zoonotic diseases in cage and aviary birds is that inapparent infections in otherwise healthy birds are common. Although birds are not a major source of zoonotic infections to humans, the list of zoonoses is continuously increasing and the potential hazards that accompany the ownership of pet birds should not be overlooked. In addition the risks can be even further reduced by the intelligent application of routine preventive measures.

Chlamydial Disease. Chlamydiosis, more commonly known as psittacosis or ornithosis, is possibly the most significant disease transmitted from cage and aviary birds to humans. The etiological agent, *Chlamydia psittaci,* has been isolated from 130 avian species. For all practical purposes all species of birds can be considered as potential reservoirs of chlamydiae (Keymer 1974; English 1982; Palmer 1982; Bell and Palmer 1983; Gough and Bevan 1983). Strains in amazon parrots are particularly virulent to humans. One particular laboratory that examined 101 parakeets and parrots recovered chlamydiae from 21 of 61 (34%) parakeets and 16 (40%) of 40 parrots (Schacter et al. 1978). Of considerable concern is the fact that most of these infections were associated with birds in the commercial flow of the pet bird industry. Avian chlamydiosis is principally an inapparent or latent infection, and it is therefore often difficult to determine the source of infection. In some areas an increase in the occurrence of chlamydiosis in pet birds has occurred, especially in psittacine birds (Panigrahy 1978a; Panigrahy et al. 1979; Palmer 1982). In humans the disease is regarded as being generally sporadic (Grimes and Panigrahy 1978; Acha and Szyfres 1980). However, a recent slight increase in the number of cases of chlamydiosis in humans has been noted (Gear 1975; Schacter et al. 1978). The disease reached epidemic proportions in Norway in 1980–1981.

Asymptomatic carriers and shedders of chlamydiae are the principal factors contributing to the transmission of the disease. Three possible modes of transmission of chlamydial agents from birds to humans are known. In order of importance, they are (1) inhalation of contaminated air; (2) direct contact with latently infected, sick, or dead birds and their feathers, feces, or oculonasal secretions; (3) bite wounds or other open skin wounds; and (4) handling of infected tissues during laboratory culture procedures (e.g., aerosols from grinding and emulsification) (Acha and Szyfres 1980; Eugster 1980).

The human respiratory tract is the most important route of entry of chlamydiae from inhalation of chlamydia-laden aerosols in a contaminated environment (Brayton et al. 1981). The source of the infective aerosols is nasal secretions and dried fecal material containing infectious organisms (Panigrahy et al. 1979; Bell and Palmer 1983). The oral route of transmission is an important means of spread in birds, but little is known in this regard concerning humans. It seems possible that the organisms might be swallowed after contamination of hands by an infected bird. Humans have never been known to contract chlamydial infection by eating infected meat or organs because chlamydiae are destroyed by heat. Although rare, person-to-person transmission has been reported (Grimes and Panigrahy 1978; Eugster 1980). Multiple cases in households have been frequently reported, but these have been mainly as a result of exposure to the same infected bird.

Human chlamydiosis should always be suspected in a patient with pneumonia who has had recent contact with a diseased or dead bird. The incubation period ranges from 1 to 4 weeks. Clinical symptomology varies greatly; many infections pass asymptomatically, while others are debilitating. Mild forms of psittacosis can be confused with common respiratory diseases and often pass unnoticed. The most serious form of the disease occurs in older persons. Nausea, vomiting, hepatitis, myocarditis, disorientation, mental depression, and even delirium may be present. Fatal cases have been recorded (Gear 1975; Acha and Szyfres 1980; Eugster 1980).

Bacterial Diseases

Salmonellosis. Salmonellosis is probably the most widespread zoonosis in the world. *Salmonella enteritidis* currently includes more than 1600 serotypes. All serotypes are potentially pathogenic to humans. Of the serotypes that infect birds, *S. typhimurium* is especially important (Williams 1980).

Birds are a common reservoir of salmonellosis, which may or may not manifest itself clinically (Komorowski and Hensley 1973; Fowler 1978; Panigrahy et al. 1979). The infection generally progresses asymptomatically. Clinical cases, especially in young birds, do occur (Schulze and Frede 1977; Williams 1980; Panigrahy and Gilmore 1983). In the subclinical form birds may become temporary or persistent carriers, shedding the agent continuously or intermittently in the feces (Acha and Szyfres 1980). With the increasing popularity of open aviaries and children's petting zoos, human salmonellosis acquired from wild animals could become a public health problem. For example, a recent outbreak of salmonellosis in an open zoo aviary was traced to the recent acquisition of a group of African Gray Parrots (Komorowski and Hensley 1973).

Humans generally acquire salmonellosis by eating contaminated food, but it can also be transmitted directly from animals to humans. Birds in close contact with humans can be the source of infection, especially in children where the bacteria is readily transmitted to a child's mouth (Williams 1980; Brayton et al. 1981). People handling infected birds can also contaminate their food. Salmonellosis of bird origin causes an intestinal infection in humans, characterized by an incubation period of 8–48 hours. The main symptoms are abdominal pains, nausea, vomiting, and diarrhea. Less commonly a localized infection can develop in any part of the body as a result of a bacteremia (Acha and Szyfres 1980).

Campylobacteriosis. Since 1977 *Campylobacter fetus* ssp. *jejuni* has become increasingly more important as a disease agent. The organism is now recognized as a major bacterial intestinal pathogen all over the world (Doyle 1981; Walder 1982). The rate of intestinal infection with *C. fetus* ssp. *jejuni* in healthy birds of all types is generally high. Information concerning campylobacteriosis has accumulated rapidly in recent years, but much remains to be learned, especially about its epidemiology. While the evidence that the infection is a cause of diarrhea in humans is convincing, the etiologic role of this organism in animals is not well established (Prescott and Munroe 1982; Symonds 1983). Further studies may determine the extent that campylobacteriosis occurs in birds and the role it plays in human infections.

The disease in humans equals or exceeds salmonellosis as a cause of bacterial diarrhea (Prescott and Munroe 1982). The mechanism of transmission of the infection from animals to humans is not clear. It is assumed that humans become infected by direct contact with infected birds or by consuming food or water contaminated with bird feces. Both food and water have been implicated as vehicles responsible for *C. fetus* ssp. *jejuni* infections. The oral route is regarded as the main mode of transmission for the disease. Based on circumstantial evidence it has been estimated that the incubation period ranges from 2 to 11 days (Doyle 1981; Symonds 1983). The disease in humans is usually characterized by moderate to severe diarrhea and is generally less acute and has a more prolonged course than salmonellosis. Protracted cases with relapses have been reported in small children. The severity of the illness varies considerably; mild cases are common, abdominal pain may persist for several days, and deaths have been reported in elderly or debilitated patients (Prescott and Munroe 1982; Walder 1982; Symonds 1983).

Avian Tuberculosis. Tuberculosis is fairly widespread in birds. *Mycobacterium avium* has been isolated from free-flying birds in captivity (Montali et al. 1976; Peavy et al. 1976; Thoen et al. 1977; Keymer et al. 1982). The incidence of avian tuberculosis reported at necropsy in zoos varies and may reach nearly 10% (Keymer et al. 1982). Clinically the disease is difficult to recognize because it tends to be chronic with a slow, insidious development during which few clinical signs appear. In a well-nourished and active bird, the illness may be completely subclinical (Peavy et al. 1976; Snyder 1979). The portal of entry of *M. avium* can either be inhalation of contaminated dust or the digestive tract (Acha and Szyfres 1980; Gough and Bevan 1983). The majority of infections follow ingestion of the organism. After natural infection, lesions are concentrated in the liver, spleen, intestines, and bone marrow rather than in the lungs. Similar infections can be induced experimentally by feeding cultures of the organisms to chickens (Falk et al. 1973). Recovery of the organisms from excreta beneath trees where starlings roosted and the association of infections in pigs with the presence of large numbers of starlings and rooks at feeding troughs supports the idea that wild birds form an important reservoir of the organisms.

Although little is known about the mechanisms of transmission of *M. avium* to humans, it is known to have caused disease primarily in patients with underlying chronic pulmonary disorders and in persons who are immunologically incompetent (Falk et al. 1973; Montali et al. 1976; Green et al. 1982; Anderson et al. 1983). Severe, life-threatening infections have been described in people with immune deficiency–type disorders. To the immunocompetent host the disease is usually of low virulence. The actual source of an infection caused by *M. avium* is usually inapparent. In one report four patients infected with *M. avium* had experienced occupational exposure to birds; other reports also indicate that bird-to-bird transmission takes place (Chapman 1980). Although human infections are rare, *M. avium* is a potential human pathogen and proper precautions should be instituted during necropsies or when handling infected birds.

Miscellaneous Bacterial Diseases. Other bacterial diseases, such as listeriosis and erysipelothrix infections, are common to humans and birds (Bowmer et al. 1980; Conklin and Steele

1980). Cage and aviary birds fortunately are not considered a primary source of infection to humans.

Viral Diseases

Arthropod-borne Viral Diseases. Numerous virus infections are biologically transmissible from animals to humans by arthropods. At present more than fifty of these types of viruses are known (Mayr 1980). Birds, even though they usually present no signs of disease when infected, play an important role in the epidemiology of some of these diseases. Birds are natural reservoirs for arthropod-borne viral diseases such as western and eastern equine encephalomyelitis; St. Louis, Japanese B, and Murray Valley encephalitis; and Sindbis and West Nile virus infections (Gear 1975). Humans can become accidental hosts when bitten by insects and are not involved in the basic cycle between birds and arthropods. Eastern equine encephalomyelitis virus can be transmitted directly from pheasant-to-pheasant by pecking (Kissling 1958). The possibility that a disease may be transmitted to humans mechanically (as among pheasants) should not be overlooked. However, the greatest risk to humans is through the bite of infected insects.

Newcastle Disease. Birds constitute the reservoir of the Newcastle disease virus. The velogenic viscerotropic virus has been repeatedly isolated in Europe and the United States from imported parrots and related birds (Pearson and McCann 1975; Acha and Szyfres 1980; Alexander et al. 1982). The disease is not very common in humans. Newcastle disease virus is spread by direct contact and aerosols. Cases can occur from handling or being in close proximity to infected birds. The clinical signs in humans consist essentially of conjunctivitis; there may also be subclinical signs.

Fungal Diseases

Histoplasmosis. *Histoplasma capsulatum* grows well in bird feces. Histoplasmosis is generally associated with soils in which there has been an accumulation of bat or bird droppings over a lengthy period (Acha and Szyfres 1980). Disturbance of such sites may release clouds of infectious spores (Ajello and Kaplan 1980). Human infection occurs almost entirely through inhalation of airborne spores; the lung is the site of primary infection (Goodwin and Des Prez 1978). Most human cases are asymptomatic. Only under very poor management conditions

do cage and aviary birds play a role in human infections.

Cutaneous Mycoses. Some of the different dermatophytes that have been isolated from the feathers and skin of cage birds are of zoonotic importance (Tudor 1983). Humans may contract dermatomycosis through direct or indirect contact with infected birds (Padhye 1980).

Parasitic Diseases

Mites. Inhalation of mite-laden dust frequently results in allergic respiratory disease. The northern fowl mite (*Ornithonyssus sylviarum*) has been shown to cause occupational asthma in poultry workers (Lutsky and Bar-Sela 1982). An infestation of this mite in a colony of Border Canaries has been recorded (Dodd 1983). In addition to allergic respiratory reactions, mites from birds may crawl onto bird handlers and cause a dermatitis.

Giardiasis. Infections with *Giardia* cause high morbidity and mortality in Budgerigars and parakeets (Panigrahy et al. 1978b, 1981). Healthy birds may acquire infection by ingestion of feed and water contaminated with the cysts. Giardiasis can be a serious problem in humans. There is no published report on human infection acquired from avian sources. However, the large number of organisms found in the intestines of pet birds with high morbidity and mortality leads one to consider possible public health implications.

Cryptosporidiosis. *Cryptosporidium* spp. are coccidian parasites usually regarded as opportunistic organisms infecting the gut of a variety of species of vertebrates. Recently *Cryptosporidium* has been associated with enteritis in calves and other mammalian species, including humans. Avian cryptosporidial infections have been reported in poultry, parrots, and quail (Tham 1982). Although human cryptosporidiosis has not been associated with avian sources, the zoonotic implications should not be overlooked.

Avian Allergens. An additional hazard associated with cage and aviary birds is that some people develop allergic reactions when exposed to avian allergens (Brayton et al. 1981). Nearly all pets are potentially allergenic, and birds are no exception. These allergies can be a major problem, especially in children.

References

Acha, N., and B. Szyfres. 1980. *Zoonoses and Communicable Diseases Common to Man and Animals.* Pan American Health Organization, Scientific Publication no. 354. Washington, D.C.

Ajello, L., and W. Kaplan. 1980. Systemic mycoses. In *CRC Handbook Series in Zoonoses,* ed. J. H. Steele. Boca Raton, Fla.: CRC Press.

Alexander, D. J., et al. 1982. Identification of paramyxoviruses isolated from birds in quarantine in Great Britain during 1980 to 1981. *Vet. Rec.* 111:571–74.

Anderson, R., et al. 1983. Immunological abnormalities in South African homosexual men. *S. Afr. Med. J.* 64:119–22.

Bell, J. C., and S. R. Palmer. 1983. Control of zoonoses in Britain: Past, present, and future. *Br. Med. J.* 287:591–93.

Bowmer, E. J., R. H. Conklin, and J. H. Steele. 1980. Listeriosis. In *CRC Handbook Series in Zoonoses,* ed. J. H. Steele. Boca Raton, Fla.: CRC Press.

Brayton, J. B., W. P. Coleman, and J. E. Johnson. 1981. Tracking down pet-associated diseases. *Patient Care* 15:18–66.

Chapman, J. S. 1980. Atypical mycobacteria. In *CRC Handbook Series in Zoonoses,* ed. J. H. Steele. Boca Raton, Fla.: CRC Press.

Conklin, R. H., and J. H. Steele. 1980. Erysipelothrix infections. In *CRC Handbook Series in Zoonoses,* ed. J. H. Steele. Boca Raton, Fla.: CRC Press.

Dodd, K. 1983. Northern mite (*Ornithonyssus sylviarum*) infestation in canaries. *Vet. Rec.* 113:259.

Doyle, M. P. 1981. *Campylobacter fetus* subsp. *jejuni:* An old pathogen of new concern. *J. Food Prot.* 44:480–88.

English, P. B. 1982. Zoonotic diseases transmitted by domestic companion animals in Australia. *Aust. Vet. Pract.* 12:68–73.

Eugster, A. K. 1980. Chlamydiosis. In *CRC Handbook Series in Zoonoses,* ed. J. H. Steele. Boca Raton, Fla.: CRC Press.

Falk, G. A., et al. 1973. *Mycobacterium avium* infections in man. *Am. J. Med.* 54:801–10.

Fowler, M. E. 1978. Infections and zoonotic diseases. In *Zoo and Wild Animal Medicine,* ed. M. E. Fowler. Philadelphia: W. B. Saunders.

Gear, J. H. S. 1975. Medical aspects of some zoonoses. *J. S. Afr. Vet. Assoc.* 46:221–25.

Goodwin, R. A., and R. M. Des Prez. 1978. Histoplasmosis. *Am. Rev. Respir. Dis.* 117:929–56.

Gough, R. E., and B. J. Bevan. 1983. Isolation and identification of *Chlamydia psittaci* from Collared Doves (*Streptopelia decaocta*). *Vet. Rec.* 112:552.

Greene, J. B., et al. 1982. *Mycobacterium avium intracellulare:* A cause of disseminated life-threatening infection in homosexuals and drug abusers. *Ann. Int. Med.* 97:539–46.

Grimes, J. E., and B. Panigrahy. 1978. Potential increase of chlamydiosis (psittacosis) in pet bird owners in Texas. *Texas Med.* 74:74–77.

Keymer, I. F. 1974. Ornithosis in free-living and captive birds. *Proc. R. Soc. Med.* 67:733–35.

Keymer, I. F., et al. 1982. A survey of tuberculosis in birds in the Regent's Park Gardens of the Zoological Society of London. *Avian Pathol.* 11:563–69.

Kissling, R. E. 1958. Eastern equine encephalomyelitis in pheasants. *J. Am. Vet. Med. Assoc.* 132:466–68.

Komorowski, R. A., and G. T. Hensley. 1973. Epizootic salmonellosis in an open zoo aviary. *Arch. Environ. Health* 27:110–11.

Lutsky, I., and S. Bar-Sela. 1982. Northern fowl mite (*Ornithonyssus sylviarum*) in occupational asthma of poultry workers. *Lancet* 2:874–75.

Mayr, A. 1980. New emerging viral zoonoses. *Vet. Rec.* 106:503–6.

Montali, R. J., et al. 1976. Tuberculosis in captive exotic birds. *J. Am. Vet. Med. Assoc.* 169:920–27.

Padhye, A. 1980. Cutaneous mycoses. In *CRC Handbook Series in Zoonoses,* ed. J. H. Steele. Boca Raton, Fla.: CRC Press.

Palmer, S. R. 1982. Psittacosis in man – Recent developments in the UK: A review. *J. R. Soc. Med.* 75:262–67.

Panigrahy, B., and W. C. Gilmore. 1983. Systemic salmonellosis in an African Gray Parrot and salmonella osteomyelitis in canaries. *J. Am. Vet. Med. Assoc.* 183:699–700.

Panigrahy, B., J. E. Grimes, and C. D. Brown. 1978a. Recent increase in incidence of chlamydiosis (psittacosis) in psittacine birds in Texas. *Avian Dis.* 22:806–8.

Panigrahy, B., et al. 1978b. Giardia infection in parakeets. *Avian Dis.* 22:815–18.

Panigrahy, B., et al. 1979. Zoonotic diseases in psittacine birds: Apparent increased occurrence of chlamydiosis (psittacosis), salmonellosis and giardiasis. *J. Am. Vet. Med. Assoc.* 175:359–61.

Panigrahy, B., et al. 1981. Unusual disease conditions in pet and aviary birds. *J. Am. Vet. Med. Assoc.* 178:394–95.

Pearson, G. L., and M. K. McCann. 1975. The role of indigenous wild, semidomestic, and exotic birds in the epizootiology of velogenic viscerotropic Newcastle disease in Southern California, 1972–1973. *J. Am. Vet. Med. Assoc.* 167:610–14.

Peavy, G. M., et al. 1976. Pulmonary tuberculosis in a Sulphur-crested Cockatoo. *J. Am. Vet. Med. Assoc.* 169:915–19.

Prescott, J. F., and D. L. Munroe. 1982. *Campylobacter jejuni* enteritis in man and domestic animals. *J. Am. Vet. Med. Assoc.* 181:1524–30.

Schacter, J., N. Sugg, and M. Sung. 1978. Psittacosis: The reservoir persists. *J. Inf. Dis.* 137:44–49.

Schulze, K., and H. Frede. 1977. Enzootic salmonelloses and mycoses in imported African Gray Parrots. *Kleintier-Praxis* 22:129–76.

Snyder, G. M. 1979. Tuberculosis and chronic demyelinating encephalitis in a parrot. *Mod. Vet. Pract.* 60:466–68.

Symonds, J. 1983. Campylobacter enteritis in the community. *Br. Med. J.* 286:243–44.

Tham, V. L., S. Kniesberg, and B. R. Dixon. 1982. Cryptosporidiosis in quails. *Avian Pathol.* 11:619–26.

Thoen, C. O., W. D. Richards, and J. L. Jarnagin. 1977. Mycobacteria isolated from exotic animals. *J. Am. Vet. Med. Assoc.* 170:987–90.

Tudor, D. C. 1983. Mycotic infection of feathers as the cause of feather-pulling in pigeons and psittacine birds. *Vet. Med. Small Anim. Clin.* 78:249–53.

Walder, M. 1982. Epidemiology of campylobacter enteritis. *Scand. J. Inf. Dis.* 14:27–33.

Williams, L. P. 1980. Salmonellosis. In *CRC Handbook Series in Zoonoses,* ed. J. H. Steele. Boca Raton, Fla.: CRC Press.

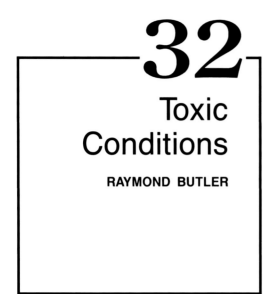

32

Toxic Conditions

RAYMOND BUTLER

THE DIFFICULTIES encountered by the practitioner trying to establish a diagnosis of toxicity in avian patients are well known. For a correct diagnosis, a comprehensive history of the patient, its environment, diet, and behavior, must be compiled.

An antemortem diagnosis of toxicity can often be made after a few well-chosen questions have been asked of the patient's owner. For instance, the veterinarian must establish the type and source of food the bird has been eating, whether any chemicals or volatile compounds have been used or applied to surfaces in the patient's immediate vicinity, whether there was adequate ventilation in the bird's environment, and what materials were used in the cage (including paint).

Detection of toxins at necropsy is often difficult or unsuccessful, particularly when small species such as finches, canaries, and Budgerigars are involved. The amount of toxic compound ingested, inhaled, or absorbed through the skin is often so minuscule that even the most sensitive laboratory tests have difficulty in detecting it in tissues or gastrointestinal contents.

Toxins from Food

Mycotoxins. The toxin produced by the fungus *Aspergillus flavus,* known as aflatoxin, may be found in cereal grains, peanuts or groundnuts, and moldy bread (Hungerford 1969; Feldman and Kruckenberg 1975). Storing grain and nuts in poor conditions (high temperature and humidity) is likely to favor the growth of the fungus.

After ingestion of aflatoxins, birds may show clinical signs of diarrhea, incoordination, depression, and anorexia. In acute poisoning

birds may die without showing any clinical manifestations.

Aflatoxin is hepatocarcinogenic when small amounts are consumed over a period of time. It also affects the hepatocyte's ability to metabolize fats. In birds intoxication is usually acute and fatal. At necropsy livers are seen to be enlarged, often showing hemorrhagic foci, necrosis, cirrhosis, and fatty infiltration. Diagnosis is difficult to make from clinical signs but can be made from demonstration of the toxin in the food, crop, or gizzard contents.

There is no specific treatment for aflatoxicosis, but supportive treatment with subcutaneous or intramuscular isotonic electrolyte solutions (1.0–1.5 ml/100 g body weight) and housing the bird in a quiet, warm environment (84–86°F, or 29–30°C) may help.

Birds should never be fed any grain or other food that shows signs of spoilage or fungal contamination. Spoiled food should be discarded and the containers cleaned well with antifungal disinfectants and dried before being used again.

Other mycotoxins produced by organisms such as *Penicillium* spp., *Claviceps* spp., and other *Aspergillus* spp. have not been reported to be important in companion birds.

(See Chapter 16 for other causes of aflatoxicosis.)

Botulin. The anaerobic organism *Clostridium botulinum* proliferates in moist, warm environments that have a high organic load (rotting animal carcasses, ponds with a high population of water birds and not much water flowing through). If food and feces are able to accumulate in such areas *Cl. botulinum* will multiply rapidly and produce one of the most potent natural toxins known.

Caged birds rarely have access to the sources of botulism that waterfowl and free-ranging domesticated species have. Omnivorous, insectivorous, and carnivorous species may ingest toxin either from the flesh of decaying animals or from maggots feeding on the flesh. Carnivorous birds (e.g., the raptors) seem to be less susceptible to the effects of the toxin.

Clinical signs result from the neurotoxic effects on the central nervous system. Muscular weakness is seen, first drooping of the head, neck, and wings; then inability to fly or walk; and finally complete paralysis. Mildly affected birds may show trembling and muscular spasms, particularly when stimulated.

Treatment can be effective if commenced early. Antitoxin, preferably administered intravenously (intramuscular injections are effective in some cases), has been helpful in larger species when continued over several days.

Type-C toxin is usually encountered in birds, so the specific type-C antitoxin should be used.

Removal of the remaining toxin from the gastrointestinal tract improves the patient's chances of survival. Mild doses of laxatives (Epsom salts or senna in weak solution) will empty the intestine. Absorbent substances following laxative treatment (chalk, charcoal, aluminium hydroxide) will help absorb any remaining toxin (Arnall and Keymer 1975).

Preventing botulism can be achieved by not allowing species at risk to consume food that may be contaminated (e.g., decaying carcasses). If waterfowl ponds are silted up with organic matter, they can be flushed out with fresh water or the silt can be removed manually.

Plants. Many outdoor and indoor ornamental plants may be toxic to hungry or inexperienced birds. Privet, wisteria, azalea, nightshade, marshmallow, castor-oil plant, and philodendron, to name a few of those more commonly grown, have been responsible for poisonings. Such plants should not be in the environment of free-flying companion birds.

Clinical signs of intoxication from most of these plants are related to nervous system disturbances (both central and autonomic) or gastrointestinal upsets such as regurgitation and diarrhea.

Treatment may be symptomatic or supportive, but specific antidotes for most plant poisonings are not of value in small birds.

Sodium Chloride. Salt poisoning can occur when salt levels of over 3% in solid food and 0.5% in drinking water (Arnall and Keymer 1975) are consumed by birds.

Symptoms include polydipsia, incoordination, loose droppings, dyspnea, and pulmonary edema.

If a diagnosis of salt poisoning is made, parenteral diuretics and access to fresh water may help dilute the salt concentration in the body.

Insecticides. The great diversity and widespread agricultural and domestic use of halogenated hydrocarbon, organophosphate, and similar compounds have created special problems in relation to food and environmental contamination of companion birds. All these compounds must be considered toxic for birds, although there are significant differences among them in lethal dose. As well as being lipotropic, most are cumulative poisons, so birds exposed to these chemicals store them in body fat depots. If for any reason fat depots are mobilized (by starvation, nonspecific stress, infections),

sufficient poison may be released into the bloodstream to cause clinical toxicity, even in apparently healthy birds having no history of recent contact with such chemicals.

Household aerosol insecticides are usually the less-toxic synthetic pyrethrins, but even these can be dangerous if used in the environments of the smaller varieties of caged domestic birds.

Agricultural insecticides usually belong to the more dangerous and longer-lasting organophosphate compounds or the halogenated hydrocarbon compounds. As these compounds are soluble in fats and fat solvents but not in water, they are more toxic when prepared in oily solutions or emulsions. Absorption from the gut is poor, but absorption of oily solutions (or as in the case of dieldrin, a dry powder) can occur through the intact skin (Papworth 1967).

The chlorinated hydrocarbons (DDT, dieldrin, gammexane, lindane, heptachlor) tend to produce stimulation of the nervous system that is seen as neuromuscular excitation.

Clinical signs include twitching, apprehension, incoordination, convulsions, and respiratory paralysis. These signs usually occur rapidly (12–24 hours after exposure) in affected caged birds; the time of onset is often dose related.

Treatment, when a diagnosis can be made from either clinical signs or history, should be directed at preventing the neuromuscular stimulation and removing the source of poison. If exposure has been cutaneous, water and mild detergent may remove residual toxin from the animal. If poisoning is by ingestion, syringe evacuation of the crop may remove residual poison.

Central nervous system depressants are used to counteract the stimulant effects of the chlorinated hydrocarbons. Nonirritant barbiturates, such as sodium pentobarbitone at 2.0–4.0 mg/100 g body weight injected intramuscularly as required, counter muscular spasms and convulsions. For best results, patients must be kept warm, preferably wrapped in a soft cloth and kept in an oxygen-rich environment.

The organophosphorous compounds (dimpylate, malathion, parathion, dichlorvos) exert their toxic effects through an ability to inhibit the enzyme cholinesterase. Acetylcholine is hydrolyzed by cholinesterase at nerve end plates, and so further passage of the nerve impulse is prevented. Acetylcholine is only present momentarily during the normal passage of an impulse, so if cholinesterase is not available to hydrolyze acetylcholine, impulses continue to pass along the nerve. Thus the toxic effects of the organophosphates are manifested as constant stimulation of the nervous system, particularly of the parasympathetic system.

The gastrointestinal tract is affected most noticeably. Intestinal hypermobility (vomiting, diarrhea), salivation, lacrimation, muscular twitching, and dyspnea due to bronchial secretion and spasm are often seen.

Many of these compounds are absorbed through intact skin as well as through the gastrointestinal and respiratory tracts. It is rare for these dangerous organophosphates to be used deliberately around companion birds. A possible source of contamination, however, is from insecticidal preparations used on domestic mammals for flea control.

Atropine is the specific antidote for organophosphate poisoning. Intravenous, intramuscular, or subcutaneous injection of atropine sulfate at 0.01–0.02 mg/100 g body weight every 1–2 hours reverses the effects of most organophosphates.

If these compounds are to be used in the environments of companion birds, adequate ventilation must be ensured. Dichlorvos pest strips should never be positioned close to caged birds, unless for a specific therapeutic purpose, such as cnemidocoptic mite treatment.

Other insecticidal preparations that are potentially toxic if used unwisely are the topical miticides. Gamma benzene hexachloride (0.1%) and benzyl benzoate (3%) can kill birds if applied too often to affected skin.

There are no specific treatments for birds poisoned by these compounds. Often they are found dead without exhibiting any clinical signs of toxicity.

Rodenticides.
Rodenticides do not pose much of a threat to companion birds unless the compounds are unwisely placed where birds may have access to them for long periods.

Anticoagulants such as warfarin are most commonly used, and most birds seem to have a fairly high tolerance to such compounds. Treatment with vitamin K or its analogues may be effective in treating warfarin poisoning when given intramuscularly. Dose rates are empirical, but a low rate of 0.01 mg/100 g body weight is effective.

Birdseed saturated with arsenic or strychnine was used as a rodenticide before the advent of the anticoagulant preparations. Such preparations are rarely used today.

Arsenical compounds have also been used as herbicides, ant poisons, and food additives and in paints and in certain medicinal preparations. Clinical signs of poisoning are mainly seen as gastrointestinal tract disturbances (vomiting, diarrhea, and anorexia). As treatment of arsenic poisoning in companion birds is of little value, such compounds should not be used in the birds'

environments.

Poisoning with strychnine usually results in neuromuscular disturbances. Muscular spasms, twitching, and respiratory failure may be seen prior to death. Again, preventing access of birds to the compound is essential. A low success rate has been claimed by treatment with methocarbamol at 14.9 mg/100 g body weight (Feldman and Kruckenberg 1975).

Miscellaneous Household Toxins. Alcohol may cause fatal toxicity in household pet birds such as Budgerigars. Birds readily drink alcoholic beverages while perching on the edge of a glass. Intoxication occurs rapidly, and signs of depression, ataxia, vomiting, and looseness of droppings are seen. Supportive treatment consisting of warmth, rest, and parenteral electrolytes may help.

Cases of nicotine poisoning from the consumption of cigarette butts or loose tobacco have been fatal. Clinical signs of weakness and depression lead to death within a short time of ingestion. No specific treatment can be offered except that the patient be kept warm and hydrated and the crop contents aspirated to remove residual nicotine.

Household cleaning products containing volatile solvents, alcohol, or hydrocarbon propellants (from aerosol cans) can be extremely toxic to small birds if inhaled. Death after exposure can be rapid with no obvious clinical signs of intoxication.

Strong disinfectant preparations (Lysol, caustic compounds, undiluted quaternary ammonium compounds) can cause severe skin burns. Care must be exercised in their use in domestic birds' environments. If used for routine cleaning of perches and cages, such compounds must be thoroughly rinsed off before the birds are replaced.

When signs of irritation are seen, the toxic substance should be thoroughly rinsed from the skin with water. For alkaline substances, mild acids (vinegar, acetic acid) can be used. Egg white or olive oil may be used as demulcents to sooth irritated membranes (Feldman and Kruckenberg 1975).

Domestic cooking gas is toxic to small birds, as are the products of gas combustion. Such pets should never be placed near gas-burning appliances.

Fumes emitted from heated polytetrafluoroethylene (nonstick) coatings on pans have been reported to cause pulmonary hemorrhage and congestion in Budgerigars (Wells et al. 1982). In fact, any compound that produces acrid or irritant products upon burning, even cooking oil, is potentially dangerous to household pet birds, as their tolerance to such compounds is low.

Treatment of suspected inhaled toxins consists of removing the patient from the source of toxin and/or ventilating the environment with fresh air. To reduce damage to irritated mucous membranes, if possible the patient should be placed in an environment where temperature, oxygen concentration, and humidity can be controlled.

Metals. The effects of heavy metal poisoning in waterfowl and other free-flying captive and wild birds are well documented (Jannsen et al. 1979; Redig et al. 1980; Elvestad et al. 1982; Kendall and Driver 1982; Locke et al. 1982; Reece and Hudson 1982; Lindsay and Dimmick 1983; Viet et al. 1983). Poisonings with metals such as lead and zinc occur in companion birds as a result of poor husbandry. Paints that contain lead, the galvanizing on some types of wire mesh, and the solder used in some welded bird meshes are all possible sources of toxic heavy metals (Butler 1981). Mercury compounds, which are often used as preservatives for stored seed grains, are toxic if consumed. Treated grains should never be fed to birds.

Clinical signs of heavy metal poisoning are usually nonspecific. A variety of presenting signs may be seen and are mainly related to gastrointestinal tract disturbances, with liver and kidney degeneration causing secondary effects. Neurological signs may show as incoordination, seizures or convulsions, and depression. Ingested lead or zinc particles may be observed in the gizzard upon radiographic examination.

Treatment for chronic lead poisoning with calcium EDTA (as in mammals) may be effective in companion birds. Intramuscular injections at 3 mg/100 g twice daily, along with removal of the lead source from the gut, is effective in some patients.

Liver lead levels of 10 ppm are considered significant at necropsy.

Iatrogenic Toxicities. Many drugs used prophylactically and therapeutically can be extremely toxic to companion birds. Not only are some drugs toxic; often the pain and trauma to tissues associated with intramuscular injection, in particular, can cause death from acute shock.

Oily injectable preparations appear to cause more adverse reactions than water-soluble preparations. For example, intramuscular injection of oxytetracycline in oily suspension has been known to kill smaller species of caged birds within seconds postinjection.

Procaine, lidocaine, procaine penicillin, streptomycin, and dihydrostreptomycin are toxic to small birds, particularly if given in high concentrations and high dose rates (Feldman and Kruckenberg 1975). Injectable drugs (the usual mammalian preparations) are best given in diluted form. Total volumes injected should be carefully monitored. The smaller psittacines and passeriforms should not be given more than 0.05 ml by injection in a single site. Larger volumes in species such as finches, canaries, and Budgerigars often result in sudden death from pain and acute shock.

Many anthelmintics are toxic to various species. Administration must be carefully controlled, but this is often difficult when drugs are given in food or water. There is a great range of species responses to the commonly used anthelmintics. For instance, levamisole phosphate administered intramuscularly to Peach-faced Lovebirds (*Agapornis roseicollis*) at 6.6 mg/100 g body weight killed birds, whereas no toxic effects were noted at 4.4 mg/100 g. In the same trial, rock doves (*Columba livia*) showed ataxia at 6.6 mg/100 g, but deaths did not result until the dose rate was increased to 11.0 mg/100 g (Robinson and Richter 1977). The author has found that Hooded Parrots (*Psephotus dissimilis*) showed central nervous system signs (ataxia, weakness, inability to stand) after subcutaneous injection with an 18.8 mg/ml solution of levamisole phosphate. They recovered completely after 1.5 hours. However, a closely related species, Golden-shouldered Parrots (*P. chrysopterygius*) showed no ill effects after subcutaneous injection with the same dose rate. Oral dosing with the same drug to Red-rumped Parrots (*P. haematonotus*) at 6 mg/100 g caused no ill effects, while deaths occurred when the drug was administered at the rate of 10 mg/100 g. Fenbendazole has been used as a broad-spectrum anthelmintic in psittacines orally for 3 days at rates varying from 2.8 mg/100 g to 5.6 mg/100 g (Harrigan 1981). However, at 1 mg/ml drinking water for 5 days, fenbendazole has been found to be toxic to California Quail (*Lophortyx californica*) and certain finch species.

Whenever an untried therapeutic drug is used in caged birds, extreme caution should be exercised in the method and rate of administration.

Anesthetics, whether injectable or inhalant, are lethal if dose rates are not carefully computed and monitored. The newer inhalant volatile liquid agents, such as halothane and methoxyflurane, are much safer than ether and chloroform. Patient monitoring is most important when general anesthetics are used.

Injectable agents, such as ketamine hydrochloride and the steroid combination alphaxalone/alphadolone acetate, are safe if injected slowly intravenously but can be rapidly fatal if high dose rates are given. If overdose is suspected, positive-pressure ventilation with pure oxygen and provision of a warm environment are the most important supportive measures.

General Principles for Treating Suspected Toxicities

1. Keep the bird restrained (wrapped in a towel or soft cloth) and warm. Maintain environmental temperature around 86°F (30°C).
2. Maintain the patient in an oxygen-rich atmosphere and turn it from side to side regularly.
3. Remove any residual toxin, either from the integument or the gastrointestinal tract. If exposure has been cutaneous, wash the bird in mild soapy water, then keep it dry and warm. If the toxin has been ingested evacuate the crop by syringe to remove any remaining material. Remove any toxin left in the bird's environment.
4. Electrolytes injected intramuscularly or subcutaneously are of great help. In some cases fluids can be given intraperitoneally, adjacent to the cloaca, although care should be taken not to insert the needle too deeply and so enter the abdominal air sacs. Hartmann's solution, standard maintenance fluid, or normal saline are all tolerated well. A dose rate of 1 ml/100 g body weight is adequate to support a debilitated bird. The subcutaneous route dorsally between the shoulders is a safe method to supply electrolyte solutions. If the intramuscular route is used, several injection sites should be chosen to avoid shock reactions.
5. Owner education is an important factor in reducing the incidence of poisoning in pet birds. Owners should be made aware that their pets require only very small amounts of what are often considered "nontoxic" household products to make them ill or kill them.

References

Arnall, L., and I. F. Keymer. 1975. *Bird Diseases: An Introduction to the Study of Birds in Health and Disease.* Neptune, N.J.: T.F.H. Publications.

Butler, R. 1981. Aviary: Problems of management in aviary and caged birds. In *Refresher Course for Veterinarians on Aviary and Caged Birds,* pp. 463–69. University of Sydney, Post-Graduate Committee in Veterinary Science, Proceedings no. 55. Sydney, Aust.

Elvestad, K., O. Karolog, and B. Clausen. 1982. Heavy metals (copper, cadmium, lead, mercury) in Mute Swans from Denmark. *Nord. Vetmed.* 34(3):92–97.

Feldman, B. F., and S. M. Kruckenberg. 1975. Clinical toxicities of domestic and wild caged birds. *Vet. Clin. N. Am.* 5(4):653–73.

Harrigan, K. E. 1981. Bird parasitism in aviary and caged birds. In *Refresher Course for Veterinarians on Aviary and Caged Birds,* pp. 337–96. University of Sydney, Post-Graduate Committee in Veterinary Science, Proceedings no. 55. Sydney, Aust.

Hungerford, T. G. 1969. *Diseases of Poultry, Including Cage Birds and Pigeons.* 4th ed. Sydney, Aust.: Angus and Robertson.

Jannsen, D. L., P. T. Robinson, and P. K. Ensley. 1979. Lead toxicosis in three captive avian species. *Proc. Am. Assoc. Zoo Vet.,* pp. 40–42.

Kendall, R. J., and C. J. Driver. 1982. Lead poisoning in swans in Washington State. *J. Wildl. Dis.* 18(3):385–87.

Lindsay, R. C., and W. Dimmick. 1983. Mercury residues in Wood Ducks and Wood Duck foods in eastern Tennessee. *J. Wildl. Dis.* 19(2):114–17.

Locke, L. N., S. M. Kerr, and D. Zoromski. 1982. Lead poisoning in Common Loons (*Gavia immer*). *Avian Dis.* 26(2):392–96.

Papworth, D. S. 1967. Organic compounds (II) pesticides. In *Garner's Veterinary Toxicology,* 3d ed. London: Baillière, Tindall and Casselle.

Redig, P. T., C. M. Stoeve, D. M. Barnes, and T. D. Arent. 1980. Lead toxicosis in raptors. *J. Am. Vet. Med. Assoc.* 177(9):941–43.

Reece, R. L., and P. Hudson. 1982. Observations on the accidental poisoning of birds by organophosphate insecticides and other toxic substances. *Vet. Rec.* 111(20):453–55.

Robinson, P. T., and A. G. Richter. 1977. A preliminary report on the toxicity and efficacy of levamisole phosphate in zoo birds. *J. Zoo Anim. Med.* 8(1):23–27.

Viet, H. P., R. J. Kendall, and P. F. Scanlon. 1983. The effect of lead shot ingestion on the testes of adult Ringed Turtle-doves (*Streptopelia risoria*). *Avian Dis.* 27(2):442–52.

Wells, R. E., R. F. Slocomb, and A. L. Trapp. 1982. Acute toxicosis of Budgerigars (*Melopsittacus undulatus*) caused by pyrolysis products from heated polytetrafluoroethylene: Clinical study. *Am. J. Vet. Res.* 43(7):1238–42.

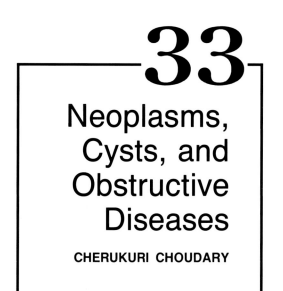

33

Neoplasms, Cysts, and Obstructive Diseases

CHERUKURI CHOUDARY

A VETERINARY practitioner must know the incidence and the general morphological characters of various tumors so that the conditions can be managed. The term "tumor" simply means a swelling, and the use of the term is usually confined to swellings that are not directly caused by inflammation. The term "neoplasm" has a roughly parallel meaning; it literally signifies a new growth, except that while it is initially developing, it may not be recognizable as a swelling or a tumor. The cells of a true neoplasm grow and multiply without the customary controls exerted by the body. The cells closely resemble the healthy cells from which they arise, but they are not arranged in any orderly fashion as they multiply, and as far as is known, they serve no useful function.

Tumors can affect any area of tissue of the body, including the blood, but a high proportion exist in or just beneath the skin and produce a noticeable swelling.

NEOPLASMS

Diagnosing neoplasia antemortem can be difficult because in many instances a bird displays little or no visible evidence of ill health until just prior to death. While there are exceptions, a bird with very advanced disease may behave normally and even initiate a reproductive cycle. Birds with advanced malignant tumors can exhibit active genitalia before the owner reports a sudden and unexpected death. The response of a bird to neoplasia differs markedly from that of mammals (Budgerigar Society 1979–1981).

Neoplasms are not uncommon in domestic fowl, but the literature supports the view that they are infrequent in the domestic duck and extremely rare in free-flying birds. Nine cases of neoplasia in free-flying wild birds have been diagnosed in more than 18,000 carcasses examined at the National Wild Life Health Laboratory, Madison, Wisconsin (Siegfried 1982).

The majority of species that are kept as cage and aviary birds are psittaciforms and passeriforms. Ratcliffe (1933), in a study of necropsies of birds and mammals at the Philadelphia Zoo, found that in general birds of the order Psittaciformes had the highest incidence of neoplasms (3.5%); in the class Aves, the Budgerigar (*Melopsittacus undulatus*) had the highest incidence (15.81%, a frequency unparalleled among other birds and mammals). On the other hand, the tumor incidence among birds belonging to the order Passeriformes was lower than that among members of any other order of either birds or mammals. Of lesions found in 257 necropsies of Budgerigars, the commonest disease was neoplasia, principally of the gonads, kidneys, and fat (Baker 1980).

Neoplasia in caged species is rare, with the exception of many benign and malignant tumors in Budgerigars, adenocarcinomas in mynahs, fibrosarcomas in amazon parrots, and lymphosarcomas and often blood cancer in canaries.

The incidence and type of tumors afflicting various organ systems, cysts, and obstructions in cage and aviary birds are detailed in this chapter. Treatment is based on body location and severity and on the age, sex, and species of bird.

Neoplasms of the Skin

Tumors of the Beak. Neoplasms, especially carcinomas, sarcomas, and osteosarcomas, can produce beak deformities. These tumors produce overgrowth of the beak, necrosis, peeling, cracking, irregular shortening, and elevation of the beak cuticle from the underlying jaw.

Most tumors causing beak deformity are malignant and should be treated by euthanasia (Altman 1969). These tumors need to be differentiated from bacterial or fungal granulomas by biopsy and also from deformity, fractures of the beak, or intralaminal hemorrhage where there is little or no bleeding. Some beak tumors may be treated by cautery or cryosurgery.

Papilloma. This tumor has been reported in amazon parrots (*Amazona ochrocephala*), African Gray Parrots (*Psittacus erithacus*), Cockatiels (*Nymphicus hollandicus*), and Budgerigars. Symptoms relate to the area of the tumor. They commonly occur on the neck, phalanxes, and uropygial gland region and over the mandible region. Pain may be evidenced by sharp screams when a bird irritates a tumor; this sometimes results in hemorrhage. Grossly the tumors appear dry and hard with an irregular crust. The cut section of the growth is fleshy, friable, and very vascular. In shape the tumor varies from a long, hornlike projection to an ulcerative, crusty, linear lesion. Microscopically the tumors consist of irregular fronds of squamous epithelium covered with a thick, dense layer of keratin. Cells in the basal part of the tumor are small and cuboidal and in the projecting fronds large and polyhedral. Occasionally small groups of cells within the fronds are keratinized. The treatment of choice is surgical excision.

Squamous Cell Carcinoma. This tumor is recorded in male Budgerigars (Petrak and Gilmore 1969), a male Military Macaw (*Ara militaris*) (Ratcliffe 1933), and also in a female Bean Goose (*Anser fabalis*). The tumor is irregular and firm and the surface often ulcerated. The cut surface is gray and smooth and microscopically consists of irregular, disorganized masses of squamous epithelium deep in the dermis. Small cysts and individual cells, some of which are keratinized, may be surrounded by fibrous stroma. The cells are generally large and varied in size. Small groups of keratinized cells sometimes occur in a slightly whorled pattern and in larger masses resembling pearls. Small tumors can be removed surgically.

Hemangioma. This tumor has only been recorded in Budgerigars (Beach 1962; Petrak and Gilmore 1969). Grossly the tumor is soft and smooth surfaced. The cut surface is uniformly red and glistening, and microscopically there are endothelium-lined spaces of varying sizes filled with blood and plasma. The interstitial spaces are separated by mature fibrous connective tissue, and often the entire mass is well capsulated. Treatment is by surgical excision.

Neoplasms of the Subcutis

Lipoma. This tumor is recorded most commonly in Budgerigars of both sexes. The majority of the tumors are located on the sternum, wings, and abdomen and rarely on the back, neck, and uropygial gland. Though lipomas are not malignant, a regrowth may be seen after excision. Symptoms depend on the location of the tumor. Sternal and cervical lipomas hamper flying, whereas those on the abdominal wall interfere with normal perching and climbing activities. Lipomas are typically globular, turgid, yellow, and well capsulated. Microscopically they consist of a mixture of a few viable fat cells and

many large cells with foamy cytoplasm. If the general health of the bird and the size and location of the tumor permit, surgical excision is recommended (Petrak and Gilmore 1969). Birds can also be treated with exogenous L-thyroxine. The results with this therapy vary, but numerous reports have demonstrated actual shrinkage of the neoplasm (Rosskopf and Woerpel 1983).

Liposarcoma. This tumor is recorded in male and female Budgerigars, arising in the sternal area and in the region of the uropygial gland. Surgical excision is the treatment of choice (Petrak and Gilmore 1969).

Hemangioendothelioma. This tumor is soft and dark red and most frequently appears as a hemorrhagic mass on the wing tip. The tumor is poorly circumscribed and highly cellular. Treatment and species incidence is seldom recorded.

Fibroma. This tumor often occurs over the wing and sternal region in male Budgerigars. It is small, globular, and firm with a dark surface. Cut sections appear firm with an intermingling of clear, glistening areas among dense white and gray areas. Microscopically the tumor is composed of mature, relatively avascular connective tissue.

Fibrosarcoma. This tumor occurs in male and female Budgerigars on many places of the body, most commonly the extremities. The tumor is globular, firm, highly cellular, and rarely capsulated (compared with fibromas). Treatment is by surgical excision.

Neoplasms of the Uropygial Gland

Adenocarcinoma. Generally, tumors of the uropygial gland are adenocarcinomas. They must be differentiated from mechanical blockage of the oil duct with inspissated material, chronic infection, granulomas, and abscessation. The organ is commonly affected in Budgerigars, presenting a change in the contour over the tail duct (Madill 1981). Blackmore (1965) recorded the tumor in a Yellow-fronted Parrot (*Chrysotis ochrocephala*). It is not reported in other bird species.

Gross clinical features of this tumor are either a globular, firm, yellow, oval, pedunculated mass or a hard, brown, cylindrical shell. Cut surfaces reveal papillary projections and striated white or white-yellow smooth masses. Microscopically the tumor consists of multiple, small, spherical nests of basophilic cells in a dense, fibrous stroma. Occasionally these are large masses of contained cells with foamy cytoplasm similar to normal sebaceous cells. Surgical treatment can be attempted if the case is not protracted.

Adenoma. Arnall (1961) recorded the occurrence of an adenoma of the uropygial gland in a canary (*Serinus canarius*), and Petrak and Gilmore (1969) recorded it in a Budgerigar. Grossly the tumor is a yellow-tan mass. A cut section reveals a thick-walled cyst containing yellow, caseated material surrounded by a soft, glossy, mottled red and tan periphery. Microscopically the tumor consists of a well-circumscribed spherical mass composed of irregular lobules of epithelial cells. There may be a large collection of lipid and necrotic cellular debris in the center of the mass. Some lobules are made up of large, foamy, polyhedral cells while others are composed of smaller basophilic reserve cells. Surgical excision is the treatment of choice.

Neoplasms of the Musculoskeletal System

Osteosarcoma. This tumor is recorded in male and female Budgerigars and in the canary. Lesions occur over the ribs, humerus, radius, and wing tip. Grossly they are firm and globular, and microscopically they consist of small irregular spicules of osteoid or poorly mineralized bones surrounded by immature osteoblasts (Fig. 33.1). There is no treatment.

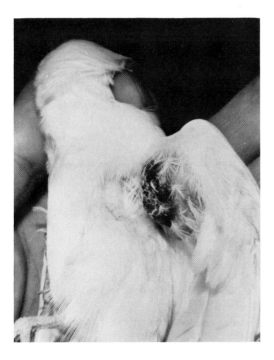

Rhabdomyosarcoma. This tumor has been recorded in the male Budgerigar in the shoulder region (Petrak and Gilmore 1969) and over the wings (Frost 1961; Beach 1962; Blackmore 1965). The tumor is poorly circumscribed, not encapsulated but intermingled with surrounding skeletal muscle. The microscopic appearance is similar to that of fibrosarcomas. Gross striations characteristic of skeletal muscle can be identified in tumor cells. Treatment is by surgical excision.

Neoplasms of the Respiratory System

Papilloma of the Larynx. Papilloma of the larynx has been recorded in an amazon parrot but is considered rare because in most bird species this organ is poorly developed. The growth was a soft, irregular mass. The cut surface resembled a hard-boiled egg in consistency and appearance. Microscopically the tumor consists of squamous epithelium with a large projecting mass of keratin and necrotic cellular debris on the surface. Surgical treatment is warranted.

Neoplasms of the Hemic and Lymphatic Systems

Cutaneous Leukosis. This form of leukosis is recorded in male Budgerigars. Clinical signs are localized feather loss and self-mutilation of skin lesions located on the head, neck, antebrachium, and foot. The affected skin is thickened, and microscopically the entire dermis is diffusely infiltrated with immature granulocytic cells or lymphocytic cells replacing the collagen. Nuclei are round and slightly vesicular. There is no successful treatment.

Visceral Leukosis. Leukosis in visceral organs is recorded in pheasants (Dren et al. 1983), canaries (Beach 1962; Petrak and Gilmore 1969), a Necklace Laughing Bird (*Turdus eriectorum*), magpies (*Pica pica*), rheas (*Rhea americana*), Budgerigars (Blackmore 1965), and cockatoos (Ratcliffe 1933). Clinical signs and symptoms include polydipsia, loose droppings, lethargy, decreased appetite, weakness, and gulping. Six cases of lymphoid leukosis were also found among 1234 necropsies of captive wild birds during a 5-year period (Wadsworth et al. 1981). Dren et al. (1983) have described an

Fig. 33.1. Osteosarcoma occurring over the humerus in a Budgerigar (*Melopsittacus undulatus*). (*Courtesy of Raymond D. Wise, Scottsdale Animal Clinic, Chicago, Ill.*)

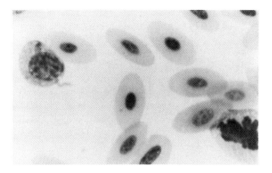

Fig. 33.2. Immature lymphocyte and one undergoing mitosis in a peachick (*Pavo cristatus*) suffering from lymphosarcoma of the liver. (*Courtesy of David J. Schultz, Hawthorn, South Australia, Aust.*)

outbreak of the lymphoproliferative phase in pheasants. Nodular or diffuse tumors were found on the head and in various internal organs. The tumors were found in the liver, spleen, heart, kidney, and lungs. Microscopically the tumors reveal either focal or diffuse infiltration of lymphoblastic cells replacing normal tissue (Fig. 33.2). The cells are undifferentiated blast cells with vesiculate nuclei. Euthanasia is usually the recommended treatment.

Neoplasms of the Spleen

Hemangioendothelioma. This tumor occurs in male and female Budgerigars. It is pink-red and soft, the cut surface irregularly mottled red and white. Because the tumor is highly vascular, surgery is seldom successful.

Leiomyoma. This tumor occurs in adult female Budgerigars. The symptoms are related to mechanical effects resulting from pressure from the mass, which is highly cellular and globular in shape. This tumor can often be removed surgically.

Leiomyosarcoma. This tumor occurs most commonly in male Budgerigars. It is oval and contains multilocular cysts filled with fluid. The tumor is highly cellular with pleomorphic nuclei. Blackmore (1965) recorded 15 leiomyosarcomas of the spleen among 168 tumors in Budgerigars. The success rate of surgery is not known.

Lymphangioma. This tumor occurs in female Budgerigars. The tumor consists of a multiloculated cystic mass lined with a single layer of endothelial cells projecting from the splenic capsule. Surgical removal is successful in some cases.

Neoplasms of the Digestive System

Fibrosarcoma of the Mouth. This tumor is recorded in Budgerigars. The gross and microscopic features are similar to skin and subcutis tumors.

Leiomyosarcoma of the Crop. This tumor resembles that occurring in the spleen.

Adenosarcoma of the Cloaca. This tumor has been recorded in female Budgerigars. Clinical features of the condition include intensive straining to defecate and loss of appetite. The neoplastic tissue originates in the mucosal epithelium and extends through the tunica muscularis to the serosa of the cloaca. Microscopically the tissue is composed of acini and tubules separated by bands of smooth muscle fibers and connective tissue. The neoplastic cells are plump, columnar, and basophilic staining, with round to oval vesicular nuclei (Beach 1962; Petrak and Gilmore 1969). Surgery can be attempted if the disease is not too far advanced.

Neoplasms of the Liver

Undifferentiated Sarcoma. This tumor was recorded in male and female Budgerigars (Petrak and Gilmore 1969), in a female ground thrush (Ratcliffe 1933), and in a canary (Lombard and Witte 1959).

Grossly the liver is usually enlarged and in the form of disseminated grayish foci (Fig. 33.3). Microscopically the cells are arranged in a compact mass with connective tissue stroma and blood vessels running through it. Mitotic figures are numerous. The surrounding hepatic tissue is fatty but otherwise unaffected. The condition is usually only diagnosed postmortem.

Fibrosarcoma. This tumor occurs most commonly in male Budgerigars (Schlumber 1957; Petrak and Gilmore 1969) and rarely in other cage birds (Arnall 1961). The liver is usually enlarged and soft, containing pale cellular tissue. Microscopically the tumor appears the same as fibrosarcomas of the skin.

Hemangioendothelioma. This tumor occurs most frequently in female Budgerigars. The liver is often pink-tan with a pink ovoid neoplastic mass. Microscopically the tumor has the same appearance as that in the subcutis.

Neoplasms of the Pancreas

Adenocarcinoma. This tumor has been recorded in a mynah bird (Rosskopf et al. 1982). Success of surgical removal is limited and probably not warranted.

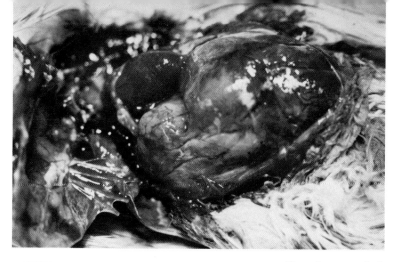

Fig. 33.3. Budgerigar (*Melopsittacus undulatus*) liver exhibiting the signs of undifferentiated sarcoma. (*Courtesy of David J. Schultz, Hawthorn, South Australia, Aust.*)

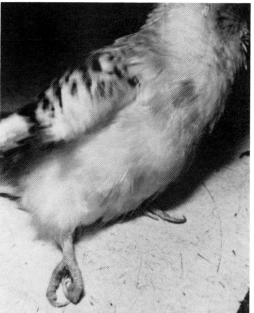

Neoplasms of the Urogenital System

Neoplasms of the Kidney

Adenocarcinoma. This tumor is recorded in both male and female Budgerigars (Fox 1923; Ratcliffe 1933; Petrak and Gilmore 1969) and in a buzzard (*Buteo buteo*) (Cooper 1978). If the tumor is on one kidney, causing pressure to the sciatic nerve, the first symptom noted will be paresis, followed by paralysis of the ipsilateral leg (Fig. 33.4). The tumor is white and may vary from irregular to ovoid in shape. Microscopically the tumor consists of small nests or masses of vesicular epithelial cells separated by varying amounts of mature or immature fibrous connective tissue (Fig. 33.5). Surgical treatment is seldom successful.

Fig. 33.4. Budgerigar (*Melopsittacus undulatus*) exhibiting paresis followed by paralysis of the ipsilateral leg. At necropsy an adenocarcinoma of the kidney was found. (*Courtesy of Raymond D. Wise, Scottsdale Animal Clinic, Chicago, Ill.*)

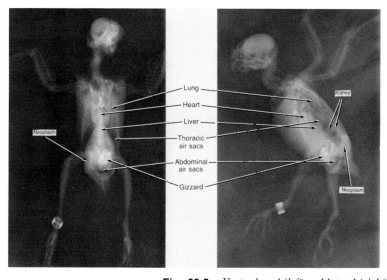

Fig. 33.5. Ventrodorsal (*left*) and lateral (*right*) radiographic projection used to diagnose renal neoplasia in a male parakeet. Histopathological examination revealed the tumor to be a cavitated adenocarcinoma. (*From Bullmore 1981, by permission*)

Embryonal Nephroma. This tumor occurs in both male and female Budgerigars. Clinical symptoms and histological features are similar to adenocarcinoma of the kidney. Acini or tubules mimic poorly formed glomeruli. Connective tissue is more abundant than in adenocarcinomas. Surgical treatment is seldom successful.

Neoplasms of the Testes

Seminoma. This tumor occurs in Budgerigars and occasionally in other bird orders (Rewell 1948; Petrak and Gilmore 1969). Symptoms are usually related to a gradually enlarging abdominal mass. Physical examination may reveal a soft, bulging abdomen and a moderate loss of condition. The tumor is firm, smooth, and whitish. The cut surface is smooth, glistening, and pale. This tumor may occupy the entire testes and is encapsulated. Microscopically it is composed of round cells of varying sizes with round hyperchromatic nuclei surrounded by a polychromatophilic cytoplasm. Narrow connective tissue trabeculae extend in an irregular pattern throughout the tumor. The seminiferous tubules often cannot be distinguished. There are also frequent mitotic figures in the neoplastic cells. Surgical removal of the tumor is indicated.

Interstitial Cell Tumor. This tumor occurs in numerous bird species. Clinical symptoms include an enlarged abdomen. The testes exhibit an irregular surface, multiple foci of necrosis, and hemorrhage. Normal testicular tissue is usually not recognized. The neoplastic cells are round to polyhedral, with small, round, hyperchromatic nuclei and finely vacuolated eosinophilic cytoplasm. Thin, fibrous trabeculae and blood vessels often divide the mass into irregular groups of cells. The tumor can be removed surgically.

Sertoli Cell Tumor. Clinical symptoms of this tumor are related to the effect of a gradually enlarging abdominal mass. The tumor is lobulated, encapsulated, and spherical to oval in shape. The cut surface is firm, glistening, and grayish. Microscopically the tumor is composed of small nests of cells separated by a moderate amount of fibrous connective tissue derived from the walls of the seminiferous tubules. Neoplastic Sertoli cells have uniform round to oval nuclei and vacuolated cytoplasm with indistinct borders. Unlike in mammals, there is little tendency for the cells in these tumors to become elongated and lie parallel within the nests. The tumors can be removed surgically.

Leiomyosarcoma. This tumor frequently occurs in Budgerigars. Clinical signs are associated with a gradually enlarging mass in the abdominal cavity. The tumor has a smooth surface, and the microscopic appearance is similar to those that occur in the spleen. The tumor can be removed surgically.

Hemangioma of the Testicular Capsule. This tumor occasionally occurs in small passerines and psittacines. Clinical symptoms are intermittent passing of bloody droppings, dyspnea, and a bulging abdomen. Grossly the tumor is an ovoid mass attached to the testes. The microscopic appearance and treatment is similar to that described for a subcutaneous hemangioma.

Neoplasms of the Oviduct

Leiomyosarcoma. The clinical symptoms, microscopic appearance, and treatment are similar to those described in the spleen.

Adenocarcinoma. A poorly differentiated adenocarcinoma of the oviduct was described in a captive Mauritius Kestrel (*Falco punctatus*). The condition is seldom reported; however, surgical intervention may be successful if the tumor is not spreading.

Mixed Cell Tumor. This tumor was recorded in a free-living Seychelles Kestrel (*Falco araca*). The tumor consisted of lymphangiomatous, epithelial, fibrosarcomatous, and chondromatous elements (Cooper et al. 1978). Surgery may be successful.

Neoplasms of the Ovary

Granulosa Cell Tumor. This tumor frequently occurs in Budgerigars (Beach 1962; Blackmore 1965; Petrak and Gilmore 1969). Birds may exhibit a marked abdominal distension and dyspnea. The tumor may be either solid or cystic. Microscopically masses of cells with round or oval and vesicular nuclei are separated by a thin band of connective tissue. The cytoplasm is often foamy and vacuolated, with indistinct borders. If the tumor is not too severe it can be removed surgically.

Adenocarcinoma. This tumor occurs most commonly in Budgerigars and Cockatiels (*Nymphicus hollandicus*) (Wadsworth et al. 1981). Abdominal distension, dyspnea, and difficulty in passing droppings are frequently seen clinical symptoms. Similar to granulosa cell tumors, these growths are solid in some and cystic in others. Metastasis to the mesentery, pancreas, duodenal loop, spleen, and liver is common (Reece 1984). Surgical intervention is seldom successful.

Arhenoblastoma. This rare fleshy tumor of the functional left ovary is occasionally found in the hyperblastic right gonad of ovariectomized pullets. The right gonad is derived from the embryonic ovarian parenchyma, which corresponds to rete testes tubules of the rete ovary. They are arranged as branching cords of columnar epithelium often two cells thick. Some tumors have a tendency to form villi. Metastasis to the liver and mesentery can occur. These tumors produce androgens and can result in virilism (Reece 1984). Surgical removal is indicated.

Epithelial Thymoma. This tumor is predominantly epithelial and possibly malignant. Budgerigars seem to be the only bird affected (Zubaidy 1980). Surgery may be successful if done before rapid growth starts.

Neoplasms of the Endocrine System

Adenocarcinoma of the Thyroid Gland. This tumor occurs equally often in both male and female Budgerigars. The clinical symptoms observed are dyspnea, trembling, and general debility. The tumors are circumscribed but poorly encapsulated. Microscopically the tumor consists of small, irregularly shaped follicles and solid nests of follicular cells separated by thin, vascular connective tissue septa. The cells are cuboidal with basophilic nuclei and granular cytoplasm. Treatment with hormones may prolong the life of the bird but seldom is completely satisfactory. Euthanasia is frequently recommended.

Follicular Adenoma. This tumor, together with cases of colloid goiter and diffuse microfollicular hyperplasia, is recorded in cage birds (Wadsworth et al. 1981). Treatment is as for adenocarcinoma of the thyroid gland.

Pituitary Tumor. This tumor occurs in numerous avian species. The common clinical symptoms seen are watery droppings and blindness.

Gross changes of the pituitary are not seen. Microscopically, however, the brain may show a poorly circumscribed growth encroaching on the hypothalamus. The tumor cells have round nuclei and are basophilic with eosinophilic cytoplasm. They are arranged in solid masses separated by thin connective tissue trabeculae. Treatment is not warranted. See Schlumber (1954, 1956).

Neoplasms of the Nervous System

Glioblastoma Multiforme. This tumor was recorded in a Budgerigar (Raphel and Nguyen 1981). Clinical symptoms of resting tremor and widely dilated pupils may be evidenced. No gross lesions occur, but microscopically lesions are seen in the diencephalon, mesencephalon, and preoptic regions of the brain. Pleomorphic cells with round nuclei and eosinophilic cytoplasm are seen in the brain. Numerous multinucleated giant cells are also seen. There is no treatment for this condition.

OTHER CONDITIONS

Cysts

Feather Cyst. Feather cysts are common in both macaws and canaries (Rosskopf 1981). They are also occasionally seen in amazon parrots. The cause is unknown. It is thought that the condition may be hereditary or viral, as they can recur in different areas of the body. Even when cysts are totally destroyed or excised, recurrences can plague a bird. Feather cysts can also result from trauma that produces misdirected feather follicles. When feather follicles do not communicate with the epidermis, this condition may produce a feather that curls within its own follicle, causing a cyst to form with the accumulation of cheesy secretions and exudate. Eventually feather cysts rupture, producing an ulcerated area with a clump of distorted feathers matted with dried exudate (Fig. 33.6).

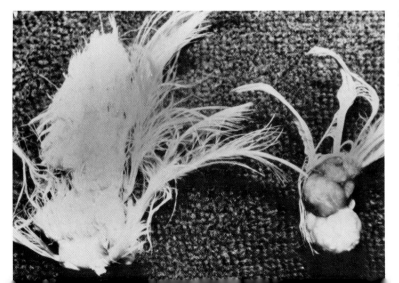

Fig. 33.6. Feather cyst easily recognized and removed surgically by curettage and chemical cauterization. (*Courtesy of Lester Mandelker, Largo, Fla.*)

In canaries, feather cysts occur mainly on wings but may affect other areas of integument. Feather cysts may become secondarily infected with bacteria. Multiple small feather cysts have been seen in Budgerigars and Peach-faced Lovebirds (*Agapornis roseicollis*) with chronic folliculitis (Perry 1984). Treatment of these cysts medically and surgically often proves futile. If the cysts are small enough, they can be treated by regular manual expression or cleaning out of the contents. If large or numerous, anesthesia is indicated to permit all cysts to be opened, emptied, and cauterized with strong iodine, phenol, or silver nitrate to destroy the follicle. Total surgical excision is frequently effective but more difficult to perform (Madill 1981). (See Chapter 6 for further information on feather cysts.)

Dermal Cyst. Dermal cysts are characterized by single or multiple tumorlike growths affecting the skin. They most frequently occur on the wings but may be found anywhere on the body. They are pedunculated or ulcerated, with yellow, granular sebaceous contents (Seneviratna 1969). It is not clear whether dermal cysts are the same as feather cysts. Epidermal cysts can be removed by surgical excision.

Obstructions

Foreign Bodies. The beaks of psittacines such as Budgerigars and Sulphur-crested Cockatoos may become impaled on bent wire hanging in the cage. This can produce a nasty, bloody wound, especially when impaled inside the upper beak. Physical removal with or without antibiotic cover is required, and treatment for shock may also be indicated (Schlumber 1957). Various sea birds (e.g., gulls) may be found with fishhooks and line lodged in their beaks. These should be handled in the least traumatic way, depending on the individual case, either by pulling or twisting the hook back out the way it went in or by cutting off the eye of the hook and forcing the barb through the beak.

Water birds with fishing line protruding from the mouth should be radiographed for the presence of a hook or lure in the gastrointestinal tract. Once hooks pass the mouth they usually lodge in the thick muscle of the gizzard, and even if they do not penetrate the peritoneal cavity, they are best removed surgically.

Cloacal Impactions. Although this condition is commonly seen in loons and grebes, it can occur in any species. The pathology consists of hard uric acid and fecal concretions that distend or obstruct the large intestine and cloaca. Dehydration and infrequent cloacal evacuation may result in excessive reabsorption of fluid from the cloaca; the concentration and precipitation of solutes causes impaction (Williams 1984). The condition may be treated with enemas, using approximately 10 ml warm water or liquid paraffin, and gently breaking up and expressing the mass. Once the bird is cleaned and behavior is normal, recurrence is rare.

Constipation. The majority of constipated birds have pasted vents, preventing the passage of feces. Occasionally (common with the finch family), the rectum becomes impacted with feces, causing the abdomen to swell. The mass in chronic cases may be palpated or seen through the abdominal wall. Urate concretions obstructing the cloaca can be differentiated from rectal impactions by auriscopic examination. Treatment is given via a crop tube with liquid paraffin at 3 ml/kg. If conservative treatment fails, exploratory surgery may be the only chance of success.

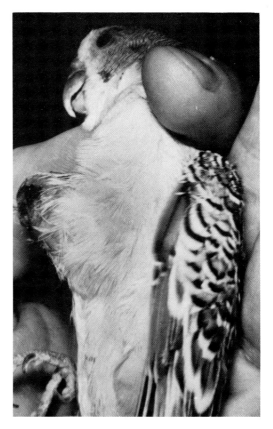

Fig. 33.7. Xanthoma occurring where there was an underlying pathological condition (lipoma). (*Courtesy of Raymond D. Wise, Scottsdale Animal Clinic, Chicago, Ill.*)

Xanthomatosis. Xanthoma of the skin is commonly seen in caged psittacines, particularly in Budgerigars (Peckham 1955). Grossly, the skin is thickened, yellowish, and quilted with many indented and nonfunctional feather follicles (Fig. 33.7). Microscopically there is an infiltration of reticuloendothelial cells or macrophages with abundant cytoplasm containing tiny lipid droplets. Predilection sites are those with underlying pathological conditions such as lipomas, hernias, chronic abscesses, or large fat deposits. Therefore the abdomen, thigh, carpus, and pectoral and tail region are most likely to be affected. The etiology and cause are unknown. It has been suggested that fat-related toxic hydrocarbons in feed can cause xanthomatosis. The pathogenesis may also involve some circulatory and metabolic disturbance to the skin, resulting in excess lipid deposition in the skin.

Treatment depends on the nature of any underlying pathology and whether or not the skin has been abraded or self-mutilated. If there is no skin damage, dieting can be a very important part of therapy because reduction in fat deposits around the area makes surgery easier. To reduce the weight of the birds, the starch-containing seeds such as millet, oat, and wheat must be reduced in quantity and some oily seeds provided. If the skin is damaged, complete removal of the xanthoma and the underlying cause is recommended. Surgical incisions heal slowly, and the tissue often will not hold tension sutures. Therefore careful appraisal of the amount of skin that can be excised without requiring tension sutures for closure is warranted prior to surgery (Perry 1981).

References

Altman, R. B. 1969. Conditions involving the integumentary system. In *Diseases of Cage and Aviary Birds,* ed. M. L. Petrak, pp. 393–451. Philadelphia: Lea and Febiger.

Arnall, L. 1961. Further experiences with cage birds. *Vet. Rec.* 73:1146–54.

Baker, J. R. 1980. A survey of causes of mortality in Budgerigars (*Melopsittacus undulatus*). *Vet. Rec.* 106:10–12.

Beach, J. E. 1962. Diseases of Budgerigars and other cage birds: A survey of postmortem findings. *Vet. Rec.* 74:10, 63, 134.

Blackmore, D. K. 1965. The pathology and incidence of neoplasia in cage birds. *J. Small Anim. Pract.* 6:217–23.

Budgerigar Society. 1979–1981. *The Budgerigar Research Digest.* The Budgerigar Society, Marlowes, Engl.

Bullmore, C. C. 1981. Renal neoplasia in parakeets. *Mod. Vet. Pract.,* pp. 863–64.

Cooper, J. E. 1978. An adenocarcinoma in a buzzard. *Avian Pathol.* 7:29–34.

Cooper, J. E., J. Watson, and L. N. Payne. 1978. A mixed cell tumor in a Seychelles Kestrel (*Falco araca*). *Avian Pathol.* 7:651–58.

Dren, C. N., E. Saghy, R. Glavits, F. Ratz, J. Ping, and V. Sztojkov. 1983. Lymphoreticular tumor in penraised pheasants associated with reticuloendotheliosis-like virus infection. *Avian Pathol.* 12:55–71.

Fox, H. 1923. *Disease in Captive Wild Mammals and Wild Birds.* Philadelphia: J. B. Lippincott.

Frost, C. 1961. Experience with pet Budgerigars. *Vet. Rec.* 73:621–26.

Lombard, L., and E. J. Witte. 1959. Frequency and type of tumors in mammals and birds of the Philadelphia Zoological Garden. *Cancer Res.* 19:127–41.

Madill, D. N. 1981. Avian surgery. In *Refresher Course for Veterinarians on Aviary and Caged Birds,* pp. 197–218. University of Sydney, Post-Graduate Committee in Veterinary Science, Proceedings no. 55. Sydney, Aust.

Peckham, M. C. 1955. Xanthomatosis in chicken. *Am. J. Vet. Res.* 16:580–83.

Perry, R. A. 1981. Unpublished data.

_____. 1984. Unpublished data.

Petrak, M. L., and C. E. Gilmore. 1969. Neoplasms. In *Diseases of Cage and Aviary Birds,* ed. M. L. Petrak. Philadelphia: Lea and Febiger.

Raphael, B. L., and H. T. Nguyen. 1981. Metastasizing rhabdomyosarcoma in a Budgerigar. *J. Am. Vet. Med. Assoc.* 177.

Ratcliffe, H. L. 1933. Incidence and nature of tumors of captive wild mammals and birds. *Am. J. Cancer* 17:116–35.

Reece, R. L. 1984. Unpublished data.

Rewell, R. E. 1948. Seminoma of the testes in a Collared Turtle Dove (*Streptopelia risoria*). *J. Pathol. Bacteriol.* 60:155.

Rosskopf, W. J. 1981. *Assoc. Avian Vet. Newsl.* 2(41):17.

Rosskopf, W. J., and R. W. Woerpel. 1983. Remission of lipomatous growth in a hypothyroid Budgerigar in response to L-thyroxine therapy. *Vet. Med. Small Anim. Clin.* 44:1415–18.

Rosskopf, W. J., R. W. Woerpel, E. M. Howard, and J. O. Britt. 1982. Pancreatic adenocarcinoma in a mynah bird. *Avian Pract.* 43:573–74.

Schlumber, H. G. 1954. Neoplasia in the parakeet. 1. Spontaneous chromophobe pituitary tumors. *Cancer Res.* 14:237–45.

_____. 1956. Neoplasia in the parakeet. 2. Transplantation of the pituitary tumor. *Cancer Res.* 16:149–53.

_____. 1957. Tumors characteristic for certain animal species: A review. *Cancer Res.* 17:823–32.

Seneviratna, P. 1969. In *Diseases of Poultry, Including Cage Birds,* 2d ed. Bristol, Engl.: John Wright and Sons.

Siegfried, L. W. 1982. Neoplasms identified in free-flying wild birds. *Avian Dis.* 27(1):86.

Wadsworth, P. F., D. M. Jones, and S. L. Pugsley. 1981. Some cases of lymphoid leukosis in captive wild birds. *Avian Pathol.* 10:499–504.

Williams, A. S. 1984. Unpublished data.

Zubaidy, A. J. 1980. An epithelial thymoma in a Budgerigar. *Avian Pathol.* 9:575–81.

INDEX